# CASE STUDIES IN
# **Trauma Nursing**

| pg. # | Correction |
|-------|------------|
| xiii | C RRN |
| XIX | CRRN |
| xiii | MTU–5 |

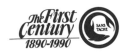

# CASE STUDIES IN
# Trauma Nursing

EDITED BY

## ROBERT H. WELTON, RN, MSN, CCRN

Clinical Nurse Specialist
Maryland Institute for Emergency Medical Services Systems
University of Maryland Medical Systems
Baltimore, Maryland

## KATHY A. SHANE, RN, BSN, CCRN, CNRN

Primary Nurse, Oncology Intensive Care Unit
University of Maryland Medical Systems
Baltimore, Maryland

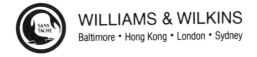

**WILLIAMS & WILKINS**
Baltimore • Hong Kong • London • Sydney

*Editor:* Susan M. Glover
*Associate Editor:* Marjorie Kidd Keating
*Copy Editor:* Melissa Andrews
*Designer:* JoAnne Janowiak
*Illustration Planner:* Ray Lowman
*Production Coordinator:* Anne G. Stewart-Seitz

Copyright © 1990
Williams & Wilkins
428 East Preston Street
Baltimore, Maryland 21202, USA

Accurate indications, adverse reactions, and dosage schedules for drugs are provided in this book, but it is possible that they may change. The reader is urged to review the package information data of the manufacturers of the medications mentioned.

*Printed in the United States of America*

**Library of Congress Cataloging-in-Publication Data**

Case studies in trauma nursing / edited by Robert H. Welton, Kathy Ann Shane.
    p.    cm.
    Includes bibliographical references.
    ISBN 0-683-08922-6
    1. Wounds and injuries—Nursing—Case studies.   2. Intensive care nursing—Case studies.   I. Welton, Robert H.   II. Shane, Kathy Ann.
    [DNLM: 1. Emergencies—nursing—case studies.   2. Wounds and Injuries—nursing—case studies.   WY 154 C337]
RD93.95.C37   1990
610.73'61—dc20
DNLM/DLC
for Library of Congress                                                                89-25062
                                                                                          CIP

                                                        90  91  92  93  94
                                        1    2    3    4    5    6   7   8   9   10

*To critical care nurses from whom I have learned and for whom I have immense respect.*

R.H.W.


*To my husband, Mark, and daughters, Amanda and Alison, for their love and encouragement throughout this endeavor, and to the staff of the University of Maryland Cancer Center Intensive Care Unit for all their patience and support.*

K.A.S.

# FOREWORD

In recent years, trauma nursing has come to be recognized as a specialty field, in collaboration with the field of traumatology in the medical profession. Hospitals across our nation have been designated as centers ready and able to admit and treat traumatically injured patients according to established standards, procedures, and protocols. Trauma care has become a refined art and a fertile field for research to improve life-saving strategies and, more importantly, to return trauma patients to a meaningful role in society.

The current texts on trauma nursing have successfully elaborated the pathophysiology of traumatic injury and nursing interventions to care for patients with specific injuries and have addressed unique populations such as pregnant or elderly trauma patients. They have also thoroughly addressed the concept that trauma nursing covers a gamut of care from resuscitation through reintegration into society. Until this time, however, little has been written to provide trauma nurses with an understanding of specific case study applications. This book attempts to do just that. Although it is vital for those providing care to these patients to understand the theoretical base underlying traumatic injury, it is even more important to be able to visualize firsthand how each individual is affected by a specific injury or injuries. This text provides this long-needed information.

Expert trauma nurses have prepared case studies that are specific, complex, and challenging. They provide the reader with a realistic application of theory in practical terms. The case study approach allows one to integrate what is known about traumatic injury and to visualize the clinical effects and responses that challenge the nurse caring for these patients on a daily basis. With increased emphasis on trauma care and the continued growth of designated trauma centers, nurses will be expected to synthesize and integrate data obtained from sophisticated monitoring systems and diagnostic maneuvers with the clinical observations and ongoing assessment findings on their patients. This text will be vital in providing the necessary link between acquisition of data and application of findings.

Trauma nursing is, and will continue to be, a growing, dynamic specialty field. Nurses providing care for the complex needs of these patients are the obvious ones to share their experience with fellow trauma nurses. Not only must we continue to integrate theory with practice in texts such as this one, but we must also broaden our scope to include ongoing research in this field. Only then will we fully understand the impact of traumatic injury on individuals and reach a more sophisticated level of trauma nursing care.

*Virginia D. Cardona*, MS, RN, CCRN
Director of Nursing Education
Maryland Institute for Emergency Medical Services Systems
Baltimore, Maryland

# PREFACE

Trauma nursing is a rapidly evolving subspecialty within critical care nursing. Several recently published trauma nursing texts provide content of varying levels of sophistication and scope on this discipline. These publications rarely offer patient care situations to which the reader may apply the principles presented. This book fills that gap between theory and practice.

This book is written for the reader who is either new to trauma care or in search of a clinical reference for unfamiliar care problems. Its purpose is to provide a clinically relevant reference on fundamental knowledge needed by practicing nurses caring for trauma patients. It provides individual patient situations that are commonly encountered by the critical care nurse. This book is not intended to be an exhaustive treatise addressing the entire body of knowledge of trauma nursing; instead, it is meant as a quick reference for information of major importance in caring for patients with specific traumatic injuries. Each case study describes a traumatic event or its sequelae to which the reader is asked to make application of theoretical content or use analytical thinking in identifying nursing diagnoses and developing appropriate plans for care. The case studies offer a wide spectrum of patient problems resulting from traumatic injuries, as well as some major complications of trauma. These case studies will provide the reader with some reality grounding and opportunities for pragmatic thinking about nursing care content presented in other trauma nursing references.

This book is organized according to a physiological systems approach. The body of the text consists of case presentations of patients with single- or multiple-system injuries. Each case study begins with a brief description of the patient's clinical presentation along with any pertinent health history and physical assessment findings. The reader is then asked a series of questions that require interpretation of the data presented and application of basic information on relevant pathophysiology and care. The following questions are presented in most of the case studies:

1. What is the pathophysiological or sociocultural basis for this patient's problem?
2. What are the nursing diagnoses of highest priority?
3. What goals of care and nursing interventions are appropriate for the nursing diagnoses identified?

The question format changes slightly in the section on special topics, to facilitate appropriate discussion of some of that unique content. No pretense is made about addressing all of a patient's potential problems; rather, the focus is on only those problems of highest priority.

The nursing diagnoses used in this text are those currently approved by the North American Nursing Diagnosis Association (NANDA). The patient situations evolve further through questions that require developing plans for nursing care. The rationale for each answer is provided, along with some guidelines for actual care that are based on the clinical experience of the authors. Integration of the family into the plan of care is addressed in selected case studies, followed by a section on selected topics and special problems encountered in the trauma patient population.

The contributing authors are clinical experts from a wide range of backgrounds and practice settings. They were selected because of their extensive experience in and knowledge of specific patient care situations. We are fortunate to have these clinicians contribute their specialized expertise.

It is our sincere intent that you find this text useful and helpful in your practice as well as a valuable addition to the prevailing literature.

*R.H.W.*
*K.A.S.*

# ACKNOWLEDGMENTS

Our gratitude is extended to Peggy Brooks and Mary-Joan McHugh, Word Processing Department, as well as Beverly Sopp, Linda Kesselring, Erna Segal, and Deborah Day, Editorial Department, Maryland Institute for Emergency Medical Services Systems (MIEMSS), for their valuable assistance in the preparation of the book manuscript. In addition, we acknowledge the staff of the Biomedical Media Resource Division at MIEMSS for their contributions of photography and artwork to this book.

# CONTRIBUTORS

**Margaret K. Aberg-Cocchia, RN, BSN**
Organ Recovery Coordinator
Washington Regional Transplant Consortium
Washington, DC

**Valerie Adair, RN, BSN**    *Unit -*
Primary Nurse III, Multitrauma *5*
Maryland Institute for Emergency Medical
  Services Systems
Baltimore, Maryland

**Adrianne E. Avillion, RN, MS, ~~CCRN~~** *CRRN*,
**CNA**
Rehabilitation Staff Development Specialist
Montebello Rehabilitation Hospital
Baltimore, Maryland

**Tom Baker, RN**
Nurse Clinician II
Hyperbaric Medicine Department
Maryland Institute for Emergency Medical
  Services Systems
Baltimore, Maryland

**Judith K. Bobb, RN, MS**
Critical Care Coordinator
Maryland Institute for Emergency Medical
  Services Systems
Baltimore, Maryland

**Ellen P. Bowers, RN, BSN**
Primary Nurse II, Multitrauma 5
Maryland Institute for Emergency Medical
  Services Systems
Baltimore, Maryland

**Carol M. Browner, RN**
Nurse Educator
Barrows Neurological Institute
Phoenix, Arizona

**Mary Elizabeth Clark, RN**
Staff Nurse, Burn Center Intensive Care Unit
Baltimore Regional Burn Center
Baltimore, Maryland

**Denise Cost, RN, CCRN**    *Unit - 5*
Primary Nurse III, Multitrauma 6, Critical
  Care Unit
Maryland Institute for Emergency Medical
  Services Systems
Baltimore, Maryland

**Christy L. Crowther, RN, MS, ANP-C,**
**CCRN**
Nurse Practitioner
Division of Infectious Diseases
Maryland Institute for Emergency Medical
  Services Systems
Baltimore, Maryland

**Barbara J. Daly, RN, MSN, CCRN, FAAN**
Assistant Director of Nursing, University
  Hospitals of Cleveland
Assistant Clinical Professor, Frances Payne
  Bolton School of Nursing
Cleveland, Ohio

**Mary T. deLauney, RN, BSN**
Primary Nurse II, Emergency Department
University of Maryland Hospital
Baltimore, Maryland

**Margaret M. Epperson-Sebour, MSW,**
**ACSW, CSW**
Department Head, Psychosocial Services
Maryland Institute for Emergency Medical
  Services Systems
Baltimore, Maryland

**Jocelyn A. Farrar, RN, MS, CCRN**
Clinical Nurse Specialist
Maryland Institute for Emergency Medical
  Services Systems
Baltimore, Maryland

**Ben Grimes, RN**
Primary Nurse III
Hyperbaric Medicine Department
Maryland Institute for Emergency Medical
  Services Systems
Baltimore, Maryland

**Robbi Lynn Hartsock, RN, MSN, CCRN**
Clinical Nurse Specialist, Admitting Area
Maryland Institute for Emergency Medical
  Services Systems
Baltimore, Maryland

**Mary Helen Hoff, RN**
Primary Nurse II, Multitrauma 5
Maryland Institute for Emergency Medical
  Services Systems
Baltimore, Maryland

**Deana L. Holler, RN, BSN**
Primary Nurse III, Admitting Area
Maryland Institute for Emergency Medical
Services Systems
Baltimore, Maryland

**Anne G. Hopkins, RN, BSN, CCRN**
Primary Nurse III, Multitrauma 6, Critical
Care Unit
Maryland Institute for Emergency Medical
Services Systems
Baltimore, Maryland

**Nancy J. Hoyt, MA, CIC**
Infection Control Officer
Maryland Institute for Emergency Medical
Services Systems
Baltimore, Maryland

**Toby A. Jardine, RN, MA**
Manager, Administration
Barrows Neurological Institute
Phoenix, Arizona

**Jane Faith Kapustin, RN, MS**
Charge Nurse, Intensive Care Unit
Montgomery General Hospital
Olney, Maryland

**Barbara J. Keyes, RN, BSN**
Primary Nurse III, Multitrauma 5
Maryland Institute for Emergency Medical
Services Systems
Baltimore, Maryland

**Kathleen Kwiatowski, RN, BA**
Primary Nurse I, Neurosurgical Intensive Care
Unit
University of Maryland Hospital
Baltimore, Maryland

**Dianne L. Mackert, RN, BSN, CCRN**
Primary Nurse II, Surgical ICU
University of Maryland Hospital
Baltimore, Maryland

**Victoria Marselek, RN, MS, CCRN**
Nurse Manager, Burn Center ICU
Baltimore Regional Burn Center
Baltimore, Maryland

**Patricia A. Moloney-Harmon, RN, MS, CCRN**
Pediatric Critical Care Specialist
Maryland Institute for Emergency Medical
Services Systems
Baltimore, Maryland

**Laurel A. Moody, RN, BSN, CCRN**
Primary Nurse III, Multitrauma 6
Maryland Institute for Emergency Medical
Services Systems
Baltimore, Maryland

**Mary Murphy-Rutter, RN, MSN**
Clinical Nurse
Montebello Rehabilitation Hospital
Baltimore, Maryland

**Alyce F. Newton, RD, MS**
Clinician Dietitian and Coordinator, Surgical
Dietetics
Maryland Institute for Emergency Medical
Services Systems
Baltimore, Maryland

**Nancy L. Palmer, RN, CCRN**
Primary Nurse III, Multitrauma 5
Maryland Institute for Emergency Medical
Services Systems
Baltimore, Maryland

**Barbara Panariello, RN, BSN**
Primary Nurse III, Multitrauma 5
Maryland Institute for Emergency Medical
Services Systems
Baltimore, Maryland

**Shirley Roth, RN, MS, CCRN**
Associate Director, Renal Nursing
Good Samaritan Hospital
Baltimore, Maryland

**Kathy L. Samuel, RN, BSN**
Primary Nurse III, Multitrauma 6
Maryland Institute for Emergency Medical
Services Systems
Baltimore, Maryland

**Mary Jane Seipp, RN, BSN, CNRN**
Stroke Nurse Coordinator
University of Maryland Hospital
Baltimore, Maryland

**Kathy A. Shane, RN, BSN, CCRN, CNRN**
Primary Nurse, Oncology Intensive Care Unit
University of Maryland Hospital
Baltimore, Maryland

**Elizabeth E. Stickles, RN, BSN**
Primary Nurse III, Neurotrauma Unit
Maryland Institute for Emergency Medical
Services Systems
Baltimore, Maryland

**Valerie May Summerlin, RN, MSN, CNAA**
Director of Nursing
Montebello Rehabilitation Hospital
Baltimore, Maryland

**Fran Swenson, RN, MSN**
Primary Nurse II, Neurosurgical Intensive Care
Unit
University of Maryland Hospital
Baltimore, Maryland

**Pamela Wachter, RN, MSN**
Primary Nurse II, Multitrauma 5, Critical Care
  Unit
Maryland Institute for Emergency Medical
  Services Systems
Baltimore, Maryland

**Joanne M. Walker, RN, MSN, CETN**
Enterostomal Therapist
Johns Hopkins Hospital
Baltimore, Maryland

**Mary Jayne Watson, RN, BSN**
Primary Nurse II, Multitrauma 6
Maryland Institute for Emergency Medical
  Services Systems
Baltimore, Maryland

**Sandra Weed, RN, MS**
Associate Director of Nursing
Maryland Institute for Emergency Medical
  Services Systems
Baltimore, Maryland

**Robert H. Welton, RN, MSN, CCRN**
Clinical Nurse Specialist
Maryland Institute for Emergency Medical
  Services Systems
Baltimore, Maryland

**Diana O. Williams, RN, MS, CCRN**
Primary Nurse III, Multitrauma 5
Maryland Institute for Emergency Medical
  Services Systems
Baltimore, Maryland

# CONTENTS

## PART 1
### Neurological Injuries/Complications

## PART 2
### Pulmonary Injuries/Complications

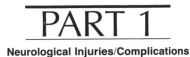

# PART 1

**Neurological Injuries/Complications**

## CHAPTER 1

# Open Head Injury Complicated by Diabetes Insipidus and Syndrome of Inappropriate Antidiuretic Hormone Secretion

Pamela Wachter, RN, MSN

## Clinical Presentation

A 26-year-old man was found unresponsive and hypotensive in a field with evidence of severe head trauma from an assault. On arrival in the emergency department, he had some spontaneous respirations but no movement of extremities. He was intubated for airway control, and mechanical ventilation was instituted. He was noted to have a large left parietal open skull fracture with no other evidence of injury. Pupils were sluggishly reactive but equal, and there was bloody fluid draining from the left ear. Following initial resuscitation, the patient was taken to the operating room where a left parietal craniectomy was performed with debridement of lacerated brain and dural repair.

Postoperatively, he was admitted to the intensive care unit (ICU), with a Richmond bolt for intracranial pressure monitoring. The opening pressure was 25 mm Hg. His vital signs were blood pressure 130/72, pulse 70, and respirations 14 via mechanical ventilation. His only response to stimulation was some withdrawal of the upper extremities. The pupils remained sluggishly reactive and equal. A right subclavian Swan-Ganz catheter, a left radial arterial line, an oral gastric tube, and a Foley catheter were in place. An admission laboratory work profile is displayed in Table 1.1, column A.

On the second day in the ICU, the patient's urinary output averaged 430 cc/hr with a specific gravity of 1.000. The patient's blood pressure was 90/60 with a pulse of 136. Laboratory work for that morning is seen in Table 1.1, column B.

The patient's morning laboratory work 4 days later is shown in Table 1.1, column C. No neurological response was elicited, except for some constant twitching of the lower extremities and some sluggish reaction of the pupils. The patient's temperature was 35°C (96°F) rectally. During the night he had several diarrhea stools and projectile emesis around the oral gastric tube. There was a weight gain of 5 lbs over the previous day, but no evidence of edema. Urinary output was approximately 60 cc/hr with a specific gravity of 1.010.

### 1. What is the pathophysiological basis for this patient's problem?

Posttraumatic diabetes insipidus (DI) is a complication of head trauma diagnosed with increasing frequency. This increase is most likely due to advancements in medical management of these patients resulting in improved survival rates, when previously they would have died from severe neurological damage (1 [p. 117]). DI is usually associated with skull and/or facial fractures, loss of consciousness, and cranial nerve dysfunction (2 [pp. 532–535]).

The clinical presentation of DI is diuresis with an onset that can range from a few

**1**

**Table 1.1.** Laboratory values

| | A<br>Baseline | B<br>DI<br>(1 day postinjury) | C<br>SIADH<br>(4 days postinjury) |
|---|---|---|---|
| Hemoglobin | 13.1 | 12.5 | 11 |
| Hematocrit | 36 | 35 | 30 |
| White blood cells | 14,800 | 13,000 | 15,000 |
| Platelets | 273 | 201 | 190 |
| Red blood cells | 5 | 4.5 | 4 |
| Sodium (serum) | 139 | 152 | 120 |
| Sodium (urine) | 200 | 10 | 75 |
| Potassium (serum) | 4.9 | 3.7 | 3.0 |
| Potassium (urine) | 66 | 7 | 26 |
| Chloride (serum) | 100 | 102 | 88 |
| $CO_2$ | 22 | 24 | 28 |
| Glucose | 119 | 154 | 160 |
| Urea nitrogen | 15 | 10 | 3 |
| Creatinine (serum) | 1.7 | 1.1 | 0.5 |
| Calcium | 8.4 | 9.4 | 10 |
| Osmolality (serum) | 275 | 322 | 254 |
| Osmolality (urine) | 606 | 145 | 890 |

hours to several months, and is caused by deficient secretion of arginine vasopressin (AVP), antidiuretic hormone (ADH) (3 [p. 22], 4, 5).

Vasopressin is produced in the hypothalamus and stored in the posterior pituitary (neurohypophysis). Its secretion is controlled by the hypothalamus in response to the intravascular blood volume and serum osmolality. Vasopressin maintains normal osmotic pressure of the plasma, stimulating the distal renal tubules and collecting ducts to increase reabsorption of water (6 [pp. 461–462], 7, 8 [pp. 313–317]).

Damage to supraoptic and paraventricular nuclei within the hypothalamus, or to the axons that travel from those nuclei to the neurohypophysis (the hypothalamo-hypophyseal tract), is necessary to produce significant DI. With head trauma there may be an actual insult to these areas, or there can be altered blood flow secondary to increased cerebral edema. For example, during a deceleration injury, the pituitary stalk may be compressed or sheared by the edge of the diaphragm sella. Hypotension or hypovolemia may also result in a decreased blood flow to these areas. The pathophysiological basis for the diabetes insipidus that insues is related to the number of vasopressin-secreting neurons that remain viable (6 [p. 463], 9, 10 [p. 66], 11 [pp. 785–796], 12).

Clinical signs of diabetes insipidus include the excretion of abnormally large quantities of dilute urine, up to 20 liters/day. In an alert patient there would also be the other cardinal symptom: polydipsia. In DI, the kidneys have lost their ability to control the amount of fluid output because of the deficit of ADH. Diagnosis is made by the use of plasma versus urine osmolality correlations. These patients have a serum sodium greater than 150 mEq/liter and a plasma osmolality greater than 290 mOsm/kg at the time of diagnosis. Urinalysis reveals an almost colorless urine with low osmolality (50 to 200 mOsm/kg) and low specific gravity (less than 1.005). Hypovolemia and hypotension may also be present; see Tables 1.2 and 1.3 (1 [pp. 129–132], 3 [p. 24], 13).

Other causes of DI include any pathology that results in a decrease or total lack of ADH production or secretion (central DI), a failure of the kidneys to respond to ADH due to osmoreceptor changes (nephrogenic DI), or as an idiopathic process. Specifically, central nervous system infection, cerebrovascular catastrophe, posthypophyseal or hypothalamic surgery, brain tumor, psychological stress, medications, renal disease, elec-

**Table 1.2.** Comparison of laboratory values in DI and SIADH

| Value | DI | Normal | SIADH |
|---|---|---|---|
| Serum osmolality | Over 295 mOsm/kg | 280–295 mOsm/kg | Under 280 mOsm/kg |
| Urine osmolality | Under 250 mOsm/kg | 300–1400 mOsm/kg | Inappropriately concentrated compared to serum osmolality |
| Serum sodium | Over 145 mEq/liter | 135–148 mEq/liter | Under 130 mEq/liter |
| Urine sodium | Normal | 130–260 mEq/liter | Over 25 mEq/liter |
| Blood urea nitrogen | Normal | 5–25 mg/dl | Under 10 mg/dl |
| Creatinine | Normal | 0.5–1.2 mg/dl | 0.4–0.7 mg/dl |
| Serum uric acid | Normal | 2–8 mg/dl | 2.9–4 mg/dl |
| Potassium | Normal | 3.8–5 mEq/liter | Normal or low |
| Hematocrit | Normal | 35–50% | Low |
| Urine specific gravity | 1.000–1.005 | 1.003–1.030 | Over 1.003 |

trolyte disturbance, and pregnancy have all been etiological factors in the development of DI (11).

Posttraumatic cases of DI may have a classic three-stage response caused by damage to the neural mechanisms that control ADH release. The pattern begins with severe DI that subsides as the patient enters the second stage during which the neurohypophysis degenerates, releasing excessive ADH into the bloodstream. Excessive ADH release is also called SIADH, which is discussed in the following paragraphs. In the third stage, permanent DI usually results (6 [p. 463], 14 [p. 170]).

The patient in this case presentation developed SIADH (syndrome of inappropriate antidiuretic hormone secretion) 5 days postadmission. In contrast to DI, it involves the

**Table 1.3.** Cardinal features of DI and SIADH

| DI | SIADH |
|---|---|
| Hypotonic polyuria of abrupt onset (over 5 liters/day) | Hyponatremia with hypo-osmolality of serum and extracellular fluid |
| Intensive polydipsia<br>  Excessive thirst for cold drinks<br>  Increased nocturnal thirst and nocturia | Continued renal excretion of sodium |
| Poor skin turgor | Absence of clinical evidence of volume depletion or edema |
| With intact thirst mechanism: dryness of skin and mucous membranes (such as dehydration of the intestinal space) | Inappropriately high urine osmolality |
| Without intact thirst mechanism: postural changes in pulse or blood pressure, azotemia, and oliguria, which would indicate dehydration of the vascular space | Normal renal function |
| Dehydration can become severe, resulting in fever, weakness, stupor, coma, and death | Normal adrenal function |
| | Thirst, impaired taste, anorexia, dyspnea or exertion, fatigue, dulled sensorium |
| | Nausea, vomiting, abdominal cramps |
| | Confusion, lethargy, muscle twitching, convulsions |

increased delivery or secretion of ADH in spite of a subnormal plasma osmolality. There is a failure in the feedback mechanisms that regulate ADH release and inhibition. Excess ADH can also be secreted by an ectopic source. This excess leads to excessive retention of water, which can progress to water intoxication. Clinical presentation includes overhydration and dilutional hyponatremia and hypochloremia. Other symptoms include weight gain without associated edema, weakness, lethargy, mental confusion, and sluggish tendon reflexes (15, 16 [p. 499]).

In SIADH the urine osmolality is elevated and serum osmolality is decreased. Expansion of the extracellular fluid volume lowers the serum hematocrit, BUN, and creatinine. Urine sodium increases to 20 mEq/liter or greater, and the urine-specific gravity is greater than 1.003. Symptoms of water intoxication include anorexia, nausea, vomiting, and diarrhea. They may progress to confusion, hostility, aberrant respirations, hypothermia, and convulsions; see Tables 1.2 and 1.3 (6 [p. 470], 17).

Since the first description of SIADH in 1957, it has progressed from a rare syndrome to a frequently seen metabolic disorder in hospitalized patients. A wide variety of disorders cause SIADH; however, most cases result from malignant or infectious disease of the central nervous system (CNS) or lungs. Overtreatment of DI with vasopressin may also lead to SIADH. Other etiologies are head trauma; drug-induced, postoperative psychiatric disorders; and idiopathic processes (14 [pp. 168–180], 18).

## 2. What are the nursing diagnoses of highest priority?

A. Alteration in electrolyte balance related to fluid volume deficit, hypernatremia, and diuresis

B. Potential for fluid and electrolyte imbalances related to fluid volume excess secondary to SIADH

## 3. What are the goals of nursing care?

### A. Nursing Diagnosis

Alteration in electrolyte balance related to fluid volume deficit, hypernatremia, and diuresis

### Goal of Care

Maintain fluid and electrolyte status.

### Nursing Interventions

- Monitor intake and output, daily weights, and urinary specific gravity.
- Monitor serum and urine electrolytes every 4 hours.
- Monitor for signs of dehydration, such as dry mucous membranes, decreased skin turgor, extreme thirst, or tachycardia.
- Monitor for CNS changes; observe for arrhythmias.
- Prevent constipation related to dehydration with bowel regimen.
- Monitor vital signs; central venous, pulmonary capillary wedge, and intracranial pressures every hour.

Management of the patient with a severe brain injury and diabetes insipidus is challenging. The circulating blood volume must be adjusted to the level needed to support tissue perfusion without elevating the intracranial pressure (ICP) (4). Patients with depressed arousal and inability to regulate their own intake will eventually lose enough fluid to lead to hypovolemia and death unless they are supplied with the correct amount of replacement. The thirst mechanism is lost as a fluid intake regulator. Enormous amounts of urine can be lost in a short period of time, which can result in hypovolemia. Electrolytes accompany the water lost by the kidneys, so they, too, must be appropriately replaced (16 [p. 515]).

The treatment for DI is fluid replacement and the administration of ADH (vasopressin). Diuresis associated with DI requires the replacement of lost water. A commonly used replacement fluid is 0.45% saline, since the total body sodium is usually low or normal. If large volumes are infused, the fluid should not contain dextrose. Hyperglycemia may occur followed by glycosuria, causing an osmotic diuresis (4, 16 [p. 515]).

In cases of severe central DI from head trauma, the treatment of choice is a continuous intravenous infusion of vasopressin (Pitressin). Pitressin's major pharmacological effects are on the kidneys and cardiovascular system. In the kidney there is an increase in water reabsorption by the distal tubules and collecting systems as the concentration of vasopressin increases. This reabsorption causes a decrease in water excretion. The effects of vasoconstriction result in decreased blood flow to splanchnic, coronary, and gastrointestinal beds including the pancreas as well as muscles and skin. The motility of the bowel is increased with the use of Pitressin (20).

Dosage is controversial. Low-dose therapy would be in the range of 0.1 to 0.6 units/minute; however, doses up to 1.5 units/minute have been used in the treatment of gastrointestinal bleeding (2, 19, 21).

Pitressin should not be used in patients with vascular disease, except with extreme caution, because of its vasoconstrictive effects. Even small doses may precipitate anginal pain, and with larger doses myocardial infarction is a threat.

Pitressin should be used cautiously in the presence of epilepsy, migraine, asthma, heart failure, or any state in which rapid addition to extracellular water may be hazardous to a potentially compromised system. Chronic nephritis with nitrogen retention contraindicates the use of vasopressin until improved renal function can be attained.

The following side effects have been reported following the administration of vasopressin: tremor, sweating, vertigo, circumoral pallor, "pounding" in the head, abdominal cramps, passage of gas, nausea, vomiting, urticaria, bronchial constriction, and anaphylaxis. Cardiac arrest and/or shock also have been observed after injection of vasopressin.

Close monitoring of all intake and output is a necessity, and an indwelling Foley catheter is required for accuracy. It is helpful to calculate and record cumulative amounts so the overall fluid balance can be easily evaluated. Hourly urine-specific gravity readings should be done, as well as urine and serum electrolytes every 4 hours. Daily body weight may serve as a guide to the state of hydration.

Vital signs should be followed closely for trends related to dehydration. The pulmonary capillary wedge pressure (PCWP) may be assessed as an indicator of intravascular volume status. ICP monitoring trends may show increases in ICP during the fluid replacement regimen that could be compromising in a head-injured patient. Because this patient is unable to respond to thirst stimuli, the nurse is solely responsible for parenteral fluid replacement via an infusion pump. Frequent mouth and skin care will promote patient comfort (8, 10 [p. 71], 11).

## B. Nursing Diagnosis

Potential for fluid and electrolyte imbalances related to fluid volume excess secondary to inappropriate antidiuretic hormone secretion

### Goal of Care

Maintain fluid and electrolyte status.

### Nursing Interventions

- Monitor urine and serum electrolytes.
- Monitor urine-specific gravity, color, composition.

- Monitor signs and symptoms of hyponatremia.
- Monitor strict intake and output.
- Restrict fluids as ordered.
- Weigh daily.
- Monitor signs of increased ICP, vital signs, and PCWP every hour.
- Monitor for neurological changes and signs of increased ICP.
- Auscultate breath sounds.
- Monitor gastric motility by assessing bowel sounds and bowel movements.

Treatment of SIADH, as does treatment of DI, depends on the underlying etiology. The etiology must be identified and treated along with the fluid and electrolyte imbalances (11).

Treatment depends on the severity of the hyponatremia, how suddenly it developed, and the severity of clinical symptoms. When the symptoms related to hyponatremia and water intoxication are mild to moderate, a fluid restriction alone of 600 to 800 ml/day may be used. Urinary and insensible water losses usually result in a negative water balance at that level. If water restriction is adequate, a steady increase in serum sodium and osmolality occurs as body weight decreases. In more severe cases, such as with a serum sodium less than 120 mEq/liter and with an acute onset, treatment must be more vigorous. A bolus of 200 to 300 cc 3% saline solution can be infused to raise the serum sodium to a level where symptoms improve. All fluid intake must continue to be restricted, perhaps as low as 500 cc/day. Hypokalemia also needs to be treated adequately. A rapid means of treating marked hypokalemia is the administration of furosemide with a saline infusion (14 [pp. 181–182], 15).

Nursing care of this patient is based on the frequent assessment of neurological and hydration status as well as the prevention of complications. Parameters included are neurological checks, intake and output, daily weight, serum electrolytes, urinary sodium, skin turgor, mucous membrane status, urine specific gravity, and PCWP (22).

As fluid restriction is the most important aspect of the treatment of the patient with SIADH, it is the nurse's responsibility to control the ordered intake. Output must also be accurately monitored.

Decreased gastrointestinal functioning can result from hyponatremia and restricted fluid intake. Monitoring for constipation and impaction needs to be done on a daily basis. Mouth care at frequent intervals will assist in keeping mucous membranes moist (11, 17).

## ASSOCIATED NURSING DIAGNOSES

A. Ineffective thermoregulation
B. Alteration in bowel elimination
C. Alterations in cardiac output
D. Potential for infection
E. Impaired physical mobility
F. Alteration in comfort related to acute pain
G. Impaired communication

**REFERENCES**

1. Moses A. Clinical and laboratory features of central and nephrogenic diabetes insipidus and primary polydipsia. In: Reichlin S, ed. The neurohypophysis. New York: Plenum, 1984.

2. Levitt MA, Fleischer AS, Meislin HW. Acute post-traumatic diabetes insipidus: treatment with continuous intravenous vasopressin. J Trauma 1984;24(6):532–535.

3. Fitzgerald P., ed. Handbook of clinical endocrinology. Chicago: Jones Medical Publication, 1986.

4. Dunham CM, Cowley RA. Shock trauma/critical care handbook. Rockville, MD: Aspen, 1986.

5. Kern KB, Meislin HW. Diabetes insipidus: occurrence after minor head trauma. J Trauma 1984;24:69–72.

6. Tindall G, Barrow D. Disorders of the pituitary. St Louis: CV Mosby, 1986.

7. Kinney MR, Dear CB, Packa DR, Voorman DMN, eds. AACN's clinical reference for critical care nursing. New York: McGraw-Hill, 1981:662.

8. Smith J. Nursing management of diabetes insipidus. J Neurosurg Nurs 1981;13:313–317.

9. Verbalis J, Robinson A, Moses A. Postoperative and posttraumatic diabetes insipidus. In: Czernichow P, Robinson A, eds. Diabetes insipidus in man. Basel: Karger, 1985:248–249.

10. Buross-Herlicky J, Gorofono CD. Identifying posterior lobe dysfunction. In: Guthrie CW, ed. Nurses clinical library: endocrine disorders. Springhouse, PA: Springhouse, 1984.

11. Germon K. Fluid and electrolyte problems associated with diabetes insipidus and syndrome of inappropriate antidiuretic hormone. Nurs Clin North Am 1987;22:785–796.

12. Swartz S. Disorders of water balance. In: Hare J, ed. Signs and symptoms in endocrine and metabolic disorders. Philadelphia: JB Lippincott, 1986:204.

13. Halloway N. Nursing the critically ill adult. Menlo Park: Addison-Wesley, 1988:538.

14. Hou S. Syndrome of inappropriate antidiuretic hormone secretion. In: Reichlin D, ed. The neurohypophysis. New York: Plenum, 1984.

15. Moses A, Notman D. Diabetes insipidus and syndrome of inappropriate antidiuretic hormone secretion. Adv Intern Med 1982;27:73–100.

16. Hudak D, Lohr T, Gallo B. Critical care nursing. Philadelphia: JB Lippincott, 1986.

17. Johndrow P, Thornton S. Syndrome of inappropriate antidiuretic hormone. Focus on Critical Care 1985;12:29–34.

18. Kannon C. The pituitary gland. New York: Plenum, 1987:565–570.

19. Hussey D. Vasopressin therapy for upper gastrointestinal tract hemorrhage. Arch Intern Med 1985;145:1263–1267.

20. Hartshorn J, Hartshorn E. Vasopressin in the treatment of diabetes insipidus. J Neurosci Nurs 1988;20:58–59.

21. Katzung B, ed. Basic and clinical pharmacology. Norwalk: Appleton and Lange, 1987:434–435.

22. Manifold SL. Craniocerebral trauma. Focus on Critical Care 1986;13:22–35.

# CHAPTER 2

## Closed Head Injury with Cerebral Edema and Intraventricular Catheter

Fran Swenson, RN, MSN

## Clinical Presentation

A 20-year-old man was admitted to the hospital following a motor vehicle accident. He was unconscious, his pupils were equal and reactive to light, and his motor response to deep pain was flexion. His vital signs were as follows: blood pressure, 100/50 mm Hg; pulse, 60 beats/minute; and respirations, 10 and labored.

He was immediately intubated with a number 8 oral endotracheal tube and placed on a volume-cycled ventilator. The ventilator settings were $FiO_2$, 0.50; tidal volume, 800 ml; positive end expiratory pressure (PEEP), 5 cm; and intermittent mandatory ventilation (IMV) rate, 12. A head computerized tomography (CT) scan showed a right temporal lobe contusion with diffuse cerebral edema. An intraventricular catheter (IVC) was placed to monitor his intracranial pressure (ICP), with an opening pressure of 20 mm Hg.

He was admitted to the intensive care unit (ICU), where a right radial arterial line measured his blood pressure as 150/70 mm Hg, with a mean arterial pressure (MAP) of 90 mm Hg. His pulse was 70 beats/minute, and his respiratory rate was 12. His ICP was 18 mm Hg, and his cerebral perfusion pressure (CPP) was 72 mm Hg. He was comatose, his pupils remained equal and reactive, and his motor response to deep pain continued to be flexion. He had a number 18 orogastric tube to low intermittent suction as well as a Foley catheter. A pulmonary artery catheter was inserted through his right subclavian vein, revealing a pulmonary artery (PA) systolic/diastolic pressure of 24/12 mm Hg, a pulmonary capillary wedge pressure (PCWP) of 13 mm Hg, and a central venous pressure (CVP) of 10 mm Hg. He was hyperventilated via the ventilator to keep his $PaCO_2$ between 25 and 30 mm Hg. His IVC was set to drain whenever his ICP was greater than 10 mm Hg.

On his sixth day, he developed bacterial meningitis. A daily culture of his cerebral spinal fluid (CSF), drawn from the IVC, grew *Staphylococcus aureus*. He was given ticarcillin (500 mg IV every 4 hours), amikacin (500 mg IV every 8 hours), nafcillin (1.5 gm IV every 4 hours), and chloramphenicol (500 mg IV every 6 hours).

His neurological status improved, and the IVC was removed on the 10th day. On the 12th day, his level of consciousness decreased, and a repeat head CT scan showed hydrocephalus. An IVC was again placed to facilitate CSF drainage until a ventriculovenous shunt could be inserted.

## 1. What is the pathophysiological basis for this patient's problem?

A closed head injury is a nonpenetrating injury to the brain with the integrity of the skull remaining intact. A brain contusion is a bruising of the brain, characterized by edema and capillary hemorrhage. Contusions may be caused by a coup injury, which occurs below the level of the impact. The movement of the semisolid brain within the cranial vault may result in bruising of the temporal lobe.

Cerebral edema is an abnormal accumulation of water and fluid within the intracellular and extracellular spaces. It is associated with increased brain tissue volume (1). There are two types of cerebral edema: vasogenic and cytotoxic. Vasogenic edema, the more

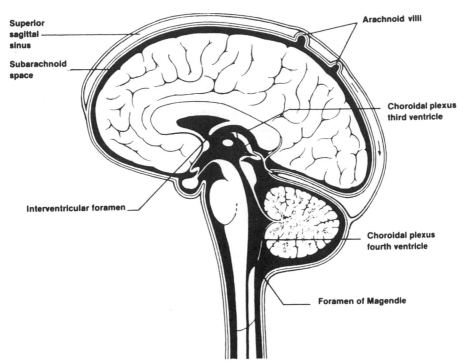

Superior sagittal sinus

Subarachnoid space

Arachnoid villi

Choroidal plexus third ventricle

Interventricular foramen

Choroidal plexus fourth ventricle

Foramen of Magendie

**Figure 2.1.** Flow of cerebrospinal fluid. (From Hickey J. The clinical practice of neurological and neurosurgical nursing. 2nd ed. Philadelphia: JB Lippincott, 1986.)

common type, occurs predominately in the white matter of the extracellular space. Cytotoxic edema occurs within the gray and white matter of the intracellular space.

Cerebral edema is associated with increased ICP. ICP is the pressure exerted by the CSF within the ventricles; the normal value is between 0 and 15 mm Hg (2 [p. 129]).

The brain is encased within a bony vault, so expansion is limited. The Monro-Kellie hypothesis states that the skull is a rigid compartment filled with essentially noncompressible contents: intravascular blood (10%), CSF (10%), and brain matter (80%) (3). If the volume of one component increases, then the other two components compensate by decreasing their volume. Increased ICP results when compensation cannot occur.

An IVC is a polyethylene catheter which is inserted (ideally) within the anterior horn of the lateral ventricle in the nondominant hemisphere. The IVC provides an accurate measurement of the ICP; it also offers the advantage of draining CSF to control ICP. (CSF is more accommodating to decreases in volume than the other two components.)

CSF cushions the brain and is formed in the choroid plexus of the ventricles. It circulates from the lateral ventricles through the foramen of Monro to the third ventricle, transverses the aqueduct of Sylvius to the fourth ventricle, and leaves the fourth ventricle and enters the cisterns via the foramina of Luschka and Magendie. It is reabsorbed into the arachnoid villi, projections from the subarachnoid space (SAS), into the dural venous sinuses (2 [p. 50]) (Fig. 2.1).

Bacterial meningitis is an infection that involves the pia and arachnoid layers of the meninges, subarachnoid space, and CSF. Because CSF circulates around the brain, the purulent exudate spreads, causing an accumulation of CSF, or secondary hydrocephalus.

Defective reabsorption can therefore result when the exudate from meningitis plugs the arachnoid villi.

There are two major types of hydrocephalus: communicating and noncommunicating. Communicating hydrocephalus occurs despite normal communication between the fourth ventricle and the subarachnoid space. The production of CSF exceeds the reabsorption rate. Noncommunicating hydrocephalus occurs when there is a blockage at any location in the ventricular system, preventing flow of CSF to the subarachnoid space. This blockage may be caused by blood, infection, edema, or other factors. Most hydrocephalus seen in trauma patients is noncommunicating.

## 2. What are the nursing diagnoses of highest priority?

A. Alteration in cerebral tissue perfusion
B. Ineffective airway clearance
C. Excess in fluid volume

## 3. What are the goals of nursing care?

### A. Nursing Diagnosis

Alteration in cerebral tissue perfusion related to cerebral edema

### Goal of Care

Maintain cerebral blood flow above 60 mm Hg and ICP at less than 15 mm Hg.

### Nursing Interventions

- Maintain head of bed at 30 to 45 degrees.
- Maintain head alignment in a neutral position; use soft collar as necessary.
- Drain the IVC for ICP greater than or equal to 10 to 15 mm Hg, as ordered by physician.
- Maintain the $PaCO_2$ between 25 and 30 with hyperventilation.

### Rationale

The patient should be positioned to facilitate venous return from the head. The best position is head elevation of 30 to 45 degrees, with the head in a neutral position. A soft collar may be used to maintain the head in this position. If the ICP remains elevated above 20 mm Hg without stimulation, the head of the bed can be further elevated 70 to 80 degrees with the patient supine (4 [p. 98]).

The patient may be turned from side to side using slow gentle motions; rapid movement increases ICP (5). Occasionally, the patient's ICP may be elevated when turned to the injured side; if this occurs, turn the patient only 10 to 30 degrees.

The physician may order the IVC to be drained at a specific level, and the nurse should position the drainage system accordingly. Improper positioning may result in rapid drainage of CSF with possible collapse of the ventricles. An intravenous (IV) pole is used to suspend the drainage system below the level of the patient. The nurse tapes the drainage system to the IV pole, with the zero point of a tape measure at the level of the ventricles. (This level is estimated by drawing an imaginary line from the patient's ear to the corner of his or her eye.) The tape is applied lengthwise and taped at 10 cm; this is the point that the drainage system should be taped to the IV pole. The IVC is connected to a stopcock that can be opened to the patient, the transducer, and the drainage system, thus allowing the CSF to drain whenever the ICP is greater than 10 mm Hg (Fig. 2.2) or as otherwise prescribed. In some cases, the neurosurgeon may order the IVC to drain continuously. If continuous drainage is ordered, the stopcocks are simultaneously opened to the patient, the transducer, and the drainage system. The nurse needs to turn the stopcock off to

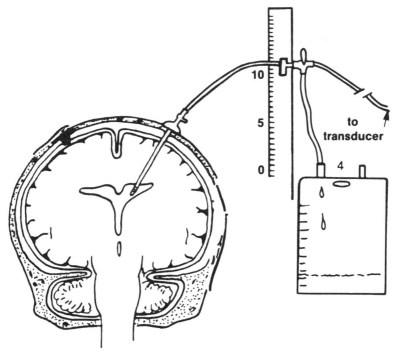

**Figure 2.2.** IVC drainage system positioning. (From Raimond J, Taylor J. Neurological emergencies: effective nursing care. Rockville, MD: Aspen, 1986.)

stop drainage when any nursing activity is performed (e.g., turning, chest physical therapy [CPT], and suctioning). These activities increase ICP, and if the system is open, CSF will drain too rapidly.

The nurse should check the CSF drainage every 2 hours and record the amount on the flowsheet as output. The IVC is a potential source of infection; therefore, a closed system should be maintained. A CSF culture is sent daily from the IVC to monitor for infection.

A reduction in the $PaCO_2$ level in the blood causes vasoconstriction of the cerebral blood vessels, which reduces cerebral blood flow and ICP (6). By lowering the ICP, cerebral perfusion is maintained. CPP is calculated by subtracting the mean ICP from the mean arterial pressure (MAP):

$$CPP = MAP - ICP$$

A CPP of 60 mm Hg is necessary to perfuse the brain adequately. A CPP below 30 mm Hg is incompatible with life (2 [p. 142]).

## B. Nursing Diagnosis
Ineffective airway clearance related to decreased level of consciousness

## Goals of Care
Maintain patient airway. Breath sounds will be clear. Chest x-ray film will be clear.

## Nursing Interventions

- Assess airway patency.
- Monitor breath sounds every 2 hours.
- Monitor chest radiograph.
- Give chest pulmonary toilet (CPT) every 4 hours.
- Suction as needed; hyperventilate and hyperinflate the patient before and after suctioning.

## Rationale

Respiratory assessment and early chest x-ray films will alert the health care team to problem areas that compromise oxygenation. When pulmonary status is poor, hypoxemia can produce poor cerebral perfusion, resulting in increased brain damage (4 [p. 97]).

Suctioning assists in the maintenance of a patent airway. The suctioning catheter should not be left in the endotracheal tube longer than 15 seconds. Extended suctioning can increase the $CO_2$ level in the blood, causing vasodilation of the cerebral arteries. CPT enhances the effect of hyperventilation and helps to treat and prevent pulmonary complications.

During suctioning, the patient will experience an increase in ICP, and lidocaine may assist in lowering it. On a physician's order, 2% lidocaine (1.5 mg/kg) may be administered intravenously before suctioning. Lidocaine suppresses the cough reflex, which increases the intrathoracic pressure, thus increasing ICP (7). The patient needs to be hyperventilated and hyperinflated for at least 20 to 30 seconds with 100% oxygen both before and after suctioning. This hyperventilation may be accomplished either by manual inflation with an Ambu bag or with the mechanical ventilator. Mechanical hyperventilation is accomplished by turning the $FiO_2$ to 1.00 and increasing the respiratory rate on the ventilator. This type of hyperventilation delivers a set volume, pressure, and rate. The nurse must remember to reset the ventilator to the ordered $FiO_2$ and respiratory rate following suctioning.

## C. Nursing Diagnosis

Excess fluid volume related to cerebral edema

## Goal of Care

Maintain a slightly dehydrated state.

## Nursing Intervention

Maintain fluid volume intake at 75 cc/hr.

## Rationale

Fluid restriction prevents extracellular volume overload. When the extracellular body volume, including that in the brain, is decreased, then the ICP is decreased. Isotonic solutions should be used because hypotonic solutions may increase cerebral edema by osmotic pull of fluids from blood to brain (2 [p. 141]).

# ASSOCIATED NURSING DIAGNOSES

A. Impaired physical mobility related to decreased level of consciousness
B. Nutritional alteration to less than body requirements related to decreased level of consciousness
C. Potential for injury related to decreased level of consciousness
D. Ineffective family coping related to hospitalization, diagnosis, and uncertainty of prognosis
E. Self-care deficit related to decreased level of consciousness

## REFERENCES

1. Hickey J. The clinical practice of neurological and neurosurgical nursing. 2nd ed. Philadelphia: JB Lippincott, 1986:251.
2. Raimond J, Taylor J. Neurological emergencies: effective nursing care. Rockville, MD: Aspen, 1986.
3. Ropper A, Kennedy S. Neurological and neurosurgical intensive care. Maryland: Royal Tunbridge Wills, 1988:9.
4. Robinet K. Increased intracranial pressure: management with an intraventricular catheter. J Neurosurg Nurs 1984;17(2):98.
5. Walleck C. Critical care of the client with increased intracranial pressure. In: Lewis S, Collier F, eds. Medical surgical nursing: assessment and management of clinical practice. 2nd ed. New York: McGraw-Hill, 1987:1517.
6. Ruby E. Advanced neurological and neurosurgical nursing. St Louis: CV Mosby, 1984:133.
7. Ruby E, Baun M, Stone K, Turner B. The relationship between endotracheal suctioning and changes in intracranial pressure: a review of the literature. Heart Lung 1986;15(5):492.

# CHAPTER 3

## Cerebral Contusion: Barbiturate Coma Therapy

Mary Jane Seipp, RN, BSN, CNRN

## Clinical Presentation

A 17-year-old man was transported to an emergency department (ED) following a motorcycle accident. He had lost control of his vehicle, hit a median strip, and was thrown several yards onto a grassy area. He was wearing a helmet. He arrived wearing a Philadelphia collar, acting lethargic, and withdrawing from pain. His pupils were equal and sluggishly reactive to light. Blood pressure was 110/60, pulse 90, respirations 12. The patient was orally intubated and was hyperventilated. Diagnostic peritoneal lavage was negative, and the entire abdominal assessment was normal. Toxicology screen was negative, and cervical films were normal. A Foley catheter and an oral gastric tube were inserted. Cervical spine films were normal; however, a head computerized tomography (CT) scan showed cerebral contusions with no evidence of hematomas or shift.

A subarachnoid bolt was inserted to monitor intracranial pressure (ICP). The patient was given 1000 mg of Dilantin intravenously over 20 minutes. Elevations in ICP (>20 mm Hg) were initially controlled with conventional therapy, such as hyperventilation, osmotic/loop diuretics, fluid restrictions, and sedation. Twenty-four hours after the accident these measures became ineffective in controlling intracranial pressure. A follow-up CT scan revealed diffuse cerebral edema.

A pulmonary artery catheter was inserted, with initial measurements showing a central venous pressure (CVP) of zero and a pulmonary capillary wedge pressure (PCWP) of 5. Colloids were given, which increased the CVP to 3 and the PCWP to 7. A pentobarbital coma was induced by intravenously administering pentobarbital at 10 mg/kg/hr over 4 hours. After instituting barbiturate therapy, ICP decreased from 26 mm Hg to 12 mm Hg within 1 hour. The maintenance dose of pentobarbital ranged from 1 mg/kg/hr to 3 mg/kg/hr based on serum drug levels and clinical findings. Coma was maintained for 5 days (see Table 3.1).

## 1. What is the pathophysiological basis for this patient's problem?

Closed head injury occurs when linear and rotational forces cause structural disruption of cranial contents. The brain is suspended in the skull; rapid acceleration-deceleration can result in a punching-bag effect. The brain is the punching bag being struck against the skull, resulting in compression, tension shearing, and rotational strains. This effect can produce structural disruption of the blood vessels, cortex, and white matter. Contusions and lacerations can result from brain displacement at the site of impact (coup), and behind, from negative pressure (contracoup). Temporal tips and the inferior surface of frontal lobes are frequent sites of injury. The extent of the primary injury depends on the extent of axon disruption and neuronal pathway interruption (1–3).

Death can occur from extensive primary brain damage or as the result of injuries to other body systems. Damage from the initial insult may not be lethal, but secondary intracranial complications, such as intracranial hypertension, may be.

ICP is a function of the relationship of blood, brain, and cerebrospinal fluid (CSF) within the cranium. Normally this pressure is 0 to 15 mm Hg. Compensatory mechanisms

14

**Table 3.1.** High-dose barbiturate therapy guidelines

| | |
|---|---|
| *Pre-Induction Care* | |
| Weight patient | Weight determines barbiturate dose. |
| Assist with insertion of invasive lines | Arterial line, pulmonary artery line, and intracranial pressure monitoring device must be inserted if not already present. |
| *Induction of Coma* | |
| Loading dose | Examine pentobarbital drips for precipitate. Do not |
| Pentobarbital | refrigerate. Incompatible with most drugs. |
| 10 mg/kg/hr × 4 hours or | Administer through large vein, preferably central |
| 40 mg/kg total dose | line. Hypotension frequently occurs. Be prepared to administer fluids and have vasopressors handy. Dopamine drug of choice. Monitor for arrhythmias. |
| *Coma Maintenance* | |
| 1–3 mg/kg/hr | Once coma is achieved, a reduction in intracranial pressure should occur. Monitoring should show decreased EEG activity. A pattern called "burst suppression," in which activity is flat or minimal, is expected. Neural activity is suppressed. Pupillary responses and cough, gag, corneal, and motor reflexes should be absent. Notify physician immediately if reflexes return, pupils change, or ICP or EEG activity increases. Monitor barbiturate levels every 6 to 24 hours. Levels of 25 to 40 μg/ml are desirable. |
| *Cessation of Therapy* | Coma duration is determined by physician. Pentobarbital is metabolized by liver and excreted by kidneys. Therefore, drug clearance depends on organ functioning. Expect to taper drug gradually. |

occur when one or more of the intracranial volumes increase. These mechanisms include displacement of CSF from the intracranial compartments to the spinal subarachnoid space, increased rate of CSF absorption, and reduction of cerebral blood volume by displacement of venous cerebral blood into the venous sinuses. Effectiveness of compensation is affected by the location and extent of injury, the rate of volume increase, and intracranial compliance.

Intracranial compliance expresses the relationship between increases in intracranial volume and the effect on ICP. Compliance is decreased when small increases in intracranial volume cause a significant sustained increase in ICP. The uninjured brain has normal compliance and can maintain normal pressure over a range of conditions. The patient with cerebral edema has decreased compliance; therefore, increases in intracranial volume, such as increased edema, blood volume, or CSF from ventricular obstruction, lead to intracranial hypertension and possibly to herniation and death.

An appreciation of factors affecting cerebral blood flow is also important when discussing ICP. Adequate cerebral blood flow is essential to meet the oxygen and metabolic needs of the brain. Cerebral blood flow is affected by oxygen and carbon dioxide levels. Hypercarbia and hypoxia cause cerebral vasodilation. Hyperventilation lowers $PaCO_2$ levels (25 to 30), which causes vasoconstriction and thereby decreases cerebral blood flow volume. In addition, the lowered $PaCO_2$ causes a correction of brain tissue acidosis, improves autoregulation, and contributes to ease of maintaining a patient on a ventilator

(4). Cerebral perfusion pressure (CPP) is an arithmetic expression of the pressure at which neuronal cells are perfused. CPP is calculated by subtracting the mean intracranial pressure (ICP) from the mean arterial pressure (MAP):

$$CPP = MAP - ICP$$

CPP should be at least 60 mm Hg for adequate cerebral blood flow. When cerebral blood flow is inadequate, brain ischemia results. If the CPP equals zero, cerebral blood flow ceases. CPP is increased by lowering ICP and maintaining adequate arterial pressures.

Autoregulation also affects ICP. Autoregulation normally maintains cerebral blood flow over a wide range of systemic arterial pressures by altering the diameter of arterioles in the brain. Brain injury impairs autoregulation, resulting in additional ischemia and damage.

Medical and nursing management are aimed at preventing secondary injury from intracranial hypertension and inadequate cerebral perfusion. Conventional therapy uses hyperventilation, glucocorticosteroids, osmotic/loop diuretics, and fluid restriction to decrease cerebral edema and prevent ischemia. Neurological findings and ICP monitoring provide information regarding efficacy of the therapy (5–7).

Barbiturate therapy may be used in cases of intractable intracranial hypertension unresponsive to conventional therapy. The exact mechanisms by which barbiturates lower ICP are not fully understood. It is believed barbiturates reduce cerebral metabolism and oxygen need, improve distribution of cerebral blood flow, stabilize cell membranes, and preserve ischemic brain cells from additional damage by oxidizing cell toxic substances (8, 9). It is clear that barbiturate therapy decreases ICP; however, there is little evidence demonstrating that barbiturates favorably alter the outcome of any disease entity (10).

Barbiturate therapy is not without risks. Profound hypotension can occur during coma induction and maintenance. Patients with intracranial hypertension for whom standard treatments have been ineffective are already dehydrated because of fluid restriction. Close monitoring of hemodynamic parameters is essential. Administration of colloids frequently is needed to prevent deleterious decreases in systemic blood pressure. Untoward decreases in systemic pressure can further compromise CPP, hence vasopressors should be readily available. The patient will require hemodynamic and ICP monitoring by experienced personnel. Daily monitoring of serum barbiturate levels is also essential. Therapeutic barbiturate levels range from 3 to 4 mg%. Dosing is adjusted based on laboratory data and clinical findings. Cardiovascular collapse and renal and liver damage can result from toxic levels (8, 9, 11).

## 2. What are the nursing diagnoses of highest priority?

A. Alteration in cerebral perfusion
B. Alteration in tissue perfusion
C. Alteration in respiratory function

## 3. What are the goals of nursing care?

### A. Nursing Diagnosis

Alteration in cerebral perfusion related to cerebral edema and ischemia

### Goal of Care

Maintain cerebral perfusion pressure greater than 50 mm Hg and intracranial pressure less than 15 mm Hg.

## Nursing Interventions

- Monitor ICP continuously.
- Calculate CPP at least hourly (CPP = MAP − ICP).
- Monitor effects of medications and fluids.
- Monitor effects of nursing care activities and environmental stimuli.
- Position patient to maximize CPP.
- Maintain $PaO_2$ and $PaCO_2$ within prescribed range.
- Monitor neurological status.

## Rationale

The patient with increased ICP is at risk for additional cerebral damage, herniation, and death. Ongoing neurological evaluation is essential. ICP monitoring and CPP calculations provide valuable information regarding the effectiveness of therapies and the patient's tolerance of nursing activities and environmental stimuli. The patient should be positioned to maximize venous return from the cranium by elevating the height of the bed 30 to 45 degrees and maintaining head alignment with the lower part of body. Extreme hip flexion should be avoided, as this increases intra-abdominal pressure, resulting in increases in ICP. The patient must be hyperventilated with 100% oxygen before and after suctioning to avoid malignant increases in intracranial pressure, secondary to vasodilation from hypoxia and hypercarbia. Nursing care activities should be planned around the response of the patient to specific interventions and rest periods incorporated into the plan of care. For example, if elevations in ICP occur following position changes, plan for a period of rest before beginning another activity that has also been identified as raising ICP (5, 6).

## B. Nursing Diagnosis

Alteration in systemic tissue perfusion related to barbiturate therapy, hypovolemia, and impaired cerebral autoregulation

## Goal of Care

Maintain adequate tissue perfusion as evidenced by a systolic arterial pressure above 90 mm Hg, urinary output at least 30 cc/hr.

## Nursing Interventions

- Hourly assessment of the following parameters:
  Systolic arterial pressure
  Pulmonary artery pressures
  Central venous pressures
  Urinary output with specific gravity
- Monitor cardiac rhythm continuously.
- Monitor EEG continuously (if available).
- Assess cardiac outputs, systemic vascular resistance, and wedges as ordered but at least every 8 hours.
- Administer intravenous fluids, vasopressors, antidiuretics, and anti-arrhythmics as ordered, and monitor effects.
- Monitor serum electrolytes, osmolarity, and barbiturate levels.

## Rationale

The proposed beneficial effects of barbiturate therapy on the brain may be complicated by systemic hemodynamic instability. The patient may be mildly dehydrated from osmotic diuretics. Prior to induction of barbiturate coma, adequate venous access and placement of pulmonary artery and arterial lines are necessary to monitor hemodynamic response to induction. Fluid boluses with colloids prior to, and during, coma are frequently given to avoid hypotension. During induction and maintenance of coma, continuous monitoring of the above parameters must be done and changes reported, as barbiturate-induced hypotension can ensue.

Vasopressors, such as dopamine and dobutamine, may be needed to raise systemic arterial pressure to provide an adequate CPP. Hypovolemic and hyperosmolar states require close monitoring of laboratory value; electrolyte disturbances should be recognized and treated promptly. Antidiuretic hormone administration may be necessary to control increased urine output, particularly if diabetes insipidus develops.

The goal of barbiturate therapy is to lower intracranial pressure by decreasing the metabolic needs of the brain. Assessment for pupillary reactivity and reflexes (cough, gag, corneals) should be performed regularly. Reflexes, if present, should be reported, as they indicate that the patient is not in coma. The neurological findings described above and the barbiturate levels are used to titrate barbiturate dose. Close monitoring is essential, since barbiturate toxicity can mimic shock with profound hypotension and cardiac arrhythmias (8, 9).

## C. Nursing Diagnosis

Alteration in respiratory function related to barbiturate therapy

## Goal of Care

Maintain normal respiratory function as evidenced by clear breath sounds bilaterally and a $PaO_2$ greater than 90.

## Nursing Interventions

- Ensure that ventilator alarms are on at all times.
- Check minimal occlusive pressure (MOP) of endotracheal or tracheostomy tube cuff every 12 hours.
- Auscultate breath sounds every 2 hours and after position changes.
- Suction oropharynx every 1 to 2 hours.
- Suction trachea as needed.
- Do not administer tracheal lavage.
- Obtain arterial blood gases as ordered.
- Administer chest physiotherapy (CPT) as ordered at prescribed height.
- Report any spontaneous respirations.

## Rationale

Once barbiturate coma is induced, the patient has complete respiratory depression. The presence of reflexes, such as a cough, gag, or spontaneous respirations, should be reported, as these signs indicate that the patient is not in coma. Frequent auscultation should be done to verify tube placement and detect changes in breath sounds. A $PaO_2$ greater than 90 is desirable. Immobility with absent protective reflexes places the patient at high risk for atelectasis and infiltrates. Oral secretions should be suctioned as needed. Saline lavage should not be instilled down the tracheal tube on patients without a cough reflex. CPT may be ordered to loosen secretions. If CPT with postural drainage is used, the patient's response to this treatment modality should be monitored. Anticipate an increase in intracranial pressure as a result of increased arterial flow and decreased venous return. Hemodynamic values may also be altered.

# ASSOCIATED NURSING DIAGNOSES

A. Ineffective thermoregulation
B. Fluid volume deficit
C. Potential for injury
D. Potential for infection
E. Family anxiety
F. Inadequate knowledge

## REFERENCES

1. Ricci MM, ed. Core curriculum for neuroscience nursing. Park Ridge, IL: American Association of Neuroscience Nurses, 1984.
2. Conway-Ruthkowski BL. Carni and Owens neurosurgical nursing. 8th ed. St Louis: Mosby, 1982.
3. Samuels MA, ed. Manual of neurological therapeutics with essential diagnosis. Boston: Little, Brown, 1978.
4. McDowell DG. Artificial ventilation in the management of the head injured patient. In: Fitch W, Baker J, eds. Head injury and the anesthetist. New York: Elsevier, 1985:149–163.
5. Mikas DL. Critical aspects of head trauma. CCQ 1987;10(10:19–43.
6. Walleck CA. Intracranial hypertension: interventions and outcomes. CCQ 1987;10(1):45–55.
7. Pollack-Latham CL. Intracranial pressure monitoring: part 1, physiologic principles. Crit Care Nurse 1987;7(5):40–51.
8. Heinemeyer G. Clinical pharmacokinetic considerations in the treatment of increased intracranial pressure. Clin Pharmacokinet 1987;13(1):1–25.
9. Eisenberg HM, Frankowski RF, Contant CF, Marshall LF, Walker MD. High-dose barbiturate control of elevated intracranial pressure in patients with severe head injury. J Neurosurg 1988;69(1):15–23.
10. Wermeling DP, Blouin RA, Porter WH, Rapp RP, Tibbs PA. Pentobarbital pharmacokinetics in patients with severe head injury. Drug Intell Clin Pharm 1987;21(50:459–463.
11. Kirsch JR, Diringer MN, Borel CO, Hart GK, Henley DF. Medical management and innovations. In: Richmond TS, ed. Brain resuscitation. Crit Care Nurs Clin North Am 1989;1(1):143–154.

# CHAPTER 4

# Epidural Hematoma with Herniation

Elizabeth E. Stickles, RN, BSN

## Clinical Presentation

A 23-year-old man was involved in a street fight and was assaulted on the head with a blunt object. At the scene he was angry, anxious, and complained of a severe headache, but was able to answer questions appropriately; pupils were equal at 4 mm and briskly reactive to light. Paramedics inserted 16-gauge angiocaths bilaterally into antecubital veins and infused normal saline solution to keep vein open (KVO). His pulse was 100, blood pressure was 150/90, and respirations were moderately deep and unlabored at 24/minute. He was transported via helicopter to the nearest hospital.

En route to the hospital, the patient became lethargic and confused, but his pupils remained equal and briskly reactive to light. His pulse was 80, BP was 158/80, and respirations were at 18/minute.

On arrival at the emergency department he uttered incomprehensible sounds, withdrew his right arm to deep pain, but was unable to move his left side. His right pupil was 5 mm and his left pupil was 3 mm; they both reacted sluggishly to light. His Glasgow Coma Scale score was 6/15. Skull x-rays revealed a right temporal linear skull fracture; cervical spine x-ray revealed no fracture. Computerized tomography (CT) scan revealed a large right epidural hematoma with a massive right-to-left shift. He was medicated with mannitol 25 gm intravenous (IV) bolus.

Physical exam revealed a midline trachea, bilateral equal chest expansion, clear lungs, and shallow respirations at 12/minute. Arterial blood gases were pH 7.45, $PaO_2$ 76, $PaCO_2$ 35, with $SaO_2$ 96%. The patient was intubated with an 8-mm oral endotracheal tube and mechanically ventilated with SIMV 16, $FiO_2$ 0.40, $V_T$ 800 ml, and PEEP 5 cm $H_2O$. Repeat arterial blood gases were pH 7.38, $PaO_2$ 123, $PaCO_2$ 28, with 99% $SaO_2$.

Electrocardiogram showed normal sinus rhythm with no ectopics. No cardiac murmurs, gallops, or rubs were auscultated. His pulse was 60 and BP was 162/78 by noninvasive automatic monitoring device. Normal saline solution was infused to KVO.

Abdominal exam revealed normo-active bowel sounds, a soft abdomen without rebound tenderness, organomegaly, or masses, and a stable pelvis. No further diagnostic studies were deemed necessary. A number 16 French Foley catheter was inserted into the urinary bladder.

The patient was immediately transported to the operating room for a right temporal parietal craniotomy with evacuation of the right EDH, ligation of a bleeding artery, and placement of a subarachnoid bolt to monitor the intracranial pressure (ICP). Opening ICP was 25 mm Hg with a cerebral perfusion pressure (CPP) of 83 mm Hg. A left subclavian pulmonary artery (PA) catheter was inserted to monitor hemodynamic status. Ringer's lactate solution was infused at KVO rate. A left radial arterial catheter was inserted to monitor blood pressure; BP was 160/90 with a mean arterial pressure (MAP) of 113.

Immediately postoperatively, both pupils were 2 mm and sluggishly reactive to light. The patient was unresponsive to pain secondary to anesthesia. Vital signs included pulse 98, BP 158/86, MAP 110, ICP 16, and CPP 94.

On admission to the intensive care unit (ICU), the patient was unresponsive to deep pain. His right pupil was 6 mm and sluggishly reactive to light; his left pupil was 4 mm and briskly reactive to light. Trace flexion of the right arm to painful stimuli was noted. Vital signs and hemodynamic parameters were stable. Normal saline with 40 mEq KCl/liter was infused to KVO.

One hour after admission, ICP increased to 30 mm Hg despite positioning of the cervical collar to maintain midline head alignment, elevating the head of the bed (HOB) to 60 degrees, and hyperventilating to $PaCO_2$ 25 to 30 mm Hg. After being medicated with fentanyl 3 cc IV, the patient's ICP immediately decreased to 25, CPP to 63, and MAP to 88. Two hours after admission, the patient was neurologically deteriorating; his pulse was 125, MAP 80, ICP 30, and CPP 50. His right pupil was 8 mm and nonreactive to light; his left pupil was 4 mm and sluggishly reactive to light with a disconjugate gaze. He abnormally extended to pain. The neurosurgeon was immediately notified of increasing ICP with decreasing CPP, widening pulse pressure with decreasing MAP, unequal pupils, and abnormal rigid posturing. After the patient was medicated with pentobarbital 50 mg IV bolus and mannitol 50 gm IV bolus to decrease ICP, he was immediately transported to CT scan.

On return from CT scan, both pupils were fixed and dilated, Doll's eyes were absent, and all extremities were flaccid. Spontaneous respirations were shallow, ataxic, and rapid at 40/minute. His pulse gradually decreased to 50 with a declining MAP to 50. CT scan and clinical exam revealed a transtentorial herniation of the brain.

## 1. What is the pathophysiological basis for the patient's problem?

An epidural hematoma (EDH) is an accumulation of blood between the skull and the dura; it may be caused by arterial or venous bleeding in the frontal or temporal regions. Most EDHs occur over the cerebral convexity, are usually overlying the temporal lobe, and result from a laceration of the middle meningeal artery caused by a skull fracture (1) (Fig. 4.1). An acute EDH is a rare injury, but it may be fatal if the bleed is arterial because ICP rises rapidly causing the brain to shift and possibly herniate.

A classic example of an EDH is the boxer who is knocked unconscious, wakes up, and is allowed to go home, and then is found dead in his bed the next morning. According to McGinnis, only 33% of the EDH cases present with this classic scenario of a lucid interval, or initial unconsciousness followed by lucidity, with subsequent unconsciousness (2). Plum and Posner describe the most common progression of an EDH: As the hematoma expands, the brain is first pushed away from the skull, then it is compressed, and then herniation occurs (3). The signs and symptoms are headache, possibly followed by a subtle change in behavior, and a decrease in level of consciousness (LOC). Symptoms accompanying the latent unconsciousness may include a dilated and fixed pupil on the same side as the injury (ipsilateral) followed by motor paralysis on the opposite side of the injury (contralateral). If the pupils are fixed and dilated for 30 minutes, survival is highly unlikely (4).

Treatment includes surgical removal of the EDH and ligation of the bleeding vessel. If a neurological emergency exists and it is impossible to surgically remove the mass, burr holes may be placed ipsilateral to the side of the dilated pupil or contralateral to the side of the motor deficit (2). Patients promptly diagnosed and treated have an excellent recovery rate.

Two potentially fatal complications of brain injury are cerebral edema and increased ICP. Brain edema is an increase in tissue volume secondary to abnormal fluid accumulation (5). Edema compresses normal adjacent tissue, increases ICP, and consequently alters cerebral blood flow (CBF). Increased ICP is the leading cause of death following severe head injury (6). The fluid within the intracranial compartments is contained in the cranium, which cannot expand. The Monro-Kellie hypothesis explains that the volume of the cranium is equal to the volume of the blood, brain, and cerebrospinal fluid (CSF);

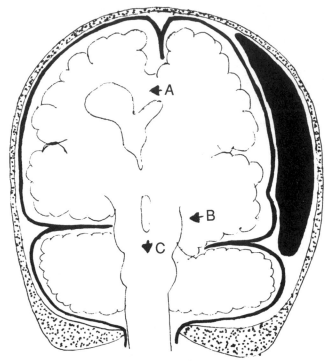

**Figure 4.1.** Types of brain herniation resulting from epidural hematoma (mass effect). **A** *Cingulate*—herniation of the cingulate gyrus of the frontal lobe below the falx cerebri; **B** *Transtentorial* or *uncal*—herniation of the uncus of the temporal lobe below the tentorium cerebelli; **C** *Central*—downward herniation of the brain stem through the foramen magnum. (Adapted from Jennett B, Teasdale, G: Management of head injuries. Philadelphia: FA Davis, 1982.)

therefore, an increase in any one of these components, without a decrease in a different component, will cause an increase in ICP.

As intracranial volume increases, ICP gradually increases. When compensatory mechanisms fail, even small increases in volume cause significant increases in ICP. Compliance is the ability of the brain to adjust to volume changes. When compliance is normal (lower end of the pressure-volume curve), a small increase in volume causes a slight, temporary increase in pressure. When compliance is abnormal (upper end of curve), the same increment in volume causes a striking increase in pressure, which does not return to baseline (4) (see Fig. 4.2).

The normal ICP is 0 to 15 mm Hg. The importance of an elevated ICP is its damaging effect on the patient's cerebral blood flow (CBF), which is closely related to the cerebral perfusion pressure (CPP):

$$CPP = MAP - ICP$$

Normal CPP is 80 to 90 mm Hg. A CPP of 50 mm Hg causes tissue ischemia and hypoxia.

Autoregulation is the brain's ability to maintain a constant blood flow despite fluctuations in arterial pressures from 60 to 150 mm Hg (7). As autoregulation fails, ICP and systemic BP increase, and CBF decreases, resulting in decreased tissue perfusion

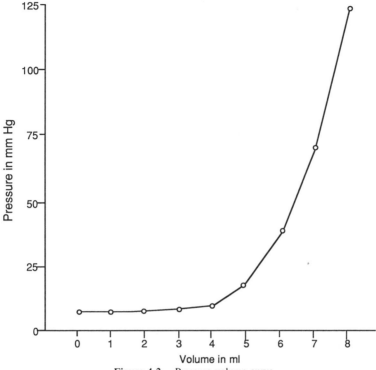

**Figure 4.2.** Pressure-volume curve.

and ischemia. The loss of autoregulation eventually leads to cerebral hypoxia, which disrupts cellular metabolism and leads to further cerebral edema. If this cerebral edema continues, the brain will herniate to relieve the increased volume and pressure.

Brain tissue may herniate because of pressure gradients caused by an increased ICP. In rapidly expanding hematomas, such as an EDH from a lacerated middle meningeal artery, herniation is usually uncal. When the temporal mass expands, volume and pressure increase, and the contents of the cranium exceed the available space in the skull. The medial aspect of the temporal lobe (the uncus) is shifted toward the midline and then over the edge of the tentorium cerebelli. This rostral-caudal progression pushes the cerebral artery down and compresses the oculomotor nerve. The temporal lobe then herniates into the tentorial notch. As the posterior cerebral artery is occluded, ischemia of the occipital lobe increases and infarction results. The brain stem is damaged by ischemia and hemorrhage (3).

Clinical signs of this uncal herniation are classic and reflect compression of the midbrain and surrounding structures; they include deterioration of the LOC, pupil abnormality, motor abnormality, brain-stem dysfunction, and alteration in vital signs, especially respiratory pattern (2, 8). Ischemia and pressure on the medullary brain structures present as Cushing's triad: increasing systolic blood pressure, decreasing diastolic pressure, and bradycardia. The presence of this triad is the terminal event (9).

## 2. What are the nursing diagnoses of highest priority?

A. Alteration in tissue perfusion
B. Impaired gas exchange

## 3. What are the goals of nursing care?

### A. Nursing Diagnosis

Alteration in cerebral tissue perfusion related to increased ICP, decreased CPP, and decreased MAP

### Goal of Care

Maintain adequate tissue perfusion.

### Nursing Interventions

- Monitor vital signs including ICP, CPP, BP, MAP, pulse, respirations, and respiratory pattern.
- Monitor neurological status including LOC, pupillary changes, and motor movement.
- Assess presence of brain-stem function including sneeze, cough, gag, and swallow reflexes.
- Position patient with HOB >30 degrees.
- Maintain normothermia.
- Medicate patient as needed with narcotics, paralytics, and/or sedatives as ordered by physician to decrease ICP prior to nursing activities.
- Administer osmotic or loop diuretics as ordered by physician.
- Monitor urinary output every hour.
- Monitor serum and urine electrolytes and osmolality.

### Rationale

Nursing interventions are directed at maintaining CBF by supporting CPP and preventing increases in ICP. Factors that affect ICP include head position, intravascular volume, serum osmolaity, $PaCO_2$, and $PaO_2$. The CPP should be calculated with each recording of vital signs to evaluate CBF. Neurological status and brain-stem function must be evaluated closely to assess for signs of neurological deterioration, including herniation. Patients should be positioned supine with HOB elevated 30 degrees to facilitate CSF drainage and venous return.

Normothermia should be maintained by the use of acetaminophen suppositories and/or a cooling blanket as ordered by the physician. Hyperthermia increases the cerebral metabolic rate.

Medications to control ICP may include narcotics, paralytics, and/or sedatives. Narcotics alter perception of pain and may include morphine or fentanyl. Narcotic analgesics decrease the sympathetic response to pain, which decreases BP and thereby reduces ICP. Paralytic agents, such as Metubine and Pavulon, and anesthetic agents, such as Pentothal, decrease motor response and prevent posturing that may cause elevations in ICP. Sedatives induce sleep and relieve anxiety; these include pentobarbital and Ativan. Medicate patients prior to providing care, which may cause elevations in ICP. If possible, group nursing actions together and then allow rest periods for the patient.

Administer osmotic and/or loop diuretics as ordered by the physician. Mannitol is an osmotic agent. It reduces cerebral edema, ICP, CSF volume, and pressure by elevating blood plasma osmolality, which results in flow of water from the brain and CSF into interstitial fluid and plasma (10). Furosemide is a potent loop diuretic. The diuresis creates a pressure gradient for edema fluid to diffuse from brain tissue into the blood. It also causes intracranial venodilation, enhancing edema reabsorption. Unlike osmotic agents, furosemide's dehydrating activity appears to be selective for traumatized brain tissue. By dehydrating only the edematous, traumatized portions, both the traumatized portions and the intact portions of the brain are protected from secondary injury (11).

Repeated use of osmotic and loop diuretics can lead to elevated serum osmolality, with a risk of seizures, renal failure, and serious fluid and electrolyte imbalances (9). Monitoring urinary output, serum and urine electrolytes, and osmolality is important to avoid these complications.

### B. Nursing Diagnosis
Impaired gas exchange related to decreased LOC, ineffective breathing patterns, and immobility

### Goal of Care
Maintain optimal oxygenation and ventilation.

### Nursing Interventions
- Monitor arterial blood gases (ABGs), maintain $PaO_2$ 80 to 100 mm Hg, and maintain $PaCO_2$ 25 to 30 mm Hg.
- Hyperventilate prior to suctioning.
- Suction every 2 hours and as needed to maintain patent airway.
- Chest physical therapy every 4 hours in Trendelenburg position, provided ICP does not exceed 25 mm Hg.
- Turn patient every 2 hours.

### Rationale
The patient with a severe head injury and altered LOC may require mechanical ventilation to maintain a patent airway and ensure adequate oxygenation. The goal of mechanical ventilation is to maintain the $PaO_2$ and $PaCO_2$ within optimal limits. $CO_2$ is a potent vasodilator; therefore, hyperventilation to maintain the $PaCO_2$ in the range of 25 to 30 mm Hg is important to constrict cerebral vessels and decrease excessive blood flow to the brain, thereby reducing ICP. Excessive hyperventilation resulting in $PaCO_2$ levels below 20 mm Hg may cause ischemia and adversely affect prognosis (2).

Pulmonary infection ranks second only to intracranial hypertension as the leading cause of head injury death; therefore, pulmonary toilet and suctioning are mandatory (2). Suctioning can produce hypoxemia, leading to vasodilation and increased blood pressure related to coughing (9). Administering prophylactic medication, hyperventilating, and preoxygenating with 100% $O_2$ prior to suctioning, as well as using intermittent suctioning and limiting suctioning to 10 to 15 seconds, can all help prevent hypoxia.

## ASSOCIATED NURSING DIAGNOSES
A. Potential for infection
B. Impaired physical mobility
C. Impaired communication

**REFERENCES**

1. Miller D, Leech P. Effects of Mannitol and steroid therapy on intracranial volume-pressure relationships in patients. J Neurosurgery 1975;42:274.
2. McGinnis GS. Central nervous system I: head injuries. In: Cardona VD, Hurn PD, Bastnagel-Mason PJ, et al, eds. Trauma nursing from resuscitation through rehabilitation. Philadelphia: WB Saunders, 1988:365–418.
3. Plum F, Posner JB. The diagnosis of stupor and coma. 3rd ed. Philadelphia: FA Davis, 1980.
4. Jorden R. Pathophysiology of brain injury. CCQ 5(3):1–12.

5. Mrsulja BB, Djuricic BM, Cvejic V. Biochemistry of experimental ischemic brain edema. In: Cervos-Navarro J, Ferszt J, eds. Brain edema: pathology, diagnosis, and therapy. Advances in Neurology, 28. New York: Raven Press, 1980:217–230.

6. Cooper P. Head injury. 2nd ed. Baltimore: Williams & Wilkins, 1987.

7. Newfield P, Cottrell JE. Neurologic-pharmacologic considerations of brain protection and resuscitation. In: Grenvik A, Safar P, eds. Clinics in critical care medicine: brain failure and resuscitation. New York: Churchill Livingstone, 1981:221–237.

8. Jennett B, Teasdale G. Management of head injuries. Philadelphia: FA Davis, 1982.

9. Mitchell P. Neurologic disorders. In: Kinney MR, Packa DR, Dunbar SB, eds. AACN's clinical reference for critical care nursing. New York: McGraw-Hill, 1988:971–1028.

10. Hartshorn J. Frequently used drugs in critical care. In: Kinney MR, Packa DR, Dunbar SB, eds. AACN's clinical reference for critical care nursing. New York: McGraw-Hill, 1988:1639–1710.

11. Tornheim PA, McLaurin RL, Sawaya R. Effect of furosemide on experimental traumatic cerebral edema. Neurosurgery 1979;4:48–52.

# CHAPTER 5

# Spinal Cord Injury: Combined Cervical and Thoracic Injuries Complicated by Spinal Shock

Jane Faith Kapustin, RN, MS
Sandra Weed, RN, MS

## Clinical Presentation

A 22-year-old man was seriously injured following a diving accident while intoxicated. On a dare from his friends, he attempted a backward flip from a rocky cliff 20 feet high into shallow water (less than 6 feet). He struck his back on a large protruding rock before entering the water and then sustained a hyperextension injury to his neck. He was immediately pulled from the water by friends and flown to the regional spinal cord injury center. On admission, he was flaccid in all extremities, with no sensation below the nipple line. He was areflexic but exhibited priapism (spontaneous penile erection). His admission vital signs were blood pressure 90/64, pulse 56, respirations 40 and very shallow, and temperature 36°C (96.8°F). He was experiencing respiratory difficulty with poor cough effort; assessment of arterial blood gases (ABGs) confirmed respiratory acidosis and moderate hypoxemia. The patient was, therefore, intubated and mechanically ventilated.

During the admitting process, cervical spine films revealed hyperextension displacement of C5, and thoracic and lumbar films showed an unstable thoracic injury at levels T6–T8. The T6 vertebral body was fractured, and the posterior ligamentous complex was interrupted. The patient was placed on a Stryker frame with Gardner-Wells tongs with 25 lbs of cervical traction for reduction of the cervical dislocation and transported to the operating room. The thoracic spine injury was stabilized using Harrington rods. The patient received 4 units of packed red blood cells intraoperatively, and vital signs were fairly stable throughout the 5-hour procedure. He was then transferred to the neurotrauma intensive care unit (ICU).

On admission to the ICU, the patient experienced a decrease in blood pressure that was treated with 500 cc of 5% plasma protein fraction (Plasmanate) and a dopamine infusion at 5 μg/kg/minute. This treatment increased his blood pressure to 110/60. He remained on the Stryker frame in cervical traction and was alert and cooperative for neurological assessments within 2 hours of ICU admission. He had an indwelling Foley cathether with adequate urine output; a pulmonary artery catheter with initial pressure readings of 30/16, with pulmonary capillary wedge pressure (PCWP) 10, central venous pressure (CVP) 5; a radial arterial line, and alternating pneumatic devices on his lower extremities. He was being warmed by an automatic warming blanket and had a nasogastric tube to low continuous suction for gastric decompression.

The back incision extended over the entire thoracic region, and there was an incision over the right iliac crest that was used for bone graft retrieval; two Hemovac drains were in place.

## 1. What is the pathophysiological basis for this patient's problem?

Spinal cord injury (SCI) can be classified according to mechanism of injury and degree of spinal cord damage. The most common mechanisms of closed cord injury include hyperflexion, hyperextension, compression, and flexion with rotation. Open injuries are usually caused by missile wounds and stab wounds. Cord damage from any injury can

27

range from the temporary effects of contusion to irreversible necrosis. Clinically, the patient will present with a variety of neurological deficits depending on the level of injury and the severity of cord damage (1).

The spinal cord is protected by the vertebral column that surrounds it, but as little as 5 mm of movement and/or compression of the vertebrae can cause permanent damage to the spinal cord. Injury to the spinal cord is classified as either complete or incomplete, depending on whether the tracts, both afferent and efferent, are totally interrupted or whether there is some sparing of fibers or tracts (see Table 5.1 and Figs. 5.1 and 5.2). In transection of the spinal cord, transient reflex depression occurs below the level of the lesion (2).

Flexion injuries with rotational forces are especially unstable because of the disruption of protective ligaments and fracture of the vertebral body. The spinal cord itself may not be severed at the time of injury; however, devastating edema and ischemic changes may follow the initial injury. Consequently, irreversible nerve destruction can develop rapidly, and neurological deficits will become permanent (1).

Spinal shock, the immediate response to SCI, usually occurs approximately 30 to 60 minutes after injury (1). This shock is characterized by temporary reflex suppression, flaccid paralysis, loss of all sensation below the level of lesion, bowel and bladder dysfunction, loss of vasomotor tone, possible priapism (abnormal, painful, continuous erection of the penis), loss of perspiration, and loss of spinal reflexes (3). Partial spinal cord transection (or cord injuries such as contusion or laceration) may result in spinal shock symptoms in those areas affected. For example, flaccid paralysis may be asymmetrical below the level of the lesion (1). Spinal shock is usually more severe for a patient with a spinal cord injury at levels T6 and above (4). Spinal shock can last from a few days to many months, although in most cases it resolves in 6 to 8 weeks, barring other complications.

Spinal cord injury also results in immediate life-threatening responses such as bradycardia, hypotension, and poikilothermia (the tendency to assume environmental temperature), all due to a loss of sympathetic outflow known as neurogenic shock; it is not seen independent of spinal shock (2). (See Table 5.2 for a comparison of spinal shock and neurogenic shock.)

Traumatic lesions to the spinal cord that interrupt the sympathetic nervous system pathways originating from the thoracolumbar region of the cord cause neurogenic shock. The sympathetic nervous system is responsible for maintaining vacular tone and increasing heart rate. When interrupted, vasodilation occurs, resulting in hypotension and pooling of blood in peripheral circulation. This ultimately results in a decrease in cardiac output (3,5). Loss of sympathetic nervous system (SNS) function is associated with an uninhibited vagus innervation of the heart, with resultant decreased heart rate and vasovagal reflex.

Priorities of resuscitation include stabilization of vital signs and prevention of further neurological deterioration. Respiratory insufficiency should be anticipated for all spinal cord injuries. Reversal of hypoxemia and hypotension is paramount to ensure adequate tissue oxygenation and cord perfusion. Immediate immobilization of suspected spinal cord injuries should begin at the accident scene and be maintained throughout the resuscitation cycle (6).

Surgical stabilization of an unstable thoracic injury is achieved by insertion of Harrington rods to realign fractures and decompress the cord. Distraction rods and hooks adequately reduce the fracture. With complete lesions, the entire affected area is usually fused. The patient usually remains on a Stryker frame for 1 to 2 weeks postoperatively.

**Table 5.1.** Incomplete cervical spinal cord injuries[a]

| Syndrome | Pathophysiology and Clinical Presentation | Etiology |
|---|---|---|
| Central cord syndrome | Cervical fibers are arranged most centrally in the cord, and sacral fibers are outermost<br>Variable degrees of sensory loss<br>Variable degrees of bowel, bladder, and sexual function<br>Motor loss in upper extremities greater than loss in lower extremities | Greatest percentage of incomplete injuries<br>Hyperextension injuries<br>Frequently associated with osteoarthritis of vertebral spinal column |
| Posterior cord syndrome | Sensory fibers are arranged in the posterior portion of the cord, motor fibers in the anterior portion<br>Loss of light touch and proprioception below level of lesion; pain and temperature sensation remain intact | Very rare occurrence<br>Hyperextension injuries |
| Anterior cord syndrome | Motor fibers are arranged in anterior portion of cord, sensory fibers in posterior portion<br>Hyperesthesias and hypalgesia below lesion level (paresthesias may be present); preservation of touch, position, pressure, and vibration<br>Complete paralysis below level of injury | Flexion injuries |
| Brown-Séquard syndrome | Hemisection of the spinal cord; clinical findings are related to where each tract decussates or crosses. The spinothalmaic tract (temperature and pain) decussates within a few segments of entry into the spinal cord and ascends on the side opposite of entry. The corticospinal tract (motor) decussates in the brain and then descends. The dorsal columns (touch and vibration) ascend on entry to the cord and decussate in the brain.<br>Ipsilateral loss of position, touch, and vibration below lesion level | Penetrating wounds to the cord |

**Table 5.1.** Incomplete cervical spinal cord injuries[a] *(continued)*

| Syndrome | Pathophysiology and Clinical Presentation | Etiology |
|---|---|---|
| Brown-Séquard syndrome *(continued)* | Contralateral loss of temperature and pain below lesion level<br>Ipsilateral motor loss below lesion level | |
| Sacral sparing | Sacral fibers are arranged in outermost portions of spinal cord and may not be damaged<br>Preservation of sensation in genital and saddle area (S3–5) even in the presence of profound motor and sensory losses<br>May retain bowel, bladder, and sexual function in varying degrees | Characteristically associated with anterior cord and central cord syndromes |

[a]*Sources*: Adapted from Richmond TS. The patient with a cervical spinal cord injury. Focus Crit Care 1985;12(12):26; and Ricci MM. Spinal trauma. In: Core curriculum for neuroscience nursing. Park Ridge, IL: American Association of Neuroscience Nurses, 1984:300–301.

The patient will then be fitted for a body cast or for a removable body jacket to decrease and/or prevent rotation and flexion of the spine (7).

## 2. What are the nursing diagnoses of highest priority?

A. Alteration in cardiac output
B. Alteration in respiratory function
C. Fear
D. Alteration in body temperature

## 3. What are the goals of nursing care?

### A. Nursing Diagnosis

Alteration in cardiac output related to hypotension, bradycardia secondary to loss of sympathetic outflow from spinal cord injury

### Goal of Care

Recognize signs of inadequate tissue perfusion.

### Nursing Interventions

- Monitor hemodynamic parameters hourly.
- Titrate inotropic drugs to maintain mean arterial pressure (MAP) >80.
- Monitor for vasovagal response and have atropine readily available.
- Monitor for cardiac dysrhythmias.
- Maintain normothermia.
- Provide for rest periods.
- Monitor intake and output closely.
- Monitor tissue perfusion (capillary refill times [CRTs] <3 sec)

### Rationale

Following spinal cord injury, the cardiovascular system endures significant change due to loss of sympathetic nervous system control. The parasympathetic nervous

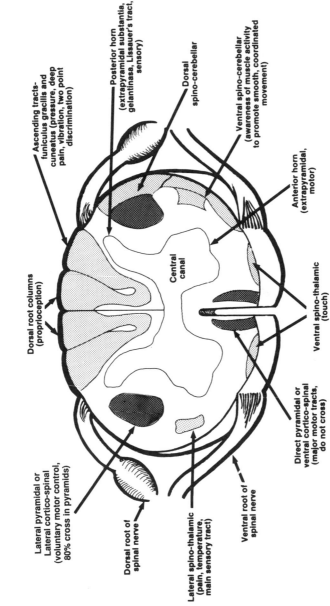

**Dorsal - primarily motor**

Ascending tracts-
funiculus gracilis and
cuneatus (pressure, deep
pain, vibration, two point
discrimination)

Posterior horn
(extrapyramidal substantia,
gelantinasa, Lissauer's tract,
sensory)

Dorsal
spino-cerebellar

Ventral spino-cerebellar
(awareness of muscle activity
to promote smooth, coordinated
movement)

Anterior horn
(extrapyramidal,
motor)

Dorsal root columns
(proprioception)

Central
canal

Ventral spino-thalamic
(touch)

Lateral pyramidal or
Lateral cortico-spinal
(voluntary motor control,
80% cross in pyramids)

Direct pyramidal or
ventral cortico-spinal
(major motor tracts,
do not cross)

Dorsal root of
spinal nerve

Lateral spino-thalamic
(pain, temperature,
main sensory tract)

Ventral root of
spinal nerve

**Ventral - primarily sensory**

Figure 5.1. Spinal tracts.

**Figure 5.1.** Spinal tracts.

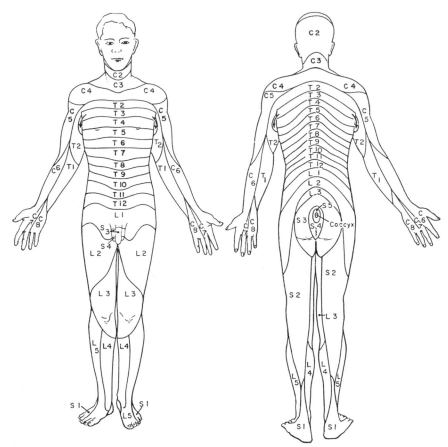

**Figure 5.2.** Cutaneous distribution of spinal nerves (dermatomes). (Reprinted with permission from Barr M: The human nervous system. New York: Harper & Row, 1972.)

system innervation dominates, resulting in hypotension and bradycardia. Damage to the spinal cord above the thoracic level of the fifth segmental section is responsible for the loss of sympathetic outflow. The loss of sympathetic outflow and interrupted communication from the brain stem to the sympathetic nervous system result in vasodilation, leading to hypotension and neurogenic shock (8).

During the acute phase, continuous hemodynamic monitoring is recommended. A pulmonary artery catheter is essential for monitoring the effects and extent of neurogenic shock, as well as differentiating hypovolemic shock from spinal shock. Following major surgery, hypovolemia for a spinal-cord–injured patient should be managed with judicious fluid and blood replacement to prevent pulmonary edema and congestive heart failure. Preload, systemic vascular resistance, cardiac output, and pulmonary artery pressures should be monitored closely for appropriate patient management. Vasopressor agents, such as dopamine or dobutamine, are titrated to maintain a MAP of 80 mm Hg (1).

The sympathetic blockade that causes hypotension is also responsible for bradycardia and associated dysrhythmias (atrial and junctional escape beats). Atropine

**Table 5.2.** Differentiating neurogenic and hypovolemic shock[a]

| | Shock Type | |
| --- | --- | --- |
| Symptom | Neurogenic | Spinal |
| Skin appearance | Warm, dry, flushed | Cool, clammy, pale |
| Blood pressure | Normal or decreased | Decreased |
| Pulse | Profound bradycardia | Tachycardia |
| Temperature | Poikilothermic | Decreased |
| Respiratory rate | Increased | Increased |
| Central venous pressure | Decreased | Decreased |
| Pulmonary capillary wedge pressure | Normal to decreased | Decreased |
| Cardiac output | Decreased | Decreased |

[a]*Source*: Adapted from Walleck CA. Central nervous system II: spinal cord injury. In: Cardona VD, Hurn PD, Bastnagel-Mason PJ, et al, eds. Trauma nursing: from resuscitation through rehabilitation. Philadelphia: WB Saunders, 1988.

should be kept at the bedside for symptomatic bradycardia or severe vasovagal responses seen in spinal-cord–injured patients. A vasovagal response, or severe parasympathetic nervous stimulation, may occur with deep endotracheal suctioning or sudden position changes. It is important to maintain the pulse at 60 or higher and the MAP at 80 mm Hg to provide adequate perfusion to all tissues, including the injured spinal cord. Nursing care should be spaced appropriately to maximize rest periods, thereby preserving cardiac functions.

## Goal of Care
Prevention of deep vein thrombosis (DVT)

## Nursing Interventions
- Apply antiembolic stockings.
- Perform passive range of motion.
- Initiate intermittent external pneumatic therapy as ordered.
- Measure calves and thighs.
- Monitor for signs of DVT and pulmonary embolism (PE).

## Rationale
Immobilization, flaccid paralysis, loss of vasomotor control, and lengthy surgical procedures contribute to the development of DVT, which increases the risk of PE in spinal-cord–injured patients. Because 15 to 20% of spinal-cord–injured patients develop DVT during the first 3 months following injury, prevention and early detection of DVT should be a major nursing goal. Other nursing measures include frequent assessments of lower extremities for redness, warmth, and edema; passive range of motion; application of thigh-high antiembolic stockings; and thigh and calf measurements daily. Stockings and Ace wraps should be applied smoothly to avoid uneven compression and should be removed every shift for hygiene and skin inspection (6).

Pneumatic compression devices are indicated for the spinal-cord–injured patient because of decreased mobility. These devices are particularly beneficial when anticoagulation is contraindicated or in the presence of lower extremity injuries (9,10).

Intermittent external pneumatic compression is thought to reduce thrombosis by avoiding stasis (11). This pneumatic compression is achieved through the use of inflatable sleeves that cover the lower leg or arm. These sleeves inflate once a minute to a pressure of approximately 50 mm Hg, lasting approximately 12 to 14 seconds. One study suggests that this compression stimulates fibrinolysis, which may contribute to the protective properties of these pneumatic devices more than do changes in actual blood flow (12).

## B. Nursing Diagnosis

Alteration in respiratory function related to immobility, hypoventilation, ineffective cough, muscle paresis, and fatigue secondary to spinal cord injury

### Goal of Care

- Achieve and maintain normal arterial blood gases (ABGs).
- Achieve and maintain clear chest x-ray (CXR).

### Nursing Interventions

- Monitor respiratory status.
  - Assess breath sounds.
  - Assess ABGs.
  - Assess rate and depth of respirations.
  - Follow chest x-rays.
  - Monitor oxygen saturation $SaO_2$ via pulse oximetry.
  - Assess ventilation parameters.
- Monitor level of consciousness.
- Provide pulmonary toilet.
  - Perform chest physiotherapy.
  - Assist with quad coughing and deep breathing.
- Maintain gastric decompression.

It is vital to monitor the patient's level of consciousness for signs of confusion, disorientation, or anxiety. These may be very important warning signs of developing respiratory distress. Respiratory monitoring parameters should be established early in the patient care process to identify potential development of problems.

When a patient has experienced a complete spinal cord lesion at the C5 level, the diaphragmatic muscles assume the primary responsibility for respiratory function, allowing for a high potential of pulmonary complications.

Pulmonary complications such as respiratory insufficiency, muscle paralysis, or pneumonia are the most serious threats to the patient with a spinal cord injury. Mortality rates from respiratory complications have been decreased as a result of early identification of high-risk patients, implementation of preventive measures, and aggressive treatment of problems (12), but respiratory failure remains the primary cause of death in acute spinal cord injury (8).

During the acute phase, hypoxemia is corrected by early intubation and mechanical ventilation to prevent further cord ischemia and hypoperfusion of vital tissue. Patients with possible aspiration, as seen with water accidents, should be treated with chest physiotherapy and pulmonary toilet at least every 2 to 4 hours. The patient on a Stryker frame can be placed in Trendelenburg's position for more effective postural drainage. The Stryker frame may cause a 25% reduction in pulmonary vital capacity when the patient is placed in the prone position. Therefore, the patient must be monitored very closely for respiratory and cardiovascular (vasovagal response) instability (4).

Vital capacity can be further compromised by gastric dilatation from paralytic ileus. Furthermore, gastric distension may lead to vomiting, placing the patient at risk for aspiration of stomach contents. The nurse should maintain decompression of gastric contents via nasogastric tube and note the return of bowel sounds (6).

Because the patient with a thoracic spinal cord injury may experience some impairment of chest and abdominal muscles required for ventilation and coughing, nursing care should include assistive "quad coughing." The heel of the hand is placed between the umbilicus and the xiphoid process, and a quick, firm upward thrust is applied during the patient's actual cough. This maneuver should be done every 2 hours to help clear secretions.

Throughout hospitalization, the patient should be assessed for signs and symptoms of infection. Breath sounds, chest x-ray reports, ABGs, nature of sputum, fever, and elevation of the white blood cell count need to be monitored very closely to prevent a potentially life-threatening respiratory infection.

Respiratory management should also include assessment for readiness to wean from the ventilator or the need for elective tracheostomy. If the patient requires endotracheal intubation for more than 1 week to 10 days, a tracheostomy may be required to avoid the risks of tracheal stenosis (9).

## C. Nursing Diagnosis

Potential for fear related to sudden loss of body function, hospitalization, invasive procedures, and prognosis secondary to acute spinal cord injury

### Goal of Care

Alleviate fear.

### Nursing Interventions

- Establish trusting relationship.
- Identify contributing factors.
- Orient to accident, injury environment.
- Establish means of communication.
- Include significant others in plan of care.
- Support normal coping mechanisms.

### Rationale

Spinal cord injury is both physiologically and psychologically devastating. The patient will experience a wide range of emotional responses from the initial injury through the rehabilitative phases. One response to sudden paralysis and potential loss of life is fear.

The critical care environment is extremely overwhelming for an already frightened patient. Unfamiliar caregivers in a seemingly noisy, chaotic setting will create further anxiety. The patient experiences this onslaught of stimuli from a confining, immobilizing Stryker frame. Fields of vision are limited to the ceiling and floor, and the patient will be unable to speak because of the ventilator.

Isolation and sensory deprivation are major concerns for the spinal-cord–injured patient. Contact with loved ones will be limited because of the critical nature of the required treatment. Hospitalization renders the patient powerless with limited territoriality. Self-concept and body image are immediately threatened by the catastrophic injury. All of these emotional responses will intensify the patient's fear (13).

Nursing interventions to alleviate fear must begin with the recognition of the profound impact this injury has had on the patient's emotional equilibrium. The patient is suddenly dependent on the health care team for most needs and must learn to trust the staff. Consistency of caregivers who follow an individualized plan of care will assist with establishing a trusting relationship (9).

During this acute phase, the patient will require information about the injury, diagnosis, and prognosis. The patient will need to be oriented frequently to the environment, invasive therapies, and his or her general status. Procedures such as turning prone on the Stryker frame into Trendelenburg position for chest physiotherapy must be explained to alleviate fear. Explanations are most effective when kept simple and given frequently.

Significant others and/or family members should be involved in this phase as soon as feasible. They will require information to regain a sense of control. When appropriate, they can participate in the care to maximize their sense of usefulness. Their mere presence should soothe and reassure the patient (13).

The inability to communicate because of mechanical ventilation can exacerbate fright. Simple means of communication should be established, such as mouthing words, blinking eyes, or gesturing if the patient is able. Most important, the patient will need a mechanism to call for assistance. The patient will need reassurance that help is readily available to overcome fear and develop confidence in the care providers (14).

During this critical phase, nurses will concentrate more on stabilizing the patient and addressing initial psychological responses. To provide holistic care for the spinal-cord—injured patient, nurses must then prepare for the patient's lengthy rehabilitative phase. The goals will shift, and independence will be fostered. The patient's emotional responses will vary during the stages of coping and adapting to this disability.

### D. Nursing Diagnosis

Hypothermia related to spinal shock

### Goal of Care

Maintain adequate body temperature.

### Nursing Interventions

- Monitor patient's body temperature.
- Monitor patient's skin integrity.
- Apply hypothermic or hyperthermic blanket if indicated.
- Apply warmed blankets and heat lamps as necessary.
- Maintain environmental temperature at 70°F.
- Maintain body temperature between 35.8°C (96.8°F) and 37.6°C (99.6°F).

### Rationale

The patient with a spinal cord injury will exhibit poikilothermia secondary to sudden autonomic dysfunction. Vasodilation and muscle paralysis are also factors that contribute to the body's heat loss. Another factor complicating this is exposure to cold prior to admission. Coupled with decreased cardiac output and prolonged surgical procedures, hypothermia may further compromise the patient's cardiovascular status. Therefore, nursing care should include measures to maintain normothermia, such as controlling room temperature, protecting the patient from drafts, warming intravenous fluids, and covering the patient as needed (9).

According to Zejdkik, however, some degree of hypothermia in spinal cord patients initially is believed to be helpful in decreasing the patient's overall basal metabolic rate, thus initially reducing oxygen requirements and the workload of breathing (3).

## ASSOCIATED NURSING DIAGNOSES

A. Impaired physical mobility
B. Alteration in patterns of bowel and urinary elimination
C. Potential for infection

D. Potential for ineffective individual and/or family coping
E. Sexual dysfunction
F. Grieving
G. Sensory/perceptual alterations
H. Alteration in tissue perfusion
I. Ineffective coping
J. Self-care deficit
K. Alterations in comfort

## REFERENCES

1. Franco L. Spinal cord injury. In: Cardona VD, ed. Trauma nursing. Oradell, NJ: Medical Economics Books, 1985:61–63.
2. VonRueden K, Walleck CA. Advanced critical care nursing: a case study approach. Rockville, MD: Aspen, 1989:185–186.
3. Zejdkik CM. Management of spinal cord injury. Monterey, CA: Wadsworth Health Sciences Division, 1983:225.
4. Buchanan LE, Nawoczenski DA. Acute care: Medical/surgical management. In: Spinal cord injury: concepts and management approaches. Baltimore: Williams & Wilkins, 1987:50–55.
5. Metcalf JA. Acute phase management of persons with spinal cord injury: a nursing diagnosis perspective. Nurs Clin North Am 1986;21(4):589–598.
6. Walleck CA. Central nervous system II: Spinal cord injury. In: Cardona VD, Hurn PD, Bastnagel-Mason PJ, et al, eds. Trauma nursing: from resuscitation through rehabilitation. Philadelphia: WB Saunders, 1988:419–448.
7. Cowley RA, Dunham CM, eds. Shock trauma critical care manual: initial assessment and management. Baltimore: University Park Press, 1982:235.
8. Nikas DL. The critically ill neurosurgical patient. New York: Churchill Livingstone, 1982:101–110.
9. Richmond TS. A critical care challenge: The patient with a cervical spinal cord injury. Focus Crit Care 1985;12:25–32.
10. Strange JM, Kelly PM. In: Cardona VD, Hurn PD, Bastnagel-Mason PJ, et al, eds. Trauma nursing: from resuscitation through rehabilitation. Philadelphia: WB Saunders, 1988:562.
11. Burrow M, Goldson H. Postoperative venous thrombosis: evaluation of five methods of treatment. Am J Surg 1981;141:250.
12. Knight MT, Dawson R. Effects of intermittent compression of the arms on deep venous thrombosis in the legs. Lancet 1972;2:1265.
13. Hickey JV. The clinical practice of neurological and neurosurgical nursing. 2nd ed. Philadelphia: JB Lippincott, 1986:380–381.
14. Richmond TS, Metcalf JA. Psychological responses to spinal cord injury. Neurosci Nurs. 1986;18:186.

# CHAPTER 6

# Brown-Séquard Syndrome

Carol M. Browner, RN
Toby A. Jardine, RN, MA

## Clinical Presentation

A 38-year-old man was reportedly drinking while fixing the roof of his home. He fell approximately 12 feet, striking his head on the sidewalk. He was unconscious at the scene, with shallow respirations, almost apneic. He was given mouth-to-mouth resuscitation by a layperson at the scene until an emergency medical team transported him to the admitting area of a Level I trauma center. C-spine precautions were maintained during transport.

On arrival at the emergency room, initial cursory examination revealed a talking, alert, and oriented individual. Length of unconsciousness at the scene was unknown. Respirations were predominantly diaphragmatic and shallow. Breath sounds were unequal, with aeration better heard on the right. His blood pressure was 110/70, and his pulse was 68 and strong. He had good movement of the left upper and lower extremities, with essentially no motor activity in the right arm and leg. No obvious signs of trauma were evident.

Further neurological examination revealed a Glasgow Coma Scale score of 14: motor = 6, verbal = 4, and eyes = 4. Pupils were equal, round, and reactive to light and accommodation. Cranial nerves 2 through 12 were intact, face symmetrical, and tympanic membranes clear. The neck was tender with no obvious deformities. Rectal tone was intact with sacral sparing present.

Sensory examination revealed a patchy picture. Position sense and response to deep pressure were present. The patient complained of burning paresthesias of the right arm and leg. Pinprick and light touch were intact through C5 on the right and decreased below. On the left side, C2 was intact to pinprick and light touch, C3 was decreased, and C4 and below were absent. Paresthesias were noted in the triceps and forearms bilaterally. Essentially, the sensory examination indicated an incomplete sensory insult at the level of C2 (Table 6.1). Reflex examination findings are shown in Table 6.2.

The abdomen was nontender, and diagnostic peritoneal lavage was negative. A Foley catheter was inserted and drained clear, straw-colored urine. The patient had no known allergies and was not currently taking any medications.

The patient continued in respiratory distress with shallow breathing; therefore, a 7-0 oral endotracheal tube was placed as a prophylactic measure. A Philadelphia collar was placed to maintain cervical alignment.

X-ray films showed a C1 Jefferson fracture through the posterior lamina. There was a C2 Hangman's fracture with bilateral pedicles fractured. The C2–C3 disk space was widened, with posterior angulation of the C2 body in relation to C3. There was a spinous fracture of C3. The odontoid was intact. Lumbar and thoracic x-ray studies were normal.

The patient was admitted with a medical diagnosis of C1–C2 fracture dislocation with a Brown-Séquard-type spinal cord syndrome.

After admission to the neurosurgical intensive care unit, the following sequence of patient management was instituted. Computerized tomography (CT) scan revealed no bone fragments in the spinal canal. Head CT scan was negative for intracranial hemorrhage. The patient was placed on a ventilator with $FiO_2$ of 0.30, intermittent mandatory ventilation (IMV) of 15, and tidal volume of 800 ml. A number 18 nasogastric tube was inserted and connected

**Table 6.1.** Findings of motor examination

| | Right[a] | Left[a] |
|---|---|---|
| Deltoid | 0/5 | 3/5 |
| Bicep | 0/5 | 4/5 |
| Tricep | 0/5 | 4/5 |
| Wrist extension | 0/5 | 4/5 |
| Wrist flexion | 0/5 | 4/5 |
| Intrinsics | 0/5 | 4/5 |
| Iliopsoas | 0/5 | 3/5 |
| Quadricep | 0/5 | 4/5 |
| Hamstring | 0/5 | 4/5 |
| Dorsiflexion | 1/5 | 4/5 |
| Plantar flexion | 1/5 | 4/5 |

[a]Codes: 0 = no movement; 1 = muscle contraction but no movement; 2 = trace movement but not against gravity; 3 = movement against gravity but not resistance; 4 = weak movement against resistance; and 5 = strong movement against resistance.

to low suction. Cardiac monitoring was initiated, and a right radial arterial line was inserted. The patient was kept flat in bed and logrolled. Two hours later a halo brace was placed because of the instability of the neck structures; follow-up x-ray films showed good alignment. A weighted feeding tube to the jejunum was inserted nasally.

During the next few days, the alignment of the cervical column changed whenever the patient was brought to a sitting position. Several halo adjustments failed to keep the neck stable. Consequently, the patient was kept on bed rest until stable enough to undergo a surgical stabilization procedure. During the next 2 weeks, the patient developed copious secretions and wheezing, required frequent suctioning, and was maintained on an IMV of 8 on the ventilator. X-ray films revealed an elevated right hemidiaphragm with a right lower lobe atelectasis. Subsequently, a tracheostomy was performed. Atelectasis then developed in the left lower lobe, and the patient had a fever of 38°C (100.5°F). Negative inspiratory force (NIF) was $-38$, forced vital capacity (FVC) was 790, and tidal volume ($V_T$) was 580. The patient was started on antibiotics following cultures. By day 12, the patient was weaned from the ventilator. Fluoroscopy confirmed a paralyzed right diaphragm.

During the remainder of the acute care stage, the patient's sensory and motor abilities improved. A fusion was performed at the C2–C3 level using an iliac crest donor site and Caspar plating. Caspar plating is a fairly new effort at providing a standardized operative technique and instrumentation to fuse and stabilize the cervical spine via an anterior approach. Because it provides firm immobilization of the injured segments after realignment and decompression, repetitive microtrauma and potential insufficient decompression are avoided. This allows earlier and safer mobility with the potential for improved recovery (1). A therapeutic bronchoscopy was performed twice to alleviate mucous plugging. The patient aspirated food when attempting to eat and therefore remained on tube feedings.

He was allowed up in a chair on day 22 postadmission. On day 29, he was transferred

**Table 6.2.** Findings of reflex examination

| | Left | Right |
|---|---|---|
| Bicep | 2+ | 0 |
| Tricep | 2+ | 0 |
| Knee | 2+ | 2+ |
| Ankle | 2+ | 2+ |
| Babinski | Negative bilaterally | |

to a spinal injury rehabilitation unit for continued therapy. His tracheostomy was removed, the feeding tube was discontinued, his swallowing improved, and his appetite returned. FVC was 1.76 liters.

## 1. What is the pathophysiological basis for this patient's problem?

The Brown-Séquard syndrome was first described in 1846 by the French physiologist and physician Charles Edouard Brown-Séquard (2). It is caused by a unilateral hemisection of the spinal cord. The Brown-Séquard syndrome is considered to be an "incomplete" spinal cord lesion with both sensation and motion being preserved to some degree below the level of the injury. It most often results from a penetrating injury due to gunshot, missile, or stab wound. Other causes have been attributed to neoplastic disease, infectious process, herniated disc, cervical spondylosis, heroin injection, trauma with fracture and dislocation of the vertebrae, and vascular compromise. Over 600 cases have been reported in the literature. The patient presents with ipsilateral motor loss, hypoesthesia or hyperesthesia, and loss of proprioceptive sensation. Contralaterally, temperature and pain sensation are lost—either analgesic or hypalgesic one or two dermatomes below the level of the lesion (3).

This mixed sensorimotor picture is due to the location of the spinal cord anatomical structures and the crossed and uncrossed tracts within the spinal cord. With Brown-Séquard syndrome, both ascending sensory and descending motor spinal tracts are interrupted, with damage to the dorsal and ventral nerve roots at the level of injury. The primary motor tract involved is the pyramidal, otherwise known as the lateral corticospinal tract. This tract descends from the cortex, crosses in the medulla, and travels down the ipsilateral spinal cord. Other motor tracts are not of clinical importance in this syndrome. The primary sensory tracts involved are the lateral spinothalamic tracts and the fasciculus gracilis and fasciculus cuneatus of the posterior columns. The posterior columns carry the sensations of proprioception, vibration, and touch and ascend uncrossed to the medulla, where they cross and ascend to the thalamus. The sensations of pain and temperature are carried upward via the lateral spinothalamic tract. These sensations enter the spinal cord via the dorsal root, ascend one or two spinal segments, synapse in the posterior horn cells, and then cross over to the contralateral side and ascend to the thalamus (Figs. 6.1–6.3). Neurological loss can be either permanent or transient, depending on the severity of the lesion. However, the Brown-Séquard syndrome carries with it a good prognosis, with some degree of returned function occurring in up to 90% of the cases reported (4).

## 2. What are the nursing diagnoses of highest priority?

A. Potential for injury
B. Ineffective breathing patterns and airway clearance
C. Impaired physical mobility

## 3. What are the goals of care and nursing interventions for the above diagnoses?

### A. Nursing Diagnosis

Potential for injury and further neurological deterioration related to instability of the supporting structures

### Goal of Care

Maintenance of vertebral alignment and absence of further motor/sensory impairment

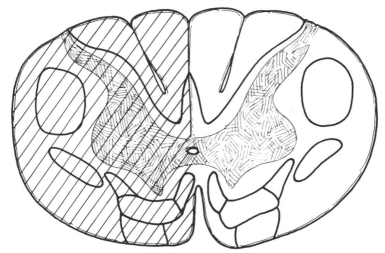

**Figure 6.1.** The Brown-Séquard syndrome is caused by damage to one side of the cord only and is usually associated with a penetrating wound or a disk or bone fragment. The patient presents with (a) loss of vibration, position, and touch sensation on the same side of the body (ipsilateral), (b) loss of motor function on the same side of the body (ipsilateral), (c) loss of pain and temperature sensation on the opposite side of the body (contralateral).

### Nursing Interventions

- Monitor sensory/motor status with hourly examination.
- Maintain proper body alignment.
- Logroll when turning patient.
- Immobilize head with cervical collar and positioning rolls or skeletal cervical traction as indicated.
- Do not extend, flex, or turn patient's head.
- Monitor intake and output accurately.
- Restrict fluids to 3000 ml/24 hr to minimize spinal cord edema and fluid overload.
- When lifting patient, use five people: one at the head, directing, and two on either side.
- Use turning bed as necessary.

### Rationale

The patient with a cervical spinal cord injury usually has vertebral column instability with disruption of the ligamentous structures, fractures of the vertebrae, or both. Injudicious movement of these structures may further compromise the neural structures within. All injuries are considered "unstable" until radiological examination proves otherwise. A spinal column injury is considered "stable" if the injured structures are able to support the damaged area well enough to prevent further deformity and progression of neurological loss.

During the first 72 hours postinjury, it is critical to accurately assess the patient's sensorimotor status hourly. Motor examination of the upper extremities should include arm elevation, elbow flexion and extension, wrist flexion and extension, and thumb and finger movement. Lower extremity examination should include hip flexion, knee extension and flexion, and foot dorsiflexion and plantar flexion. Motor power can be described simply by recording absent, present, or present against resistance or gravity. Motor function of the trunk can be established by observing

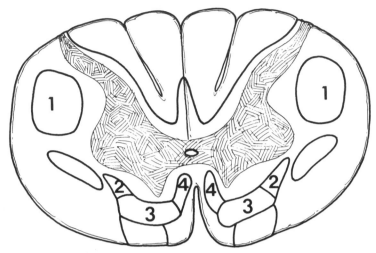

**Figure 6.2.** Major descending (motor) tracts in the spinal cord. *1*, Lateral corticospinal tract. Voluntary motion for opposite side. *2*, Lateral reticulospinal tract. Mainly facilitatory influence on motoneurons to skeletal muscle. *3*, Medial reticulospinal tract. Mainly inhibitory influence on motoneurons to skeletal muscle. *4*, Ventral corticospinal tract. Voluntary motion for same side.

breathing patterns, chest movement, and the patient's ability to elicit a forceful cough. Note whether the patient's breathing mechanism involves the intercostal muscles or the diaphragm alone. Monitoring spontaneous ventilatory parameters is helpful in this assessment, including measuring forced vital capacity, tidal volume, and negative inspiratory force.

Sensory examination is less objective but no less important and is easily monitored by marking the last normal level on the body with a felt pen. Sensory examinations can be limited to the sensations of position sense, pinprick, and light touch using a safety pin and cotton swab as tools. The patient should be reminded to keep his or her eyes closed during the examination. Both sides should be tested, working upward from the areas of impaired sensation to the areas of normal sensation.

Proper alignment is maintained by immobilization in skeletal traction with Gardner-Wells tongs and weights, a cervical collar or brace of choice, or positioning rolls. Flexion, extension, and rotation must be avoided by turning the patient as a whole. Some facilities use a Stokes-Manville or Roto-Rest bed to help maintain alignment when turning. These beds are designed to provide the means to turn the patient frequently or continuously without manual manipulation of the patient or the established stabilization. The patient is "padded" into place to prevent any slippage and turned on a regular schedule or continuously at an established angle. Because of the frequent postural changes, lung secretions are mobilized, physiological body function is improved, and better respiratory exchange occurs (5). Every patient should be turned every 2 hours as soon as stability is established. If alignment is being maintained with skeletal traction, it is imperative to keep the specified poundage of traction constant. The free-hanging weights should not be removed unless traction is maintained by manual pull by a physician. The patient should be reminded not to shake his or her head when answering questions. The patient with a head injury should be observed closely for restlessness and unsafe movements.

Secondary injury to the spinal cord is caused by edema and vascular compromise.

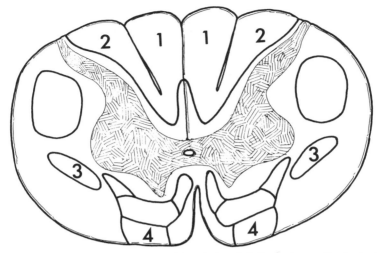

**Figure 6.3.** Major ascending (sensory) tracts of the spinal cord. *1*, Fasciculus gracilis. Carries impulses from receptors in muscles, tendons, and joints in the lower areas of the body for proprioception, vibration, passive motion, joint and two-point discrimination, and deep touch and pressure. *2*, Fasciculus cuneatus. Same as fasciculus gracilis except for upper thoracic and upper extremities. *3*, Lateral spinothalamic tract. Transmits pain and temperature; is possibly the pathway for tickle, itch, and muscle fatigue; transmits sensation of fullness of bladder; and conveys sexual sensations. *4*, Ventral spinothalamic tract. Transmits sense of light or crude touch from opposite side. (From Barrow Neurological Institute, Phoenix, AZ, 1989.)

Monitoring fluids to prevent cord edema and further neurological damage is essential. It is not uncommon to mistake spinal shock for hypovolemic shock in the very acute stages, but administering fluids to help elevate the blood pressure may only complicate the situation and result in further neurological deterioration. Accurate intake and output measurements should be made hourly.

Skilled nursing assessment and management are vital to prevent further neurological insult and to achieve the best functional outcome for these patients.

## B. Nursing Diagnosis

Ineffective breathing patterns and ineffective airway clearance related to diaphragm, intercostal or abdominal muscle paralysis/paresis, hypoventilation, and impaired gas exchange

### Goals of Care

- Arterial blood gases within normal limits
- FVC 60–75 ml/kg body weight
- Adequate ventilation of the aveoli with normal chest expansion
- Absence of atelectasis and infection
- Normal color
- Normal breath sounds
- Absence of secretion retention
- Clear chest x-ray film
- Absence of aspiration
- Improvement of cough force
- Establishment of respiratory muscle-strengthening exercises

## Nursing Interventions

- Assist in establishing an airway.
- Keep suction readily available; suction as necessary.
- Observe breathing patterns.
- Auscultate breath sounds.
- Assist with intubation if necessary.
- Obtain pulmonary history.
- Avoid fluid overload.
- Manually cough when necessary.
- Incorporate postural drainage and percussion routinely.
- Observe for signs of respiratory fatigue.
- Observe for further neurological deterioration.
- Observe for signs of respiratory infection.
- Insert nasogastric tube.
- Administer oxygen as indicated.
- Assist with chest x-ray studies.
- Humidify air.
- Allow for frequent rest periods.
- Reassure frightened patient.
- Teach patient how to cough effectively.
- Use incentive spirometer hourly while the patient is awake.
- Culture sputum as indicated.
- Assist with bronchoscopy as indicated.
- Administer antibiotics as indicated.
- Have patient deep breathe several times per hour.
- Reposition patient frequently.
- Incorporate use of abdominal binder.
- Facilitate respiratory treatments being performed in a timely fashion.

## Rationale

The patient who has suffered a fractured neck with compromise to the cervical spinal cord will immediately have problems with the respiratory system. Injury to any cervical segment or to the high thoracic segments will cause denervation to the muscles of respiration, either partially or totally. These muscles may include the diaphragm, external and internal intercostals, accessory muscles, and abdominal muscles. Nerve impairment to any or all of these muscles will compromise the patient's inspiratory capacity and expiratory force; the patient will not be able to take a deep breath or produce an effective cough. If the damage is above C3, all of these muscles will be paralyzed and the patient will be ventilator dependent. Damage to C3 through C5 segments will hinder the diaphragm's function, but the patient will breathe "abdominally" with the diaphragm alone, resulting in a greatly diminished FVC. Forced vital capacity is a commonly used measurement of lung function. It is the volume of gas expired after maximal inspiratory and expiratory effort. It is significantly reduced when the respiratory muscles weaken or fatigue (6). For this reason, serial readings are important in monitoring the patient for decreasing respiratory capacity and potential respiratory failure or distress. The level of lesion will determine the degree of inspiratory/expiratory dysfunction. Lesions of the cord from C1 to T12 will affect this mechanism, with the lower thoracic lesions being less threatening. Partial or "incomplete" spinal cord lesions will cause partial paralysis to these muscles.

The first emergency department intervention may be intubation. It is vital to prevent further damage to the compromised vertebral column and the delicate spinal cord. Intubation must be done carefully, avoiding any hyperextension of the neck. The jaw thrust or chin-lift methods of intubation or blind nasal intubation will prove safer for the patient. Passing the endotracheal tube with a fiberoptic bronchoscope can aid greatly in safe intubation.

Associated chest trauma or head injury could complicate the picture. Did the injury happen in or near water, and did the patient aspirate water or vomitus? Does the patient have fractured ribs or sternum or a hemothorax or pneumothorax? Is the patient in shock? In the prehospital setting, was the patient overloaded with fluids that could lead to respiratory complications?

Respiratory assessment is warranted at this time by checking important pulmonary parameters: Forced vital capacity, tidal volume, negative inspiratory force, and blood gases should be evaluated to determine if mechanical ventilation is necessary to assist the patient in breathing adequately. Assessment will also include respiratory rate and the rhythm and quality of chest and abdominal movement. Chest x-ray films will aid in diagnosis.

Nursing measures in the intensive care unit are aimed at preventing further complications. A thorough pulmonary history should be obtained. Is the patient a smoker? Is there a history of asthma, allergies, or a recent upper respiratory infection? Oxygen should be administered to the patient. Auscultation of breath sounds will help detect secretion retention and determine if the lower segments of the lungs are being ventilated adequately. Hypoventilation can lead to alveoli collapse and atelectasis. The use of intermittent positive pressure breathing (IPPB) will help aerate the alveoli. The patient should be encouraged to practice with an incentive spirometer every hour and encouraged to deep breathe frequently. Family members can be taught to help the patient with these tasks.

The patient will have difficulty clearing the airway and coughing because the respiratory musculature is weakened. Suctioning the patient will help remove the retained secretions. "Manually coughing" (quad cough) the patient is essential each time the patient is obstructed. This is accomplished by delivering an abdominal thrust, with one hand just below the xyphoid process, inward and upward toward the patient's head. This allows for enough expulsive force to move the secretions from the airways. Family members should be taught this technique early. Patients with abdominal trauma or chest trauma and those who have just eaten a large meal should not be manually coughed.

Other methods of clearing retained secretions include postural drainage and percussion. These should be incorporated as part of the treatment regimen and are effective methods of clearing atelectasis and secretions in the lower segments of the lungs. Repositioning the patient every 1 to 2 hours may also help mobilize secretions. Placing a patient on a special bed to facilitate turning and repositioning will be of benefit. Humidifying the air and using saline when suctioning will keep secretions loose and easier to remove.

If appropriate, the patient can also receive small volume nebulizer treatments with bronchodilator medications. Bronchoscopy may be necessary to clear any mucous plugs. Signs of respiratory fatigue should be acted on quickly, for a quadriplegic patient can easily advance into respiratory failure in only a few days after admission. Fatigue is the main causative factor of respiratory failure in the patient working hard to breathe with diminished muscle function. Frequent rest periods between activities and treatments will help combat fatigue and failure. Reassuring a frightened, anxious patient is always a positive force. It is imperative that the nurse be a skilled observer of signs of respiratory failure. If these are identified early and treated aggressively, the patient can be spared a tracheostomy.

A nasogastric tube should be placed to keep the abdomen from becoming overdistended. Distension will put undue pressure on the diaphragm and further impede movement. Decreased movement will diminish the patient's inspiratory capacity and could lead to respiratory failure. Consequently, when the patient is helped to a sitting position, an abdominal binder should be applied to aid diaphragm movement. The abdominal binder substitutes for loss of abdominal tone that would hinder movement of the diaphragm.

Vigilant and aggressive nursing management of the patient's real and potential respiratory problems cannot be overstated. Fear and anxiety are decreased with early education and active patient participation and can also improve long-term outcome. Preventing further compromise or complications can significantly decrease the expense of care, the length of hospital stay, and additional trauma to the patient.

## ASSOCIATED NURSING DIAGNOSES

A. Activity intolerance
B. Impaired adjustment
C. Anxiety
D. Alterations in bowel elimination
E. Altered comfort: acute pain
F. Impaired verbal communication
G. Fear
H. Grieving
I. Hopelessness
J. Knowledge deficit
K. Impaired swallowing
L. Alterations in nutrition: less than body requirements
M. Powerlessness
N. Impaired gas exchange
O. Self-care deficit
P. Impairment of skin integrity
Q. Alterations in patterns of urinary elimination
R. Disturbances in self-concept
S. Sexuality pattern alterations

**REFERENCES**

1. Caspar W. Anterior cervical fusion and interbody stabilization with the trapezial osteosynthetic plate technique. Federal Republic of Germany: Aesculap-Werke AG, 1986:1–52.
2. Bartolomei FJ, Georgeoff RM Jr. Pedal manifestation of Brown-Séquard syndrome. J Am Podiatr Med Assoc 1985;75(11):603–606.
3. Koehler PJ, Kuiters RRF. Brown-Séquard syndrome caused by a spinal subarachnoid hematoma due to anticoagulant therapy. Surg Neurol 1986;25:191–193.
4. Leech RW, Shuman RM. Neuropathology: a summary for students. Philadelphia: Harper & Row, 1982.
5. Rudy EB. Advanced neurological and neurosurgical nursing. St Louis: CV Mosby, 1984:394–425.
6. Harvey A, Johns RJ, McKusisk VA, Owens AH, Roff RS. The principles and practice of medicine. 20th ed. New York: Appleton-Century-Crofts, 1980:360–362.

## SUGGESTED READINGS

Alvarez SE, Peterson M, Lunsford BR. Respiratory treatment of the adult patient with spinal cord injury. Phys Ther 1981;61(12):1737–1745.

Braun SR, Giovannoni R, O'Conner M. Improving the cough in patients with spinal cord injury. Am J Phys Med 1984;63(1):1–10.

Browner CM, Hadley MN, Sonntag VKH, Mattingly LG. Halo immobilization brace care: an innovative approach. J Neurosci Nurs 1987;19(1):24–29.

Carpenito LJ. Nursing diagnosis: application to clinical practice. Philadelphia: JB Lippincott, 1983.

Chusid JG. Correlative neuroanatomy and functional neurology. 15th ed. Los Altos, CA: Lange, 1973.

Drake TR, Walls RM, Marx JA. Case report: Brown-Séquard's syndrome associated with histiocytic lymphoma. J Emerg Med 1987;5:1–4.

Herr RD, Barrett J. An unusual presentation of Brown-Séquard syndrome. Ann Emerg Med 1987; 16(11):1285–1288.

Kennedy EJ. Spinal cord injury—the facts and figures. Birmingham, AL: University of Alabama, 1986.

Koehler PJ, Endtz LJ. The Brown-Séquard syndrome: true or false? Arch Neurol 1986;43:921–924.

Little JW, Halar E. Temporal course of motor recovery after Brown-Séquard spinal cord injuries. Paraplegia 1985;23:39–46.

Morrison ML. Respiratory intensive care nursing. Boston: Little, Brown, 1978.

Ricci MM, ed. Core curriculum for neuroscience nursing. Vol II. Park Ridge, IL: American Association of Neuroscience Nurses, 1984.

Saxon M, Snyder HA, Washington JA Jr. Atypical Brown-Séquard syndrome following gunshot wound to the face. J Oral Maxillofac Surg 1982;40(5):299–302.

Traver GA, ed. Respiratory nursing: the science and the art. New York: Wiley, 1982.

Zejdkik CM. Management of spinal cord injury. Boston: Jones & Bartlett, 1983.

# PART 2

Pulmonary Injuries/Complications

# CHAPTER 7

## Pulmonary Contusion Associated with Rib Fractures

Kathy L. Samuel, RN, BSN

## Clinical Presentation

A 30-year-old man was admitted to the hospital after being struck on his bicycle from behind by an auto traveling at moderate speed. He was thrown 20 feet, landing on his back on the hood of a parked car. The patient had been in excellent physical condition and without significant health history prior to this accident. He arrived in the emergency department awake, alert, and oriented, without history of loss of consciousness. He was able to move all extremities, and there was no apparent evidence of limb fracture. His complaints were of moderate abdominal pain, severe chest discomfort, and shortness of breath. His blood pressure was 120/60 and heart rate was 100 with shallow, moderately labored respirations at 30 to 35. Arterial blood gas (ABG) analysis on room air revealed the following: $PaO_2$ 65, pH 7.32, $PaCO_2$ 49, and $O_2$ saturation 88%. An upright chest film revealed bilateral rib fractures with bilateral diffuse cloudy opacities. Hemoglobin and hematocrit were 9.2 and 28.8 respectively. Diagnostic peritoneal lavage was positive, and the patient was taken to the operating room for exploratory laparotomy, during which liver lacerations were repaired.

Postoperatively the patient was taken to the intensive care unit (ICU) for hemodynamic monitoring and ventilatory support. He was mechanically ventilated on a volume-cycled ventilator through a number 8 cuffed endotracheal tube. His ventilator settings were $FiO_2$ of 0.40, tidal volume of 800 ml, synchronized intermittent mandatory ventilation (SIMV) rate of 12/minute, and positive end-expiratory pressure (PEEP) of 8 cm. Peak inspiratory airway pressures (PIP) averaged 42 cm $H_2O$. In addition, there was a Swan-Ganz catheter in the right subclavian vein, a right radial arterial line, a nasogastric tube to suction, and a Foley catheter. Hemodynamically monitoring revealed the following: pulmonary artery pressure (PAP) of 41/23 mm Hg, mean PAP of 31 mm Hg, and pulmonary capillary wedge pressure (PCWP) of 8 mm Hg. Pulmonary vascular resistance was calculated at 300 dynes/sec/cm$^{-5}$. A postoperative chest radiograph revealed diffuse bilateral infiltrates. This finding, coupled with deteriorating blood gases and poorly controlled chest pain, prompted the initiation of more aggressive ventilator therapy, inotropic support with intravenous infusions of dopamine and dobutamine, and a continuous intravenous infusion of morphine sulfate for pain management.

Within 24 hours, his oxygenation improved. Further improvement in his pulmonary status over the next several days permitted weaning of inotrope infusions, removal of the Swan-Ganz catheter, and some weaning of ventilator settings. Progress continued over the next week with pain control and spontaneous ventilatory effort. On the 14th day the patient was extubated without problems. During the next week the morphine drip was weaned and discontinued, all invasive lines were discontinued, and an oral diet was started. The patient was transferred to a subacute area for further convalescence and was discharged to home at the end of four weeks.

## 1. What is the pathophysiological basis for this patient's problem?

A pulmonary contusion, or bruising of the lung, occurs after penetrating or blunt chest trauma. Pulmonary contusion resulting from penetrating trauma occurs when a foreign body, such as a bullet, knife, or impaling object, moves through the thoracic cavity causing localized hemorrhage and edema (1). Major causes of pulmonary contusions from blunt chest trauma are compression-decompression injuries from steering wheels and handlebars of motorcycles and bicycles. Contusions may also result from falls, explosions, industrial and farm accidents, or contact sports (2,3 [p. 145]). Some estimate that between 30 and 75% of blunt trauma victims sustain pulmonary contusions (4). Pulmonary contusion has been described as one of the most common potentially lethal chest injuries seen in this country, as well as one of the most underestimated problems confronting trauma care providers (5).

The pathophysiology of pulmonary contusions starts with the initial damage to the lung parenchyma caused by the chest trauma. This damage causes alveolar capillary damage with interstitial and intra-alveolar extravasation of blood and interstitial edema. The accumulation of edema and cellular debris obstructs air flow through the small airways and alveoli and decreases pulmonary blood flow. Gas exchange becomes impaired, resulting in decreased $PaO_2$ and elevated $PaCO_2$. This pathological mechanism is summarized in Figure 7.1.

The severity of the initial traumatic event determines the degree of parenchymal damage and the extent of involvement. When parenchymal damage is minimal, there is little alteration in pulmonary function because of minimal intra-alveolar hemorrhage and focal

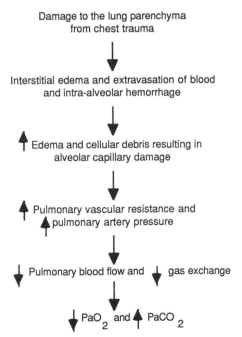

**Figure 7.1.** Basic pathophysiology of pulmonary contusion.

areas of interstitial edema (6,7). When the injury is severe, there is widespread damage to the lung and the classical "wet lung" is seen on autopsy (4).

Trauma to the chest increases mucous production, and the patient may not be able to cough because of pain from the chest injury. Atelectatic lung areas do not provide effective gas exchange, and a reflex tachypnea and tachycardia develop. Resistance to air flow in the conducting airways is increased. Pulmonary compliance is diminished, and the work of breathing is increased, resulting in an oxygen deficit because the lungs cannot meet the heightened demand caused by the effort to breathe (4).

Information about mechanism of injury may be helpful in anticipating and establishing early diagnosis of injury, as radiographic evidence of pulmonary contusion can be delayed as long as 72 hours (8). The chest x-ray may show patchy, irregular, ill-defined densities or homogeneous consolidations (9). The patient should be assessed for symptoms, such as cyanosis, dyspnea, tachypnea, poor chest excursion, contusion and abrasion of the chest wall, crepitus, and hemoptysis. Subjective complaints will reveal pain on inspiration and shortness of breath. Arterial blood gas analysis will reveal hypoxia and hypercapnia resulting from impaired gas exchange and hypoventilation. Alveolar hemorrhage occurs after pulmonary contusion because of capillary damage. A localized area of inflammation precipitates a cellular response to injury, which causes increased extravascular lung water as a result of changes in capillary permeability. This edema may be compounded by shock and fluid resuscitation related to the pulmonary contusion and other injuries (2 [p. 431]).

## 2. What are the nursing diagnoses of highest priority?

A. Impaired gas exchange
B. Altered comfort
C. Potential for infection

## 3. What are the goals of nursing care?

### A. Nursing Diagnosis

Impaired gas exchange related to tissue injury, consolidation, and edema

### Goal of Care

Improve oxygenation and reduce hypercapnia.

### Nursing Interventions

- Monitor clinical parameters: skin color, breath sounds, chest excursion, arterial blood gas, and chest x-ray findings.
- Assist in ventilator therapy.
- Monitor peak airway pressure and measure pulmonary compliance.
- Maintain PEEP.
- Maintain accurate intake and output records.
- Reposition frequently.
- Perform chest physiotherapy.
- Monitor pulmonary secretions.

### Rationale

Bleeding, edema, and atelectasis associated with lung trauma impair the exchange of oxygen and carbon dioxide. Some patients with minimal chest trauma may be able to cough effectively, clear secretions, and maintain adequate ventilation via a natural airway. In such instances, supplemental oxygen may be delivered by face

**Table 7.1.** Indications for mechanical ventilation

Vital capacity <10 ml/kg body weight
Arterial pH <7.25
Alveolar-arterial oxygen tension difference >350 mm Hg
$PaO_2$ <50 mm Hg breathing room air
$PaCO_2$ <50 mm Hg
Apnea

mask, face tent, or nasal cannula, depending on patient need, preference, and tolerance. Patients with more severe lung contusions and greater pain due to rib fractures may have poor lung ventilation and cough effort. Patients with severe lung injuries may have a continuous wet cough from copious, thick mucoid sputum and occasional bloody secretions that they are unable to clear effectively. Dyspnea and tachypnea are common in these patients, and their ABG values should be monitored closely to identify progressive declines in arterial $PaO_2$ and pH. These patients may require intubation and mechanical ventilation. Indications for mechanical ventilation are listed in Table 7.1. A primary goal of therapy is to prevent systemic hypoxia by restoring adequate oxygenation with the lowest possible $FiO_2$ (10). Airway pressures, spontaneous effort, volumes, pulmonary compliance, and ABG values should be monitored frequently and trends identified. Progressive increases in peak airway pressures and decreases in measured pulmonary compliance are evidence of significant pulmonary contusions. Positioning may be used to perfuse healthy lung tissue maximally and expand damaged and atelectatic areas. The patient may be positioned with healthy lung segments in dependent positions with the goal of increasing blood flow to those areas and subsequently promoting exchange of oxygen and carbon dioxide (11 [p. 485]). Fluids must be administered judiciously to prevent exacerbation of lung edema (3 [p. 446]).

## Goal of Care
Establish and maintain patent airway.

## Nursing Interventions
- Assess cough effort and ability to maintain airway.
- Maintain proper airway position and cuff seal.
- Monitor airway pressures.
- Suction airway when clinically indicated.
- Institute and maintain safety measures.

## Rationale
The patient's cough effort and ability to maintain a patent natural airway may be impaired because of neurological injury, intoxication, or sedation. In such instances it may be necessary to establish an artificial airway with an endotracheal tube. Endotracheal tube position should be checked frequently and the cuff seal maintained to prevent loss of tidal volumes. Minimal occlusive volume (MOV) should be used to maintain the cuff seal, and the intracuff pressure should be maintained at less than 20 mm Hg. An increase in airway pressure may signal mucous plugging, which could result in airway obstruction. Suction the endotracheal tube and upper tracheobronchial tree to remove those secretions and reduce this hazard. The endotracheal tube must be securely taped and the patient restrained in accordance with hospital policy to prevent inadvertent extubation. Intubation equipment should be available close by and a spare airway kept at the bedside, should accidental extubation occur or emergency intubation be required (11 [p. 458]).

## B. Nursing Diagnosis

Altered comfort with potential for ineffective breathing patterns

### Goal of Care

Alleviate/minimize discomfort.

### Nursing Interventions

- Administer analgesia.
- Assist with intercostal nerve block or epidural administration.
- Administer TENS therapy.
- Provide for periods of rest.
- Use other comfort measures.

### Rationale

Pain associated with rib fractures may be quite severe, making adequate ventilation difficult and cough ineffective. A variety of pain-control strategies exist that may be used with these patients. Conventional intermittent parenteral administration of narcotics may be used but with caution, as the systemic effects may further suppress respirations. In some centers, a continuous narcotic infusion has been found to provide relief, often with lower doses of medication (3 [pp. 149–150]). Patients reported increased comfort that may be related to steady-state drug levels and the ability to titrate dosage for pain control. Intercostal nerve block is another pain-control approach and may be achieved by injection (by a physician) above and below rib fracture sites with 0.25 to 0.5% bupivacaine (Marcaine). Intermittent doses of preservative-free morphine (Duramorph) administered by an anesthesiologist via a thoracic epidural catheter have been useful with some patients (3 [pp. 149–150]). The patient's respiratory rate should be documented every hour, as delayed respiratory depression may occur. Transcutaneous electrical nerve stimulation (TENS) is a useful pain-control strategy with some chest trauma patients. The precise mechanism of action of TENS is unknown; however, there are several theories, one of which suggests that endorphin production is stimulated by TENS (12). TENS is one example of noninvasive pain management techniques that may be useful in the acute and intermediate stages of trauma. Other noninvasive physical or sensory techniques are cutaneous stimulation with pressure, massage, cold, heat, contralateral stimulation, and breathing exercises, all of which are gaining interest by nurses and patients alike (13). As with any therapy, patient response to care measures must be assessed on an individual basis and therapy adjusted accordingly.

## C. Nursing Diagnosis

Potential for infection related to atelectasis and therapies associated with pulmonary contusion

### Goal of Care

Facilitate mobilization of secretions and prevent retained secretions.

### Nursing Interventions

- Assess breath sound frequently.
- Provide aggressive pulmonary toilet measures:
  - Turning, positioning
  - Coughing, deep breathing, incentive spirometry
  - Postural drainage and, in some instances, chest physiotherapy
  - Suctioning
- Encourage early mobilization, ambulation.
- Provide humidification.
- Monitor character of secretions.

## Rationale

Atelectasis develops as a result of accumulated blood, fluid, and cellular debris, and is compounded by the patient's inability to clear secretions because of pain. An artificial airway bypasses the body's natural pulmonary defense system; therefore, measures must be taken to prevent pulmonary infection. Asepsis in managing the airway will help to reduce the incidence of nosocomial infection. Early mobilization and ambulation may be difficult or impossible with some multitrauma patients. Patients on ventilators without other restrictions can be ambulated with assistance, using a portable oxygen tank and Ambu bag for manual ventilation. Frequent position changes and postural drainage will move secretions into the tracheobronchial tree, where they can be removed by suctioning. The use of chest percussion in the acute stage of severe pulmonary contusions is controversial, as it may exacerbate bleeding, particularly if a coagulopathy exists. Secretions must be monitored with respect to color, amount, tenacity, and odor, as these may provide early evidence of pulmonary infection. Once the patient is able, coughing and deep-breathing exercises should be established. Incentive spirometry will provide information about the efficacy of a patient's own ventilatory capacity.

## ASSOCIATED NURSING DIAGNOSES

A. Potential fluid volume deficits
B. Nutrition: less than body requirements
C. Anxiety
D. Altered coping
E. Interruption of skin integrity

### REFERENCES

1. Corpening J. Cardiothoracic trauma. In: Mann JK, Oakes AR, eds. Critical care nursing of the multi-injured patient. Philadelphia: WB Saunders, 1980:64.
2. Budassi SA, Barber J. Mosby's manual of emergency care: practices and procedures. St Louis: CV Mosby, 1984.
3. Dunham CM, Cowley RA. Shock trauma/critical care handbook. Rockville, MD: Aspen, 1986.
4. Chopra PS, Kroncke GM, Berkoff HA, et al. Pulmonary contusion: a problem in blunt chest trauma. Wis Med J 1977;76:51–53.
5. Trunkey DD. Thoracic trauma. Advanced trauma life support course for physicians. Chicago: American College of Surgeons, 1985:78.
6. DeMuth WE, Smith JM. Pulmonary contusion. Am J Surg 1965;109:1819.
7. Fulton RL, Peter ET. The progressive nature of pulmonary contusion. Surgery 1970;67:499.
8. Condon RE, Nykus LM, eds. Manual of surgical therapeutics. 2nd ed. Boston: Little, Brown, 1972:25.
9. Roscher R, Bittner R, Stockmann U. Pulmonary contusion: clinical experience. Arch Surg 1974;109:510.
10. Corpening J. Cardiothoracic trauma. In: Mann JK, Oakes AR, eds. Critical care nursing of the multi-injured patient. Philadelphia: WB Saunders, 1980:64.
11. Hurn PD. Thoracic injuries. In: Cardona VD, Hurn PD, Bastnagel-Mason PJ, et al, eds. Trauma nursing: from resuscitation through rehabilitation. Philadelphia: WB Saunders, 1988.
12. Porter J, Jick H. Addiction rare in patients treated with narcotics. N Eng J Med 1980;302:123.
13. Schott BE, Luff S. Pain management in the trauma patient. In: Cardona VD, Hurn PD, Bastnagel-Mason PJ, et al, eds. Trauma nursing: from resuscitation through rehabilitation. Philadelphia: WB Saunders, 1988:333.

# CHAPTER 8

## The Patient with Adult Respiratory Distress Syndrome

Kathy L. Samuel, RN, BSN
Valerie Adair, RN, BSN

## Clinical Presentation

A previously healthy 27-year-old man involved in a single-car collision was admitted to a regional trauma center. Paramedics found the man trapped in his car, unbelted, and pinned against the steering wheel. They immobilized his neck with a Philadelphia collar and started intravenous lines in both forearms prior to helicopter transport to the hospital.

On admission, he was awake but disoriented and combative. Initial vital signs were blood pressure 160/88, pulse 128, and respirations 36, with retractions. Oxygen was administered at 100% via a nonrebreather face mask. Physical examination revealed lacerations on the face and anterior trunk. Blood was obtained for an arterial blood gas (ABG), complete blood count, electrolytes, and toxicology screen. Despite efforts to reassure the patient, he remained uncooperative and aggressively refused all treatment and further examination. Pavulon and fentanyl were administered intravenously, and the patient was orally intubated with a 8-mm endotracheal tube. During intubation the patient vomited and experienced bronchospasm. A post intubation chest x-ray film indicated correct airway placement and revealed diffuse interstitial and alveolar infiltrates consistent with adult respiratory distress syndrome (ARDS). The results of ABGs sampled during this patient's admission are summarized in Table 8.1.

Because of difficulty in achieving adequate oxygenation in this patient, the health care team agreed to increase positive end-expiratory pressure (PEEP) to 10 cm, which resulted in an increased $PaO_2$ of 221 mm Hg (Table 8.1). The patient was transported to the intensive care unit (ICU) for continued monitoring and ventilatory management. During his 8-week hospitalization, he was treated with several ventilatory modes. These modes, ventilatory parameters, and subsequent ABG results are presented in Table 8.2. Ventilatory support was discontinued, and the patient was placed on a trach collar 44 days after admission. After a 10-day period of convalescence in the intermediate care unit, he was discharged home.

## 1. What is the pathophysiological basis for this patient's problem?

The incidence of ARDS in this country is estimated to be greater than 150,000 cases annually, with a mortality rate of approximately 50% (1). A scenario of initial lung injury (trauma, contusion, aspiration, sepsis) followed by lung edema, altered gas exchange, shunting, and poor compliance is typical of ARDS. Clinical presentation includes dyspnea, rales or rhonchi, hypoxemia refractory to high concentrations of inspired oxygen, and diffuse interstitial infiltrates on chest x-ray film (2). In addition, pulmonary compliance is reduced and functional residual capacity decreases with alveolar collapse, causing pulmonary shunting and a mismatch of ventilation and perfusion (3). A number of predisposing factors have been associated with the development of ARDS (Table 8.3). Attempts to describe the syndrome have led to the use of numerous synonyms for ARDS; Table 8.4 lists some of the terms most commonly used.

The basic mechanism or pathway responsible for ARDS is extremely complex and not completely understood. Most investigators agree that some catastrophic event pre-

**Table 8.1.** Admission ABG results[a]

| | Time (minutes) | | | | | | |
|---|---|---|---|---|---|---|---|
| | 30 | 60 | 90 | 120 | 135 | 150 | 180 |
| $O_2$ delivery route | Mask | Mask | ETT | ETT | ETT | ETT | ETT |
| Ventilator mode | — | — | SIMV | SIMV | SIMV | SIMV | SIMV |
| $FiO_2$ | 100 | 100 | 100 | 75 | 100 | 100 | 100 |
| PEEP | 0 | 0 | 5 | 5 | 5 | 10 | 10 |
| $PaO_2$ | 164 | 151 | 280 | 102 | 173 | 198 | 221 |
| $PaCO_2$ | 44 | 42 | 33 | 35 | 36 | 43 | 42 |
| pH | 7.33 | 7.32 | 7.44 | 7.44 | 7.44 | 7.35 | 7.35 |

[a]*Abbreviations:* ETT, endotracheal tube; SIMV, synchronized intermittent mandatory ventilation; PEEP, positive end-expiratory pressure.

cipitates the syndrome and that the general pathophysiology follows the scheme in Figure 8.1.

The diffuse infiltrates seen on x-ray studies are thought to be a consequence of pulmonary edema of a noncardiogenic origin. Pulmonary edema occurs when the hydrostatic pressure in the pulmonary capillaries exceeds the intravascular osmotic pressure (also called cardiogenic pulmonary edema) or when a change occurs in the permeability of the alveolar capillary membrane, resulting in the leakage of fluid into the interstitial spaces (noncardiogenic pulmonary edema). Normally the alveolar capillary membrane is able to restrict the diffusion of plasma protein into the interstitium, and pulmonary lymphatics act to prevent fluid accumulation in the lungs (4,5). In ARDS, pulmonary capillary permeability increases and these protective mechanisms become compromised (6), evidenced in part by elevated protein content in the edema of ARDS patients (7). Increases in both fluid and protein movement occur from the capillary space to the interstitial and intra-alveolar spaces at normal to low hydrostatic pressures (5). Interstitial alveolar fluid accumulation causes a diffusion deficit as a result of the increase in the distance gases must travel for exchange. As the syndrome progresses, alveolar flooding occurs, which further impairs gas exchange (6).

Cellular changes may be a result of microvascular injury caused by the release of toxic humoral substances such as lysosomal proteases, complement, and oxygen-free radicals (8). Although the precise mechanism is unclear, these substances are known to damage cells (9). The resulting inflammatory response causes leaking of protein and fluid into interstitial and alveolar spaces, thereby impeding gas diffusion.

Overall, increased extravascular lung water reduces functional residual capacity (FRC), the lung volume at which inspiration begins (10). Collapsed alveoli fill with fluid, further reducing lung volume. Ventilation-perfusion abnormalities occur as blood passes through partially or nonventilated areas of the lung. Blood is therefore shunted through the lungs and returns to the arterial system without being oxygenated, resulting in hypoxemia (10).

Another element in the pathophysiology of ARDS involves surfactant. Surfactant is produced in the alveoli by type II pneumocytes, which become injured in ARDS (3). The role of surfactant is to stabilize surface tension within the alveolar walls and prevent alveolar collapse (11). If surfactant is not present in sufficient amounts, surface tension and airway resistance increase. The ARDS patient is unable to overcome this increased resistance; therefore, tidal volume ($V_T$) is reduced and atelectasis ensues. In addition, remnants of surfactant, cellular debris, and fibrin aggregate to form hyaline membranes (11). Pulmonary compliance, the degree of elasticity of the lungs, is reduced as the lungs become "stiff" because of increased amounts of lung water, fibrotic changes, and loss

**Table 8.2.** Compilation of ventilatory modes, ventilatory parameters, and arterial blood gas measurements[a]

| | Day 1 | Hour 1 | Hour 2 | Hour 3 | Day 7 | Day 14 | Day 21 | Day 28 | Day 28 | Day 30 | Day 32 | Day 33 | Day 34 | Day 35 | Day 36 | Day 37 | Day 39 | Day 41 | Day 43 | Day 44[b] |
|---|---|---|---|---|---|---|---|---|---|---|---|---|---|---|---|---|---|---|---|---|
| Ventilator mode | SIMV | SIMV | PC | PC | PC | PC | PC | SIMV/PS | PC | PC | PC | PC | PC | PC | PC | PC | PC | SIMV/PS | PS | PC |
| Set rate | 10 | 8 | 10 | 12 | 16 | 12 | 12 | 16 | 16 | 16 | 16 | 14 | 12 | 12 | 10 | 12 | 12 | 12 | 0 | 8 |
| Pressure support | — | — | 30 | 30 | 65 | 62 | 55 | 60 | 55 | 58 | 60 | 58 | 50 | 40 | 34 | 34 | 30 | 26 | 8 | |
| Set PEEP/effective PEEP | 10/18 | 12/20 | 12/21 | 12/21 | 20/24 | 20/23 | 22/26 | 18/22 | 22/25 | 20/24 | 22/25 | 20/24 | 18/24 | 16/20 | 10/16 | 10/14 | 8/12 | 5 | 5 | |
| $FiO_2$ | 100 | 70 | 70 | 50 | 50 | 45 | 45 | 45 | 55 | 55 | 55 | 55 | 55 | 50 | 50 | 40 | 40 | 40 | 35 | |
| PIP | 70 | 70 | 40 | 41 | 78 | 69 | 66 | 78 | 65 | 60 | 62 | 62 | 60 | 56 | 52 | 46 | 44 | 42 | | |
| Plateau | 38 | 39 | 40 | 41 | 78 | 69 | 66 | 66 | 65 | 60 | 62 | 62 | 60 | 56 | 52 | 46 | 44 | 29 | 19 | |
| MAP | ? | ? | 29 | 29 | 45 | 35 | 38 | 32 | 35 | 35 | 37 | 35 | 34 | 30 | 26 | 20 | 14 | 10 | 8 | |
| $PaO_2$ | 244 | 188 | 235 | 176 | 122 | 135 | 112 | 140 | 130 | 135 | 144 | 112 | 98 | 112 | 100 | 122 | 138 | 124 | 116 | 90 |
| pH | 7.45 | 7.46 | 7.40 | 7.41 | 7.40 | 7.47 | 7.40 | 7.41 | 7.44 | 7.40 | 7.42 | 7.47 | 7.44 | 7.46 | 7.40 | 7.38 | 7.42 | 7.39 | 7.42 | 7.43 |
| $PaCO_2$ | 33 | 35 | 35 | 36 | 35 | 35 | 40 | 36 | 35 | 37 | 35 | 40 | 44 | 47 | 42 | 44 | 41 | 40 | 42 | 49 |

[a]Abbreviations: SIMV, synchronized intermittent mandatory ventilation; PC, pressure control; PS, pressure support; PEEP, positive end-expiratory pressure; IPI, peak inspiratory pressure; MAP, mean airway pressure.
[b]Patient placed on a trach collar on day 44.

**Table 8.3.** Predisposing factors for ARDS[a]

| | |
|---|---|
| Trauma | Multiple transfusions |
| Shock | Fluid overload |
| Sepsis | Disseminated intravascular coagulation |
| Burns | Drug overdose |
| Smoke inhalation | Near-drowning |
| Oxygen toxicity | Acid aspiration (gastric) |

[a]*Source*: Adapted from Rinaldo JE. Adult respiratory distress syndrome. In: Shoemaker WC, Ayres S, Grenvik A, Holbrook PR, Thompson WL, eds. Textbook of critical care. Philadelphia: WB Saunders, 1989:615–636.

of FRC. The alveolar membrane becomes thickened, which impairs gas exchange, resulting in hypoxemia.

A number of nursing diagnoses were addressed in planning care for this patient with ARDS. This chapter will focus only on problems with hypoxemia and ventilator management and on interventions directed toward supporting and improving alveolar ventilation and oxygen transport.

## 2. What is the nursing diagnosis of highest priority?

Impaired gas exchange

## 3. What are the goals of nursing care?

### Nursing Diagnosis

Impaired gas exchange related to interstitial edema, alveolar congestion, and ineffective breathing patterns

### Goal of Care

Monitor and assist in measures to achieve effective gas exchange.

### Nursing Interventions

- Monitor:
  - Vital signs and hemodynamic parameters: HR, RR, BP, CVP, pulmonary capillary wedge pressure (PCWP), cardiac output (CO)
  - Breath sounds
  - Ventilatory parameters: airway pressures, $V_T$, minute ventilation
  - Arterial and mixed venous blood gases values
- Maintain accurate records of intake and output.
- Collaborate with physician to adjust ventilator therapy to maximize gas exchange and hemodynamic function.

Care of the ARDS patient is complex and requires the collaborative efforts of a multidisciplinary team. Overall, goals of care are to

**Table 8.4.** Synonyms for ARDS[a]

| |
|---|
| Shock |
| Wet lung |
| Traumatic wet lung |
| White lung |
| Congestive atelectasis |
| Adult hyaline membrane disease |
| Posttraumatic pulmonary insufficiency |
| Noncardiogenic pulmonary edema |
| Da-Nang lung |

[a]*Source*: Adpated from Taylor RW, Norwood SH. The adult respiratory distress syndrome. In: Civetta JM, Taylor RW, Kirby RR, eds. Critical care. Philadelphia: JB Lippincott, 1988:1057–1068.

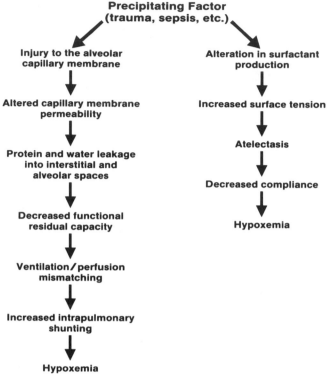

Figure 8.1. Pathophysiology of ARDS.

(1) Treat the underlying disease process
(2) Provide cardiopulmonary support to achieve optimum gas exchange and tissue perfusion
(3) Prevent complications

Patients in pulmonary failure are often critically ill and require aggressive therapy to achieve these goals. In addition, astute nursing assessment and intensive monitoring are necessary to determine the effects of and patient response to such aggressive therapies.

Supplemental oxygen is often administered in an attempt to correct hypoxemia. If ARDS is not diagnosed until late in its course, it may be necessary to use high concentrations (FiO$_2$ greater than 0.5) to maintain acceptable PaO$_2$ values. Yet, prolonged therapy with high oxygen concentrations can lead to a type of lung damage, referred to as oxygen toxicity. Although the precise mechanism of oxygen toxicity is not entirely clear, it probably involves the generation of a variety of free radicals that are produced during the reduction of molecular oxygen (12). The lung can metabolize these radicals to a certain extent, but once the required enzyme system is exhausted, lung injury results (11). Additionally, hypoxemia associated with ARDS may become refractory to oxygen therapy, even at high concentrations. Therefore, the goal of care is to decrease the concentration of inspired oxygen (FiO$_2$) to below 0.50 as soon as possible (14).

One of the most effective strategies for improving oxygenation with reduced FiO$_2$

is the use of positive end-expiratory pressure (PEEP). Goals of PEEP therapy are an increase in functional residual capacity (FRC) and alveolar recruitment. The FRC, the amount of gas remaining in the lung at the end of a normal expiration, is reduced in ARDS. The use of PEEP produces a continuous increase in the airway and alveolar pressures. This continuous positive distending pressure keeps a greater number of airways open throughout the respiratory cycle and re-establishes the patency of closed or atelectatic alveoli. The FRC increases, which allows more gas to be available to more alveoli. The increase in the FRC and the recruitment of previously closed alveoli improve ventilation of gas exchange units (13). The net effect is increased $V_T$ volume and improved compliance and arterial oxygenation.

To prevent recurrence of alveolar collapse and loss of FRC, it is important to maintain PEEP as much as possible while providing airway care. When manual ventilation may be necessary (e.g., prior to suctioning), an Ambu or ventilating bag with a PEEP valve should be used to maintain PEEP during this presuctioning hyperoxygenation. Patients receiving PEEP therapy at levels greater than 10 cm $H_2O$ may be suctioned through the suctioning port of the airway adapter connected to the ventilator tubing. Hyperoxygenation also may be achieved by increasing the ventilator $FiO_2$ setting to 1.00 for three to four breaths before and after each attempt at endotracheal suctioning (3).

Set and effective PEEP must be considered with reduced lung compliance. As the lungs stiffen, the actual or effective level of PEEP may be greater than the level of PEEP the ventilator is set to deliver to the patient. In addition, PEEP therapy has been associated with a reduction in cardiac output. Therefore, it is recommended to use an optimum level of PEEP (also referred to as best PEEP), which is the PEEP level that reduces shunt fraction with the least impingement on cardiac output (14).

Respiratory function in ARDS is usually severely impaired, and the patients are unable to maintain adequate ventilation. In these circumstances, endotracheal intubation and positive pressure ventilation (PPV) with a mechanical ventilator become necessary.

The patient described in this case report was intubated and managed on a Servo 900C ventilator. During the course of his ICU stay, the following modes were used:

(1) Pressure support (PS)

(2) Synchronized intermittent mandatory ventilation (SIMV)

(3) Synchronized intermittent mandatory ventilation with pressure support (SIMV/PS)

(4) Pressure control (PC)

Figure 8.2 illustrates airway pressures and air flow for each of these modes.

PS can be used as a ventilator mode to assist patients with poor ventilatory effort. This mode supports the respiratory muscles by enhancing the spontaneous $V_T$ while maintaining the patient's own intrinsic respiratory rate and flow pattern (15). When the patient initiates a breath, gas is delivered rapidly at a predetermined pressure, which is maintained throughout inspiration; therefore, a greater $V_T$ and minute ventilation may be achieved, improving FRC and gas exchange. This is accomplished by adjusting the PS level until the desired $V_T$ is achieved (16). Gas flow ceases when the patient begins to exhale, and airway pressure returns to the predetermined PEEP level.

PS is particularly helpful during the weaning process, espcially for those patients who have experienced lengthy ventilator therapy. Such patients may have weak respiratory muscles because of disuse atrophy and may benefit from supported ventilation until they become strong enough to resume spontaneous ventilation.

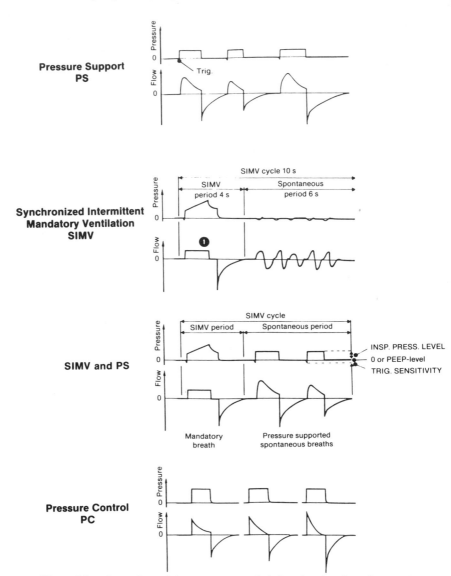

**Figure 8.2.** Comparison of airway pressure and air flow in selected ventilator modes.

The PS level is reduced gradually, over a period of days to weeks, with careful attention to $V_T$ and respiratory rate. Reduced $V_T$ and dyspnea and/or tachypnea indicate that the patient is not ready for further weaning from PS.

SIMV is used frequently for patients requiring mechanical ventilation. $V_T$ is initially determined by the patient's weight, with 10 to 15 ml/kg commonly used to calculate normal $V_T$. The rate is set to produce minute ventilation necessary to maintain $PaCO_2$ between 35 and 45 mm Hg (7). The patient may breathe spontaneously; the synchronized mode prevents a ventilator breath from occurring when a patient initiates a breath.

A difficulty encountered in using SIMV is that spontaneous $V_T$ may be small (e.g., 200 to 300 cc) because of weak respiratory muscles or poor ventilatory effort. Spontaneous $V_T$ can be improved by adding PS. The PS level can be adjusted until spontaneous $V_T$ approximates delivered $V_T$.

At times these conventional ventilator modes are not effective in achieving adequate gas exchange. ARDS may result in profound airway resistance, which may be compounded by PEEP and PPV. When airway pressures exceed 60 cm $H_2O$ or more, the risk of barotrauma to the lungs increases markedly (17). PC may be a ventilator mode for this patient population because it achieves adequate volume ventilation with controlled and reduced peak inspiratory pressures (PIP) (18).

Gas is delivered at a constant pressure during a predetermined inspiratory time; once this preset pressure is achieved, the gas flow rate decelerates to maintain that pressure. Decelerating gas flow reduces PIP, often dramatically in comparison with that associated with SIMV. The constant pressure results in an increase in mean airway pressure. Higher mean airway pressure allows alveoli with higher surface tensions (i.e., decreased surfactant) to remain open and prevents their collapse. Ultimately, more alveoli are opened and available for ventilation and gas exchange. Some clinicians advocate mean airway pressure rather than PEEP as a major determinant of gas exchange (19).

The length of time for gas delivery on the PC mode is preset and is referred to as a percentage of the ventilatory cycle. Normal inspiratory time, such as that used with SIMV, is 33%, which corresponds to an inspiratory to expiratory ratio (I:E) of 1:2. Inspiratory time during PC generally is initiated at 50% (I:E = 1:1) and may be increased to 67% to 80%, reversing the I:E ratio. This prolonged inspiratory time allows more time for gas exchange across healthy as well as damaged membranes and may prove beneficial for those patients with increased airway resistance and reduced compliance (20).

The use of PPV and PEEP has two potential complications: decreased cardiac output (CO) and barotrauma (8). The main mechanism by which CO is decreased is a reduction in venous return (preload) due to increased intrathoracic pressures produced by pressure from the ventilatory circuit. Other mechanisms contributing to decreased CO include abnormal ventricular compliance and increased pulmonary vascular resistance (21). Most of the undesirable hemodynamic effects of positive pressure breathing are prevented or corrected by optimizing preload with careful intravascular fluid management (22) and by avoiding high PIP.

Barotrauma refers to trauma caused by pressure. In the lung, the source of this pressure may be the result of increased airway resistance due to lung injury or positive pressure therapy. As previously mentioned, when PIP exceeds 60 cm $H_2O$, there is an increased incidence of barotrauma (19). Barotrauma may present as pneumothorax, pneumomediastinum, or subcutaneous emphysema (15). Pneumothorax and pneumomediastinum may result in severe hemodynamic compromise; therefore, decompression of the affected lung or correction of the displaced mediastinum is of paramount importance. The nurse must frequently monitor for changes in airway pressures, ventilatory volumes, and breath sounds. In addition to signaling a possible complication of PPV, these assessment parameters provide data to evaluate airway patency and the need for or effectiveness of pulmonary toilet measures.

Hemodynamic monitoring with an arterial line and pulmonary artery catheter is recommended to assess the efficacy of fluid therapy and cardiac function. It is important to maintain CO sufficient to provide tissue perfusion. Adequate intravenous fluid therapy usually achieves this goal; however, inotropic support may be necessary to augment fluid therapy. Oxygen delivery to tissues is also dependent on hemoglobin concentration. The hemoglobin level should not be permitted to fall below 10 gm%, and many clinicians recommend that this level be kept near 12 gm% (13). Care must be taken to avoid fluid volume overload, which may result in further increased lung edema. Inotropic agents and diuretics may help to improve renal function and reduce excess fluid volume (23).

Placement of arterial and pulmonary artery catheters permits direct sampling of arterial and mixed venous blood, the results of which indicate the degree of arterial and tissue oxygenation. ABG analysis is important to determine response to therapy and the need for changes as appropriate. Noninvasive measures such as pulse oximetry and $SaO_2$ monitoring may be used to assess oxygenation and minimize blood sampling. Arterial $O_2$ and $CO_2$ levels, though valuable, are not infallible measures of patient status. The wise clinician will use ABG results in conjunction with other parameters as well as the total clinical presentation to completely assess, plan, and evaluate patient care.

## REFERENCES

1. Shoemaker WC. Pathophysiology and fluid management of postoperative and post-traumatic ARDS. In: Shoemaker WC, Ayres S, Grenvik A, Holbrook PR, Thompson WL, eds. Textbook of critical care. Philadelphia: WB Saunders, 1989:615–636.
2. Petty TL. Adult respiratory distress syndrome. In: Kryger MH, ed. Pathophysiology of respiration. New York: Wiley, 1981:89–102.
3. Bradley RB. Adult respiratory distress syndrome. Focus Crit Care 1987;14:48–59.
4. Parker RE. Secondary pulmonary edema. Semin Respir Med 1983;4:279–284.
5. Taylor RW, Norwood SH. The adult respiratory distress syndrome. In: Civetta JM, Taylor RW, Kirby RR, eds. Critical care. Philadelphia: JB Lippincott, 1988:1057–1068.
6. Brigham KL. Primary (high permeability) pulmonary edema. Semin Respir Med 1983;4:285–288.
7. Rogers M, ed. Textbook of pediatric intensive care. Vol 1. Baltimore: Williams & Wilkins, 1987.
8. Taylor RW: The adult respiratory distress syndrome. In: Kirby RR, Taylor RW, eds. Respiratory failure. Chicago: Year Book Medical Publishers, 1986:208–244.
9. Robbins SL, Angell M, Kunmar V. Basic pathology. Philadelphia: WB Saunders, 1981:369–420.
10. Mecca RS. Respiratory: essential physiologic concerns. In: Civetta JM, Taylor RW, Kirby RR, eds. Critical care. Philadelphia: JB Lippincott, 1988:1023–1037.
11. Demling RH. Respiratory failure from trauma and sepsis (ARDS). In: Zuidema GD, Rutherford RB, Ballinger WF, eds. The management of trauma. 4th ed. Philadelphia: WB Saunders, 1985:137–167.
12. Taylor AE, Matalon S, Ward PE, eds. Physiology of oxygen radicals. Baltimore: Williams & Wilkins, 1986.

13. Shapiro B. General principles of airway pressure therapy. In: Shoemaker WC, Ayres S, Grenvik A, Holbrook PR, Thompson WL, eds. Textbook of critical care. Philadelphia: WB Saunders, 1989:505–515.
14. Suter PM, Fairly HG, Isenberg MD. Optimum end-expiratory pressure in patients with acute pulmonary failure. N Engl J Med 1975;292:284.
15. Toben BP, Lewandowski V. Nontraditional and new ventilatory techniques. CCQ 1988;11(3):12–27.
16. MacIntyre NR. Pressure support ventilation: effects on ventilatory reflexes and ventilatory-muscle workloads. Respir Care 1987;32:447–453.
17. Bone RC, Francis PB, Pierce AK. Pulmonary barotrauma complicating positive end-expiratory pressure. Am Rev Resp Dis 1975;11:921.
18. Tharatt RS, Roblee PA, Abertson TE. Pressure controlled inverse ratio ventilation in severe adult respiratory failure. Chest 1988;94(4):755–762.
19. Gallagher TJ, Banner MJ. Mean airway pressure as a determinant of oxygenation. Crit Care Med 1980;8:244.
20. Dammann JF, McAslan TC, Maffeo CT. Optimal flow pattern for mechanical ventilation of the lungs: 2. The effect of a sine wave versus square wave flow pattern with and without an end-inspiratory pause on patients. Crit Care Med 1978;6:293.
21. Pick PA, Handler JB, Murata GH, et al. The cardiovascular effects of positive end expiratory pressure. Chest 1982;82:345–350.
22. Walkinshaw M, Shoemaker WC. Use of volume loading to obtain preferred levels of PEEP: a pulmonary study. Crit Care Med 1980;8:81.
23. Hemmer M, Suter PM. Treatment of cardiac and renal effects of PEEP with dopamine in patients with acute respiratory failure. Anesthesiology 1979;50:399.

# CHAPTER 9

## Smoke Inhalation

Ben Grimes, RN
Tom Baker, RN

## Clinical Presentation

A 72-year-old woman was watching television at home when suddenly her television set picture tube exploded, causing a fire and rendering her unconscious. She regained consciousness when moved outdoors by the paramedics. She was flown by helicopter to the emergency department of a university-based medical center.

On arrival she was awake, but having some difficulty breathing. Her face, upper extremities, and clothing were covered with soot. She was vomiting carbonaceous fluid, and there was soot in the oropharynx. She had first- and second-degree burns on the face and upper extremities. The patient had equal breath sounds with bilateral wheezing. There was no stridor, but because of labored breathing and increased secretions she was orally intubated with a number 8 endotracheal tube (ETT). A direct bronchoscopy was performed, revealing an erythematous trachea with thick carbonaceous material covering the bronchial walls. A small amount of irrigation resulted in increased edema, so further irrigation was not performed. Initial arterial blood gas (ABG) on an $FiO_2$ of 100% showed $PaO_2$ 365, pH 7.31, $PaCO_2$ 46, oxygen saturation 76%, and carboxyhemoglobin (HbCO) 23.3%.

Psychometric testing could not be done because the patient was intubated and heavily sedated. Because the patient had loss of consciousness at the scene and her HbCO was 23.3%, it was decided to treat her with hyperbaric oxygen (HBO). An ear, nose, and throat physician performed bilateral myringotomies and inserted pressure equalization (PE) tubes, as the patient could not clear her ears because of intubation. The nurse and the respiratory therapist agreed that tracheal edema was such that a seal had been achieved and no cuff inflation was necessary. There was no air leak, and breath sounds could be heard equally throughout. The patient's HBO treatment was carried out uneventfully.

Posthyperbaric oxygen treatment HbCO was 3.3, but because of her compromised pulmonary status she remained intubated and was admitted to the intensive care unit (ICU) in stable condition. HBO therapy was continued to treat her first- and second-degree burns. She was given a total of 10 treatments each, consisting of 90 minutes of HBO at 33 feet of sea water. The remainder of her hospital treatment consisted of respiratory management, chest physiotherapy, serial x-rays and ECGs, and additional HBO.

On the fifth day of hospitalization she was successfully extubated. Her diet was slowly advanced to a mechanical soft diet and ambulation was begun.

Her burns were treated locally with bacitracin ointment and were 50% healed at time of discharge. Follow-up clinic visits showed good resolution of inhalation injury and complete healing of burns.

## 1. What is the pathophysiological basis for this patient's problem?

One of the most common causes of postburn respiratory injury is smoke inhalation. Smoke inhalation generally refers to injury to the pulmonary system by inhalation of thermal gaseous or particulate products of combustion. Smoke is a complex mixture of particulate matter, consisting of large carbon particles coated with organic acids and aldehydes that cause toxic effects in the bronchioles. A variety of gases are produced

**Table 9.1.** Toxic products that may be obtained from combustible materials[a]

| Toxic Gas or Vapor | Source Materials |
|---|---|
| Carbon dioxide | All combustible materials containing carbon |
| Carbon monoxide | |
| Nitrogen oxide | Cellulose polyurethane |
| Hydrogen cyanide | Wool, silk, or plastics containing nitrogen |
| Formic acid | Cellulosic materials, cellulosic plastics, rayon |
| Acetic acid | |
| Sulphur dioxide | Rubber, thiokolis |
| Halogen acids | Polyvinyl chloride, fire-retardant plastics, fluorinated plastics |
| Ammonia | Melamine, nylon, urea, formaldehyde resin |
| Aldehydes | Phenol formaldehyde, wood nylon, polyester resins |
| Benzene | Polystyrene |
| Phenol | Phenol formaldehyde |
| Azo-bis-succino-nitrite | Foamed plastics |

[a]*Source*: Winter Emergencies Workshop literature. Maryland Institute for Emergency Medical Services Systems, 1983.

from the combustion of various materials, all of which are pulmonary irritants that have a direct effect on lung tissue (see Table 9.1). In low concentrations they cause bronchoconstriction; however, in high concentrations they produce pulmonary edema and possible hemorrhage (1). Among the important considerations when treating a patient exposed to smoke is carbon monoxide (CO) poisoning. Inhaled CO combines readily with hemoglobin to form HbCO, a compound that is 200 times more stable than oxyhemoglobin (2). The production of HbCO within the body has two major effects. First, it effectively blocks the transport of oxygen from the lungs to the tissues because oxygen cannot bind with or be transported by HbCO. Second, it shifts the oxygen dissociation curve to the left, which facilitates the binding of oxygen on the unaffected hemoglobin in the lungs, but severely impairs oxygen release to the tissues. CO intoxification therefore induces a nonischemic hypoxia. Recent studies also suggest that CO binds with the iron-containing proteins of the intracellular cytochrome oxidase systems, thereby directly inhibiting cellular respiration (3).

This patient presented with a history of loss of consciousness; an HbCO level of 23.3%, which is a moderate CO poisoning level (see Table 9.2); and first- and second-degree burns of the face and arms. The rationale for use of HBO is that it effectively displaces CO from hemoglobin and cytochrome systems in accordance with the law of mass action. HBO provides increased amounts of available oxygen, the ratio of oxygen to CO is increased, and CO is displaced from the hemoglobin and the cytochrome more rapidly than breathing oxygen via a face mask at normal atmospheric pressures (2). The elimination of CO results in an exponentially decreasing HbCO level that is commonly referred to as HbCO half-life (3). The HbCO half-life when breathing room air is approximately 5 hours, as compared to breathing 100% oxygen in a hyperbaric chamber at three atmospheres, which would decrease the half-life of HbCO to 23 minutes.

The patient would be placed in either a large multiplace chamber or a monoplace (one-person) chamber. In the multiplace chamber, 100% oxygen would be delivered via face mask, head tent, or artificial airway, such as endotracheal tube or tracheostomy tube.

If the monoplace chamber were to be used, the chamber would be compressed with 100% oxygen, thus making the ambient environment one of pure oxygen.

**Table 9.2.** Carbon monoxide effects[a]

| CO Blood Level | Indications | Manifestations |
|---|---|---|
| 0.3–0.7% HbCO | Endogenous | Produced in the process of hemoglobin breakdown |
| 1–10% HbCO | Normal | Increased blood flow to vital organs<br>Increased threshold to visual stimuli<br>Decreased angina threshold in persons with existing cardiovascular disease |
| 10–20% HbCO | Mild poisoning | *CNS symptoms*: Headache, decreased cerebral function, decreased visual activity<br>*Cardiopulmonary symptoms*: slight breathlessness |
| 20–40% HbCO | Moderate poisoning | *CNS subjective symptoms*: Headache, tight forehead, ringing in ears, diminished vision, nausea, aching limbs, weakness, vertigo<br>*CNS objective symptoms*: Altered mental status, confusion, irritability, hyperreflexia, vomiting, yawning, dilated pupils, Cheyne-Stokes respirations<br>*Cardiopulmonary symptoms*: Decreased blood pressure, increased pulse, ST segment depression, atrial and ventricular arrhythmias, pale to reddish-purple skin color |
| 40–60 HbCO | Severe poisoning | *CNS symptoms*: Coma with convulsions, cardiopulmonary instability, and arrhythmias |
| 60–80% HbCO | Usually fatal | |

[a]*Source*: Unsworth IP. Acute carbon monoxide poisoning. Anesthesia and Intensive Care (Nov) 1974;2:329–333.

## 2. What are the nursing diagnoses of highest priority?

A. Potential for ineffective airway clearance
B. Potential for impaired gas exchange
C. Potential for infection

## 3. What are the goals of nursing care?

### A. Nursing Diagnosis

Potential for ineffective airway clearance related to the artificial airway, altered state of consciousness, and the secondary effects of inhaled heated toxic agents

### Goal of Care

Restore and maintain a patent airway.

### Nursing Interventions

- Observe and report signs of respiratory distress.
- Assemble and ensure proper functioning of the necessary equipment to perform emergency intubation or surgical cricothyroidotomy.
- Suction established airway as needed during the acute phase.
- Restrain according to hospital policy, and administer prescribed sedation as needed during the acute phase to prevent self-extubation.

### Rationale

The patient subjected to large concentrations of smoke in an enclosed area generally has sustained some degree of respiratory burn. This type of burn is more commonly designated as a chemical event because of the toxic compounds forming smoke, and it can be classified as a toxic pneumonitis. Toxic agents of combustion damage the pulmonary structures on contact, including the alveoli (1). The common scenario in a patient diagnosed with severe smoke inhalation is upper airway obstruction, bronchospasm, plugging of airways, and pulmonary edema followed by potential bacterial pneumonia. The latter problem develops 48 or more hours postinhalation. The health care team must assume that any patient who has inhaled smoke has also inhaled toxic gases and must anticipate pulmonary and systemic complications (see Table 9.2).

## B. Nursing Diagnosis

Potential for impaired gas exchange related to decreased transport, release, and use of oxygen secondary to toxic levels of CO and other potential toxic agents

### Goal of Care

Restore and maintain adequate gas exchange.

### Nursing Interventions

- Administer 100% oxygen via the artificial airway to the unconscious patient; assist respiratory status with mechanical ventilation and positive and expiratory pressure as ordered.
- Auscultate breath sounds regularly; provide optimal pulmonary hygiene, including frequent suctioning, turning, and positioning in semi-Fowler's unless contraindicated.
- Administer sedation as ordered to prevent patient from inadvertently dislodging the artificial airway.
- Prepare the patient for HBO treatment to include assisting with myringotomies if necessary; inflating the endotracheal tube or tracheal tube cuff with fluid (sterile water); and obtaining consent for hyperbaric therapy from significant others if available. Send serial arterial blood gases to include HbCO levels to lab as ordered.

### Rationale

Hypoxia is the most common consequence of inhalation events regardless of the toxic inhalant. Oxygen competes with CO for the same binding sites on the hemoglobin molecule. Increased arterial oxygen tensions mean that an increased number of dissolved oxygen molecules are competing for the hemoglobin sites occupied by CO. Increasing the arterial $PaO_2$ is the single most important factor in CO elimination along with meticulous pulmonary toilet. Early administration of 100% oxygen begins the CO washout process and increases capillary oxygen availability. Common practice is to do serial arterial blood gases and HbCO levels until the HbCO level is under 5% for two consecutive samples drawn 1 hour apart. Return of normal cilia action, assisted by bronchoscopy irrigation and suctioning, will aid in removal of carbonaceous exudate from the lungs, thus improving adequate gas exchange. HBO is a useful therapeutic tool in the rapid elimination of CO, since an arterial $PaO_2$ of 1500 mm Hg can be achieved (3). The half-life of CO ranges from 45 to 80 minutes when 100% oxygen is breathed. The half-life of CO is shortened even further (20 minutes) when 100% is breathed at hyperbaric pressures (three atmospheres) (4).

## C. Nursing Diagnosis

Potential for infection related to the secondary effects of toxic smoke inhalation and the disruption of skin as a result of first- and second-degree burns

## Goal of Care

Reduce the risk of infection.

## Nursing Interventions

- Observe strict sterile technique when providing pulmonary hygiene.
- Obtain cultures and administer prescribed antibiotics.
- Observe strict compliance to institution's protective isolation policy.

## Rationale

Infection, which has the potential to progress to sepsis, poses a constant threat to the smoke inhalation/burn victim. Pneumonias in this type of patient are usually secondary to nosocomial gram-negative bacteria and are often polymicrobial (4). Aspiration, inactivated bronchial cilia, and plugs of thickened mucus obstruct the lesser bronchioles, providing a perfect medium for bacterial growth. Removal of pulmonary secretions reduces the risk of lung infection and other pulmonary complications. The adherence to proper sterile technique reduces the risk of burn area contamination and the likelihood of infection.

# ASSOCIATED NURSING DIAGNOSES

A. Potential alteration in respiratory function
B. Potential alteration in tissue perfusion
C. Anxiety
D. Impaired communication

**REFERENCES**

1. Ewers D. Smoke inhalation: Assessment and management. JEN (Jan/Feb) 1979;5:5–7.
2. Davis JC, Hunt TK. Hyperbaric oxygen therapy. Undersea Medical Society, 1977:177–190.
3. Mesnick PS. Smoke inhalation. In: Roy D, Shapiro BA, eds. Case studies in critical care medicine. Chicago: Year Book Medical Publications, 1985.
4. Marzella L, Myers RAM. Carbon monoxide poisoning. Am Fam Phys 1986;34(5):83–93.

# CHAPTER 10

# Flail Chest with Intercostal Bleeding

## Mary Jayne Watson, RN, BSN

## Clinical Presentation

Mr. J., a 39-year-old construction worker, fell approximately 35 feet from a scaffolding onto soft earth and was admitted to an emergency department 18 hours after injury. On arrival he was assessed and found to be in respiratory distress with severe chest pain, asymmetric chest excursion, absent breath sounds on the left, and a midline shift of the trachea. He had large areas of bruising on the left upper torso and shoulder. The chest x-ray film revealed a left hemopneumothorax and fractures in ribs 3 through 7. The arterial blood gases showed a $PaO_2$ of 55, a $PaCO_2$ of 50, and a pH of 7.32 on 100% $O_2$ via nonrebreathing mask. He was agitated, uncooperative, and tachycardic, with a heart rate of 120 and blood pressure of 180/90.

Initial management included endotracheal intubation with mechanical ventilation, placement of a left chest tube connected to a Pleur-evac drainage system with 20 cm $H_2O$ suction, and insertion of invasive lines. Mr. J.'s initial blood loss was assessed at 1500 ml at the time of chest tube placement, and replacement fluids were Plasmanate and Ringer's lactate.

Mr. J. was transferred to the intensive care unit (ICU) for management approximately 2 hours after admission. His medical diagnoses were flail chest with intercostal bleeding; hemopneumothorax (left); and possible contusions to the heart, kidney, and left lung.

### 1. What is the pathophysiological basis for this patient's condition?

Flail chest results from multiple fractures of two or more adjacent ribs, which produces a loose section of chest wall (1). This disrupted section of chest wall moves inward when the rest of the chest wall is expanding on inspiration and pushes outward when the chest is contracting on expiration. This paradoxical movement is generally referred to as "flailing." The structural integrity of the chest wall is disrupted, which affects the ability of the chest to generate the pressure gradient needed to exchange air. Ventilation is painful and less efficient, and more effort is required to move the air in and out of the lungs (1–4).

Consideration must always be given to the mechanism of injury when evaluating blunt trauma. The mechanism of injury may alert the caregiver to the potential scope of injury to be expected (3). An acceleration-deceleration mechanism, as Mr. J. experienced when he fell 35 feet onto soft ground, can be described in terms of a series of internal events. The chest wall abruptly stops, stressing the ribs and causing fractures and chest wall damage; underlying soft tissue structures move forward until they hit the interior chest wall. After this initial impact, the organ bounces back, striking the opposite side, and the force of the rebound produces trauma to the side of the organ opposite the original impact (4). The force wave of the impact transmits energy through the chest wall to the internal tissue structure beneath, producing a diffuse injury to the lungs, heart, and vascular structures in the chest (4,5). Not only can the chest wall be disrupted, but also a shock wave may be transmitted to the tissue, capillaries, and small airways of the lung itself. Inside the lung tissue, capillaries, small airways, and alveoli may be ruptured, and a self-perpetuating cycle leading to respiratory failure, and possibly adult respiratory distress syndrome (ARDS), can be set in motion (1,5). After impact, the alveolar capillaries, ruptured by the rapid deceleration, begin to hemorrhage into the alveolar and interstitial spaces, resulting in interstitial edema (6).

The major physiological alterations resulting from this injury are intra-alveolar hemorrhage with extravasation of blood and interstitial edema, leading to a decrease in gas exchange, lung compliance, and functional residual capacity and increasing physiological shunt (7). The obvious manifestation of this is progressive hypoxia (1). A cycle is established as the blood now present irritates the mucosa and increasing amounts of bronchial secretions are produced. Accumulating secretions in the small airways will further interfere with oxygen exchange, producing hypoxia; significant hypoxia leads to increased capillary permeability, which produces still more secretions (1). A number of major factors are now at work, all of which contribute to hypoxia.

When assessing and observing patients who have sustained a blunt injury to the chest, the first sign of lung injury is a drop in the $PaO_2$, not an increase in the $PaCO_2$, because $CO_2$ is 20 times more diffusible than $O_2$ (8). It is also important to remember that flailing may not be observable at the time of initial assessment because of muscle spasms in the chest wall. It may appear later after narcotics have caused relaxation (1).

A number of important pathophysiological factors need rapid consideration when the care for this type of patient is planned. These are the amount or extent of damage to the lung tissue, degree of pain from the fractures, volume of retained secretions and edema, and the hemopneumothorax (9).

Other factors include potential alteration of cardiac output, fear/anxiety, urinary complications secondary to myoglobin release, deep vein thrombosis from immobility, alteration of the nutritional status, and psychological implications of the sick role for this patient and the family.

## 2. What are the nursing diagnoses of highest priority?

A. Potential for impaired gas exchange and infection
B. Potential for decreased tissue perfusion
C. Potential for impaired gas exchange

## 3. What are the goals of nursing care?

### A. Nursing Diagnosis

Potential for impaired gas exchange and infection related to lower airway obstruction and atelectasis secondary to flail chest with loss of chest wall integrity

### Goal of Care

Maintain patent airway to facilitate gas exchange.

### Nursing Interventions

- Monitor patient's inspiratory and expiratory volume and airway pressure.
- Suction endotracheal tube as needed.
- Monitor arterial blood gases frequently.
- Prevent self-extubation with soft restraints (according to hospital policy) and/or mild sedation.
- Monitor intake and output closely.
- Maintain patency of naso-orogastric tube.

### Rationale

Depending on the severity of injury, patients with flail chest may need endotracheal intubation. In the case of Mr. J., who experienced significant injury and respiratory distress, endotracheal intubation was necessary. The artificial airway then becomes a nursing responsibility of high priority. Because of the loss of chest wall integrity, the decrease in lung compliance, and the increase of airway exudate, it is vitally important to be constantly aware of any alterations in either volumes or airway pressures. For Mr. J., it became necessary during the first 2 hours in the ICU, because of increasing airway pressures, to change from the volume-cycled ventilator to a time-cycled ventilator using the pressure control mode to allow for more precise volume control.

A volume-cycled ventilator will automatically switch to the expiratory phase when a present pressure is achieved. This becomes an obvious problem with a patient such as Mr. J., who had a very high (greater than 50 cm $H_2O$) airway pressure during inspiration (1,10). The ventilator will cut off the inspiration at the preset pressure irrespective of the volume delivered, and the patient can become more hypoxic from being underventilated (1,10).

Another factor that should be considered is the need to maintain consistently the amount of positive end expiratory pressure (PEEP) that has been ordered by the physician. PEEP is used to prevent atelectasis, which results from the underlying pulmonary contusion (1).

Endotracheal suctioning is also important in the care of flail chest patients. Suctioning assists in preventing or resolving atelectasis that may result from exudate production (11). However, it also permits monitoring of the appearance of secretions, which can indicate the progress and/or resolution of an underlying lung contusion (5).

Frequent monitoring of arterial blood gases (ABGs) is another important factor in the care of these patients. A primary problem associated with flail chest is hypoxemia, which, if left untreated, will lead to systemic hypoxia. Ventilator adjustments may be necessary to stabilize and maintain the patient within acceptable parameters. A $PaO_2$ of 80 to 100 mm Hg and a $PaCO_2$ of 30 to 40 mm Hg, using a fractional inspired oxygen ($FiO_2$) of 0.5 or less, is considered an acceptable range for arterial blood gases (8).

Prevention of self-extubation is of the utmost importance with any patient requiring mechanical ventilation. The flail chest patient is suffering a significant compromise of a very basic life-supporting function, and self-extubation would only further compromise his or her status. Appropriate use of restraints, in accordance with hospital policy, and in combination with mild sedation and reassurance, is the most common method of dealing with this problem. It is appropriate to keep intubation equipment and spare endotracheal tubes close at hand to allow rapid reintubation should it become necessary.

Close monitoring of patient intake and output is also important. A controversy prevails over whether patients with significant pulmonary insult should be given replacement fluids (crystalloids and colloids), but proponents of each theory generally agree that replacement should be conservative (11). The lung is already bruised and edematous, and excessive amounts of fluid may facilitate the development of ARDS (1).

Maintaining patency of the naso-orogastric tube may be seen as minor in view of the patient's overall condition, but it is an important consideration in any intubated patient. Gastric distension, which could cause respiratory embarrassment for the patient, and the threat of aspiration can be greatly diminished by a functional gastric drainage tube (11).

## Goal of Care
Prevent secretion retention and infection.

## Nursing Interventions

- Perform chest physiotherapy (CPT) and postural drainage.
- Administer prescribed antibiotics.
- Administer prescribed bronchodilators.

## Rationale

Pulmonary toilet is of major importance in the flail chest patient. Postural drainage should be started early and considered a priority treatment for this patient. Chest percussion should be used selectively with flail chest injuries. A comprehensive respiratory care regimen should be individualized for each patient to help minimize or avert atelectasis and decrease the time the patient requires mechanical ventilation. A patient with significant pulmonary injury requiring mechanical ventilation may be given prophylactic antibiotics. This patient has a bruised edematous lung under the flail segment, and the normal mechanism for clearing bacteria is significantly compromised by the endotracheal tube, thus increasing his risk for pneumonia (6).

Bronchodilators may also be ordered for this patient to alleviate wheezing and facilitate the removal of secretions in atelectasis (13). Anyone administering these medications should be aware of the safe dosage range and the expected side effects. For example, when administering metaproterenol (Alupent) to a patient who is already tachycardic and experiencing arrhythmias, the potential benefits must be weighed against the possible risks (13).

## B. Nursing Diagnosis

Potential for decreased tissue perfusion related to fluid volume deficit as a result of bleeding into the pleural space secondary to multiple rib fractures with intercostal vessel damage

## Goal of Care

Decrease risk of hypotension due to blood loss from the chest injury.

## Nursing Interventions

- Monitor chest tube drainage every 30 to 60 minutes for color, amount, and bubbling.
- Monitor central venous pressure (CVP), blood pressure (BP), pulse, and urine output closely.
- Monitor hemoglobin and hematocrit levels closely.

## Rationale

Close monitoring of chest tube output cannot be overemphasized for this type of patient. Although the majority of hemothoraces can be managed conservatively there is the possibility that the patient may begin to hemorrhage and require a thoracotomy (13). Obviously, the earlier the bleeding is detected, the earlier the patient can be treated aggressively and the complications of shock avoided. This potential complication is particularly important for the patient who is already at risk for developing ARDS (1).

Monitoring the CVP, BP, pulse, and urinary output at frequent intervals also provides a valuable guide to the patient's status. In a healthy young patient, a blood loss of 15 to 25% would need to occur before the blood pressure might begin to drop: A persistent tachycardia may be the first indication of volume depletion (15). The CVP is an important tool in monitoring the blood volume because the increased pulmonary vascular resistance of the injured lungs causes an automatic increase of the pulmonary artery pressure and therefore does not accurately reflect the blood volume (11). The adequacy of tissue perfusion can be monitored in patients with normal renal function by observing the urinary output, which should be greater than 30 ml/hr (14).

Monitoring hemoglobin and hematocrit is important because tissue oxygenation requires sufficient hemoglobin and will be compromised if the level is allowed to drop. In general, a hematocrit of less than 30% may warrant a transfusion (5,11).

### C. Nursing Diagnosis

Potential for impaired gas exchange related to ineffective breathing patterns secondary to pain resulting from flail chest

### Goal of Care

Promote effective breathing patterns through appropriate pain management.

### Nursing Interventions

- Administer prescribed narcotic analgesics as needed.
- Administer prescribed neuromuscular blockers as needed.

### Rationale

Pain from fractured ribs caused by movement of the chest wall during natural or mechanical respiration or coughing will cause the patient to "splint," curtailing the inspiration or cough. Splinting is an attempt by the patient to prevent or minimize chest pain by self-limiting chest wall movement. Chest percussion accompanied by postural drainage and endotracheal suctioning will be intolerable for this patient unless adequately medicated for pain. The use of narcotic analgesia is necessary with trauma patients not only for pain caused by the injury but also for the pain caused by all the treatments necessary for recovery (11).

For general pain management, Mr. J. received morphine sulfate intravenously in frequent small doses to minimize the blood level fluctuation (11). A combination of pancuronium bromide (Pavulon: a rapid-acting nondepolarizing muscle relaxant) and fentanyl (Sublimaze: a rapid-acting narcotic analgesic) was used for respiratory treatments (CPT and suctioning) (11,13). Between respiratory care sessions, Mr. J. was comfortable and relaxed with the morphine, and he was still able to communicate by writing notes to his wife and the staff.

## ASSOCIATED NURSING DIAGNOSES

A. Potential for anxiety/fear
B. Potential for impaired urinary elimination
C. Potential for alteration in peripheral tissue perfusion
D. Potential for alteration in nutrition
E. Potential for impaired adjustment

**REFERENCES**

1. Brenner BE, ed. Comprehensive management of respiratory emergencies. Rockville, MD: Aspen, 1985.
2. Hoyt KS. Chest trauma assessment. Trauma Q 1986;2:1–7.
3. Shackford SR. Blunt chest trauma: the intensivist's perspective. J Intensive Care Med 1986;1:125–136.
4. Andrews JF. Patterns in blunt trauma. Trauma Q 1987;3:1–5.
5. Cardona VD, Hurn PD, Bastnagel-Mason PJ, Scanlon-Schilpp AM, Veise-Berry SW, eds. Trauma nursing: resuscitation through rehabilitation. Philadelphia: WB Saunders, 1988:472–473.
6. Hinton-Hart L. Hidden chest trauma in the head-injured patient. Crit Care Nurse 1986; 6:51–55.

7. Hughes JM. Postoperative pulmonary care: past, present and future. CCQ 1983;6(2):67–71.

8. Garg V, Peck M, Savino JA. Respiratory monitoring in trauma. Trauma Q 1987;3:32–44.

9. Hoyt KS. Flail chest: a case study. Trauma Q 1986;2:57–63.

10. Bushnell SS. Respiratory intensive care nursing. Boston: Little, Brown, 1973.

11. Kirsh MM, Sloan H. Blunt chest trauma: general principles of management. Boston: Little, Brown, 1977.

12. Thomas R, Hudgins C, Markey WF. Pharmacologic considerations in pulmonary trauma. Trauma Q 1986;2:21–32.

13. Dunham CM, Cowley RA. Shock trauma/critical care handbook. Rockville, MD: Aspen, 1986.

14. Govani LE, Hayes JE. Drugs and nursing implications. 3rd ed. New York: Appleton-Century-Crofts, 1978.

15. Worth MH, ed. Principles and practice of trauma care. Baltimore: Williams & Wilkins, 1982.

# CHAPTER 11

## Pulmonary Embolism

Laurel A. Moody, RN, BSN, CCRN

## Clinical Presentation

A 35-year-old obese woman was admitted to the emergency department after a motor vehicle accident in a small compact car. She arrived awake, alert, and oriented, complaining of severe left leg pain. Upright chest x-ray revealed normal lungs and normal mediastinal anatomy. Her vital signs were blood pressure (BP) 112/50, pulse 120, and respirations 24. An arterial blood gas (ABG), complete blood count (CBC), and serum electrolytes were drawn on admission. She was moving both arms and her right leg spontaneously and admitted to weighing 300 pounds. There was pronounced swelling of the left thigh. A left femoral fracture was suspected; orthopedic surgeons were consulted.

X-rays of the left leg revealed a closed distal fractured femur. Laboratory results were $PaO_2$ 96, $PaCO_2$ 37, pH 7.40, $O_2$ saturation 99% on room air, hematocrit 30%, hemoglobin 9.0 gm/100 ml, potassium 3.8 mEq/liter, sodium 140 mEq/liter, glucose 112 mg/dl, white blood cells 7200, chloride 109 mEq/liter, blood urea nitrogen 9 mg/dl, creatinine 0.4 mg/dl. The patient was transported to the operating room for closed reduction and internal fixation with intramedullary nailing of her femur fracture. The patient's vital signs remained stable throughout the surgery; postoperatively she was transferred to the intermediate care unit.

On the first day after the operation her vital signs were BP 120/70, pulse 120, respirations 20, and temperature 37.2°C (99°F). Two Hemovac drains placed surgically were patent and draining moderate amounts of serosanguinous fluid from the left leg. She complained of left leg pain and was receiving intramuscular analgesics every 4 to 6 hours. She remained on bed rest.

The patient continued to progress without much difficulty for the following 4 days. Surgical drains were discontinued on the third postoperative day. The nursing staff began to mobilize the patient by standing her and pivoting her into a chair until she was strong enough to learn crutch walking. Ambulation and mobilization of this patient was difficult because of her lethargy and fatigue, complicated by her obesity. On the fifth postoperative day, the patient complained of chest pain on deep inspiration. She verbalized fear and became extremely agitated and restless in bed. A stat chest x-ray was unremarkable, and a stat electrocardiogram (ECG) showed sinus tachycardia without ectopy. Arterial blood gas results were $PaO_2$ 65, $PaCO_2$ 34, pH 7.35, and $O_2$ saturation 80% on room air. other laboratory results were within normal limits. The patient was transferred into the intensive care unit for further observation and a workup to rule out pulmonary embolism (PE).

## 1. What is the pathophysiological basis for this patient's problem?

PE is an acute respiratory complication and a major cause of unexpected death in hospitalized patients. The incidence of PE in the United States in approximately 600,000 cases/year with an estimated annual mortality of 200,000. Ten percent of patients die within the first hour before any treatment has been initiated (1).

Pulmonary embolism occurs when a thrombus detaches from a vessel wall, travels through the systemic circulation, and lodges in the pulmonary circulation. Distal branches

74

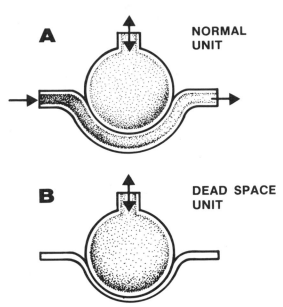

A — NORMAL UNIT

B — DEAD SPACE UNIT

**Figure 11.1.** The theoretical respiratory unit. **A** Normal respiratory unit = normal ventilation, normal perfusion; **B** Dead space unit = normal ventilation, no perfusion. (*Source*: Shapiro BA, Harrison RA, Walton JR. Clinical application of blood gases. 3rd ed. Chicago: Year Book Medical Publishers, 1982.)

of the pulmonary arteries at the periphery of the lung are the usual sites of thrombus obstruction. In normal oxygenation states, ventilation of each alveolus is accompanied by adequate perfusion of the alveolus by an arteriole. In the presence of a PE there is normal ventilation of the alveolus but inadequate perfusion due to the presence of the clot obstructing the blood flow through the arteriole (2). The alveolus becomes a dead space unit, and the ventilation is referred to as "wasted" and therefore gas exchange is ineffective. Eventually, as the symptoms persist, the cumulative effect of this "wasted ventilation" is hypoxemia. Figure 11.1 illustrates the normal respiratory unit and the dead space unit (3).

The severity of hemodynamic and respiratory complications resulting from PE depends on the size of the embolus and the patient's previous cardiopulmonary status (4). Emboli might be small in size and several in number. They frequently occur without significant impact on the cardiovascular system. Massive emboli can produce immediate circulatory and respiratory compromise (5).

Pulmonary embolism frequently develops as a complication of deep vein thrombosis (DVT). Thrombi present in the deep veins of the legs and pelvis are especially susceptible to becoming pulmonary emboli. In 1846 Virchow identified three major elements that contribute to venous thrombosis: hypercoagulability, venous stasis, and injury to vessel wall (6). Table 11.1 outlines clinical states associated with these elements. Other risk factors include fractures of the lower extremities and pelvis, age greater than 40, and a past history of thrombophlebitis or thromboembolism. In addition, the incidence of clot formation in patients undergoing orthopedic surgery has been reported to be as high as 70% (1).

Patients with PE will often experience varying degrees of symptoms, from mild to severe. Diagnosis of the PE is often difficult on clinical assessment alone even though

**Table 11.1.** Virchow's triad: major elements promoting venous thrombosis[a]

| Stasis | Injury to Veins | Hypercoagulability |
|---|---|---|
| Immobilization | Surgery | Carcinoma |
| Hospitalization | Trauma | Polycythemia |
| Obesity | Burns | Hemolytic anemia |
| Varicose veins | Venipuncture | Splenectomy |
| Congestive heart failure | Additives to IV fluids | Smoking |
| Pregnancy | | Oral contraceptives |
| Incompetent vein valves | | Systemic infection |
| Dehydration | | Blood dyscrasias |
| | | Cigarette smoking |

[a]*Source*: Modified from: Doyle J, Johantgen M, Vitello-Cicciu J. Vascular disease. In: Kinney MR, Packa DR, Dunbar SB, eds. AACN's clinical reference for critical care nursing. New York: McGraw-Hill, 1988:749.

there are several characteristic symptoms. Table 11.2 lists symptoms that should be further investigated to rule out the presence of a PE.

There are no specific laboratory tests to confirm the diagnosis of PE; however, the initial workup for PE may include arterial blood sampling, chest x-ray, and an ECG. A PE should be suspected in any trauma patient who develops a sudden unexplained drop in arterial oxygen (4). In a patient without pre-existing disease, a $PaO_2$ of 80 or lower may indicate presence of PE with "wasted ventilation" (2). Chest x-ray results are normal initially but may later show regional atelectasis, pleural effusion, and an elevated diaphragm. ECG results are usually normal except in the presence of massive PE when right ventricular failure has developed (7). The ECG may be used to differentiate between a PE and acute myocardial infarction.

The patient may undergo a pulmonary perfusion/ventilation (also called a $\dot{V}/\dot{Q}$) scan. This noninvasive scan assesses both pulmonary perfusion and lung ventilation. The procedure for the scan has the patient breathe air tagged with radioactive isotopes then the lung fields are scanned. This ventilatory component is followed by an intravenous injection of isotopes. The lung fields are again scanned to show the distribution of the radioactive isotopes within the pulmonary circulation. If an embolism is present, the scan will display decreased or absent blood flow in the part of the pulmonary artery occluded by the embolus. This decreased blood flow is called a perfusion defect. The ventilation component looks at the distribution of air through the airways; if the airway is obstructed, the scan will demonstrate decreased distribution of the radioactivity in obstructed areas of the lungs. Because a PE obstructs blood flow, not air flow, the ventilation component should be relatively normal and the perfusion component abnormal or showing a perfusion defect. Scans showing perfusion defects are highly suggestive of a PE in a patient without pre-existing lung pathology (1). Despite the normal ventilation scan, the nonperfused area of the lung does not carry out normal gas exchange, which ultimately affects overall oxygenation.

Questionable results from a $\dot{V}/\dot{Q}$ scan may necessitate pulmonary angiography, which

**Table 11.2.** Early symptoms associated with PE

Sudden unexplained dyspnea and cough
Chest pain, diffuse chest discomfort or substernal discomfort
Apprehension and anxiety
Tachycardia, tachypnea
Diaphoresis
Hemoptysis (rare finding)

is considered the only definitive diagnostic tool for the detection of pulmonary embolus (8). This invasive study involves cannulation of the pulmonary arteries by right heart catheterization and injection of a radiopaque dye into the pulmonary circulation under fluoroscopy. Obstruction of the dye flow within the pulmonary artery provides fairly clear evidence of filling defects in the pulmonary circulation. This study carries with it risks of cardiac arrhythmias, allergic reactions to the dye, bleeding from the cannula insertion site, ischemia in the extremity distal to the insertion site, and possible infection.

## 2. What are the nursing diagnoses of highest priority?

A. Potential for decreased tissue perfusion
B. Potential for impaired gas exchange
C. Anxiety

## 3. What are the goals of nursing care?

### A. Nursing Diagnosis

Potential for decreased tissue perfusion related to mechanical obstruction secondary to pulmonary embolism.

### Goal of Care

Maintain adequate pulmonary perfusion and prevent clot extension.

### Nursing Interventions

- Institute continuous cardiac monitoring.
- Assess vital signs frequently.
- Administer anticoagulant therapy as ordered.
- Monitor coagulation profiles.
- Monitor hemoglobin and hematocrit.
- Auscultate heart sounds frequently.

### Rationale

Treatment of a patient with a PE is considered "supportive care," since there is no cure for embolism once it has already occurred (6). The goal of treatment is to prevent reoccurrence of the emboli and to maintain adequate pulmonary perfusion. Prevention is aimed at reducing all elements of Virchow's triad: hypercoagulability, venous stasis, and vessel damage (6). Strategies used are active and passive exercises for patients at bed rest, early ambulation, leg elevation, use of compression stockings, or treatment with pneumatic compression devices (9). The effects of in-bed exercises are believed to last about 1 hour (8); therefore, it is recommended that these exercises be performed for at least 5 minutes every hour (10). The use of pneumatic compression devices is thought not only to reduce venous stasis but also to promote release of thrombolytic substances.

Anticoagulant therapy with heparin is most commonly used to prevent extension of an existing clot or the formation of a new embolus. A bolus dose of 10,000 units followed by continuous infusion of 500 to 1500 units/hr of intravenous heparin is considered standard therapy (1,5–8). A therapeutic dose elevates the patient's partial thromboplastin time (PTT) two to three times the baseline PTT. The patient usually continues on the heparin infusion for 7 to 14 days. Coumadin therapy, an oral anticoagulant, is usually started 3 to 5 days before heparin therapy is discontinued. Patients frequently remain on Coumadin for 8 to 12 weeks following cessation of the heparin infusion (8). Thrombolytic agents, such as streptokinase and urokinase, have been used for early, rapid lysis of the emboli, usually within 12 to 24 hours; however, because of their serious side affects of bleeding and allergic reactions, these agents are often reserved for patients at high risk of death. Also, this therapy is contraindicated in any patient who has undergone recent surgery or has sustained significant contusion to vital organs.

Pulmonary embolectomy requires major thoracic surgery, and it involves placement of a catheter into the femoral vein, passing into the right heart, and into the pulmonary artery. This procedure also carries great risk and is reserved for the acutely hemodynamically unstable patient. In those patients in whom anticoagulant therapy is contraindicated, or in the case of chronic reoccurrence of emboli, placement of a filter device in the inferior vena cava may be necessary to prevent embolism. This procedure is very serious and poses risks to the patient (1). If the embolus is not reduced or dissolved, it may lead to further obstruction of the pulmonary circulation. Pulmonary hypertension may develop in patients with massive PE and result in increased pulmonary vascular resistance, increased pulmonary artery pressures, and eventual increased right ventricle workload (4).

A patient with suspected PE should remain under close observatin in a critical care setting with continuous cardiac monitoring and frequent vital sign assessment. In addition to the administratin of the anticoagulant therapy, the nurse should continually assess the patient's coagulation profiles and hemoglobin and hematocrit values, observing for early signs of bleeding. Assessment of urine and stool specimens for blood, as well as inspection of intravenous puncture sites for hematomas, should be incorporated into the patient's plan of care. Along with frequent vital sign assessment, the nurse should assess the patient's heart sounds for murmurs and gallops that may signal early signs of cardiac compromise (5).

## B. Nursing Diagnosis
Potential for impaired gas exchange related to mechanical obstruction secondary to pulmonary embolism

### Goal of Care
Maintain optimal conditions for oxygenation.

### Nursing Interventions
- Frequent chest assessment with auscultation of breath sounds
- Aggressive pulmonary toilet
- Administration of oxygen
- Complete bed rest
- Analgesics administered as ordered

### Rationale
In the presence of a PE, the patient develops dead space ventilation, also known as wasted ventilation, which occurs when the patient is adequately ventilating but there is inadequate lung perfusion to complete the gas exchange process at the cellular level (1). The patient will become hypoxemic, hypocarbic, and dyspneic. Prolonged hypocarbia will cause vasoconstriction of the alveoli and further decrease gas exchange (1). When the alveoli become constricted, there will be a decrease in the production of surfactant that is necessary to prevent total collapse of the alveoli.

Respiratory care is of paramount importance to these patients. Frequent assessment of the patient's chest is necessary, observing for asymmetry with respirations and auscultating for the presence of adventitious breath sounds such as rales, wheezing, pleural friction rub, or decreased breath sounds (2). Treatment consists of aggressive pulmonary toilet using cough and deep-breathing exercises, chest physiotherapy, and postural drainage to maintain a clear airway. Retained secretions will further tax an already compromised system. The patient should be instructed to take slow, deep breaths for deep inflation of the lungs, thereby promoting retention of carbon dioxide and reducing hypocarbia (5). Administration of oxygen by mask or endotracheal tube is necessary to relieve hypoxemia and promote tissue oxygenation. Frequent monitoring of arterial blood gases assists in determining the effectiveness of treatment. The patient may remain on bed rest to reduce the workload of the heart and lungs (7,11). The patient should be placed in a semi-Fowler's position with head elevation to facilitate breathing. Analgesics may be necessary to relieve chest discomfort; however, narcotics should be used with caution, as their effects may further depress respirations.

## C. Nursing Diagnosis

Anxiety related to lack of knowledge of hospital environment and fear of further injury

### Goal of Care

Decrease anxiety and promote adequate coping mechanisms.

### Nursing Interventions

- Assess patient's level of anxiety.
- Assess patient's knowledge of the complication and provide information as needed.
- Explain diagnostic procedures and medical treatments to patient and family.
- Provide opportunities for patient to verbalize questions, fears, and anxieties.

### Rationale

In addition to the anxiety experienced during an unplanned hospitalization, a patient suffering a PE has special psychosocial needs. The patient may experience fear from the sudden onset of symptoms, particularly shortness of breath and dyspnea. Because of the fairly common incidence of PE, the patient may be aware of the severity of this complication and fear further clot formation with increased destruction to the respiratory system or even sudden death (7). The nurse should anticipate these concerns early. It is often necessary to use sedatives and analgesics to relieve pain and anxiety. Explanation of diagnostic procedures and medical treatments to both patient and family will decrease fear of the unknown and provide accurate information for the patient and family to integrate into their thinking. Allow family members to be supportive and encourage their participation in any discussions with the patient. This intervention will also decrease the anxiety family members may be experiencing. Patients with PE usually have prolonged hospitalization, causing further stress to both patient and family. It is important that the nurse be available for the patient to verbalize questions, fears, and anxieties about his or her situation.

## ASSOCIATED NURSING DIAGNOSES

A. Potential for decreased cardiac output
B. Potential for fluid volume deficit
C. Potential for infection

**REFERENCES**

1. Spence TH. Pulmonary embolization syndrome. In: Civetta JM, Taylor RW, Kirby RR, eds. Critical care. Philadelphia: JB Lippincott, 1988:1081–1101.
2. Williams SM. The pulmonary system. In: Alspach JG, Williams SM, eds. Core curriculum for critical care nursing. Philadelphia: WB Saunders, 1985:1–100.
3. Shapiro BA, Harrison RA, Walton JR. Clinical application of blood gases. 3rd ed. Chicago: Year Book Medical Publishers, 1982:65.
4. Silvergleid A. Thromboembolism diagnosis and treatment. West J Med 1974;120(3):219–225.
5. Roberts SL. Pulmonary tissue perfusion altered: emboli. Heart Lung 1987;16:128–137.
6. Doyle J, Johantgen M, Vitello-Cicciu J. Vascular

disease. In: Kinney MR, Packa DR, Dunbar SB, eds. AACN's clinical reference for critical care nursing. New York: McGraw-Hill, 1988:751.

7. Thomas M. Acute pulmonary embolism. Focus Crit Care 1983;10:21–28.

8. Dunham CM, Cowley RA. Shock trauma/critical care handbook. Rockville, MD: Aspen, 1986:453–457.

9. Chamberlain SL. Low dose heparin therapy. Am J Nurs 1980;80:1115–1117.

10. Husni E, Ximenes J, Gayette E. Elastic support of the lower limbs in hospital patients: a critical study. JAMA 1970;214(8):1456–1462.

11. Groer ME, Shekleton ME. Basic pathophysiology. A conceptual approach. St Louis: CV Mosby, 1979:460–461.

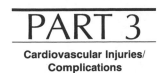

# PART 3

**Cardiovascular Injuries/ Complications**

# CHAPTER 12

# Myocardial Contusion

Laurel A. Moody, RN, BSN, CCRN

## Clinical Presentation

A 29-year-old man was admitted to the hospital following a head-on collision in which he was the driver; he had not worn a seat belt. He arrived awake, alert, and oriented, complaining of left-sided chest pain. He was moving all four extremities and denied abdominal pain. His blood pressure was 110/60 mm Hg, pulse 120 beats/minute, and respirations 30/minute. Several small lacerations were noted around the bridge of his nose and lower lip. There was obvious deformity of the nasal septum. A large circular abrasion was noted on the patient's anterior chest.

A myocardial contusion was suspected along with probable nasal fracture. Computerized tomography (CT) scan of the head was normal. Upright chest x-ray revealed normal lungs with no obvious rib fractures and normal aortic and mediastinal anatomy. Electrocardiogram (ECG) revealed sinus tachycardia with no ectopy. Cardiac enzymes, specifically creatine phosphokinase (CPK) with MB fraction, were drawn with arterial blood gas, hemoglobin, hematocrit, and serum electrolytes. The patient was transported to the intensive care unit (ICU) for continuous cardiac monitoring and further observation.

On admission to the ICU, the patient was awake, alert, and oriented. His vital signs were 120/70, pulse 130, respirations 26/minute, and his temperature was 99°F (37.2°C) orally. His cardiac monitor displayed sinus tachycardia without ectopy. The patient had a peripheral intravenous catheter in his right forearm and face mask oxygen at $FiO_2$ of .35. An ice pack was placed on the nasal splint. Lab results were hematocrit 48, hemoglobin 15.8, $PaO_2$ 136, pH 7.42, $PaCO_2$ 39, sodium 139, potassium 4.6, glucose 103, chloride 100, $CO_2$ 29, blood urea nitrogen (BUN) 13, creatinine 1.1, Osmo 287. Other lab results were pending.

## 1. What is the pathophysiological basis for this patient's problem?

Myocardial contusion is a potentially lethal injury that commonly occurs as a result of blunt chest trauma. One source estimates that the occurrence of myocardial contusion ranges from 10% of patients with any form of blunt chest trauma to 76% of patients with severe multisystem trauma (1). Unfortunately, the diagnosis of myocardial contusion is often overlooked because it may not produce immediate cardiac dysfunction or it is overshadowed by more dramatic injuries.

The heart is suspended in the chest cavity by the aorta and pulmonary tree. It is susceptible to injury when an impact or force compresses it against the sternum or thoracic vertebrae. The most common cause of a myocardial contusion is a high-speed motor vehicle accident when there is direct impact to the anterior chest from a steering wheel, causing the heart to strike against the sternum (see Fig. 12.1). Other causes include direct blows to the chest, such as animal kicks, falls from great heights, or industrial

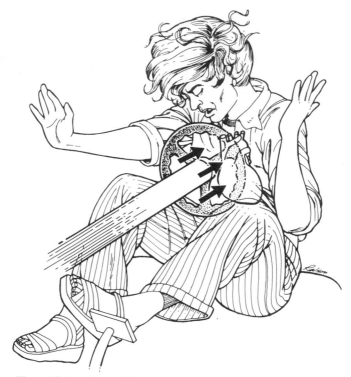

**Figure 12.1.** Myocardial contusion from impact of steering wheel.

crush injuries. A myocardial contusion may be associated with other blunt chest injuries, such as rib fractures, sternal or clavicular fractures, and pulmonary contusions.

Myocardial contusion is a result of hemorrhage into the interstitial space of the myocardium with fibril disruption, as well as neutrophil and macrophage influx (2). It may range from small areas of subepicardial ecchymosis to full-thickness injury with fragmentation and necrosis of muscle fibers. If a large area of the myocardium is damaged, the patient's cardiac output may decrease and arrhythmias may occur. Extensive injury could subject a patient to the same complications seen in an acute myocardial infarction: cardiac failure, aneurysm formation, and cardiac rupture. The right ventricle is most often affected because of its proximity to the sternum.

The diagnosis of a myocardial contusion involves a variety of clinical and laboratory data. Several sources suggest that the health care team needs initially to develop an "index of suspicion" based on the mechanism of injury and the associated injuries or symptoms (3–5). A common symptom is chest pain that may radiate to the arm, similar to that seen in angina. This type of pain differs from angina in that it is not relieved by coronary vasodilators, such as nitroglycerin. ECG results are often abnormal. Sinus tachycardia is common, with nonspecific ST-segment and T-wave changes. Several other rhythm disturbances may be seen, such as premature atrial or ventricular contractions, atrioventricular blocks, ventricular tachycardia, or fibrillation. Elevated serum cardiac enzymes are often seen in patients with myocardial contusion. CPK is separated into three isoenzymes, labeled as CPK-MM, CPK-BB, and CPK-MB. The myocardium contains MB fraction as well as some MM fraction. An elevated MB fraction that is greater than 5% of the total CPK level is a specific indicator of myocardial injury (6). A multiple-gated acquisition (MUGA) scan is often used to evaluate cardiac performance. This nuclear imaging scan provides information about ventricular wall motion and ejection fraction. The ejection fraction, an indicator of ventricular strength, is the percentage of blood ejected from the ventricle with each cardiac cycle. Normal ejection fraction for the left ventricle is greater than 55% and for the right ventricle is greater than 45% (7). In myocardial contusion, decreased wall motion and decreased ejection fractions are seen. A two-dimensional echocardiogram may also be used to evaluate cardiac structure and motion.

## 2. What are the nursing diagnoses of highest priority?

A. Potential for decreased cardiac output
B. Potential for discomfort
C. Anxiety

## 3. What are the goals of nursing care?

### A. Nursing Diagnosis

Potential for decreased cardiac output related to pump insufficiency and possible electrical disturbances secondary to myocardial contusion

### Goal of Care

Maintain adequate cardiac output and prevent arrhythmias.

### Nursing Interventions

- Establish continuous cardiac monitoring.
- Monitor cardiac enzyme values and serial ECGs.
- Monitor patient for signs and symptoms of hypovolemia and hypoxia.
- Assess vital signs frequently.
- Administer humidified oxygen.
- Assist physician with management of arrhythmias.
- Delay surgeries for non-life-threatening conditions.

### Rationale

The patient with a myocardial contusion is at risk for the development of life-threatening complications. Early recognition and prompt treatment of symptoms is essential. Continuous cardiac monitoring with frequent vital-sign assessment is necessary to detect subtle changes in the patient's cardiovascular status. Often, ECG changes may not be present until 24 to 48 hours postinjury. Therefore, serial ECGs should be obtained for 3 to 4 days after admission. The cardiac enzyme levels, specifically the CPK-MB, rise within 4 hours of injury and peak by 24 hours post-injury. Therefore, serial cardiac enzymes should be monitored from the time of admission and repeated every 8 hours ($\times$ 3). Hypovolemia, hypoxia, and electrolyte imbalances increase the myocardial oxygen demand and predispose the heart to develop arrhythmias. Adequate fluid replacement, administration of supplemental oxygen, bed rest, and correction of electrolyte imbalances decrease the cardiac workload. Elective surgeries involving general anesthesia should be delayed because the effect of anesthesia increases myocardial irritability (3). If a patient requires surgery during the early postinjury period, a pulmonary artery catheter should be placed to monitor the patient's cardiovascular status adequately. A cardiology consult should also be considered preoperatively.

## B. Nursing Diagnosis

Potential for alteration in comfort related to chest pain secondary to a myocardial contusion.

### Goal of Care

Promote comfort.

### Nursing Interventions

- Assess patient frequently for signs and symptoms of pain.
- Monitor serial ECGs.
- Monitor heart sounds frequently.
- Administer analgesics as indicated.
- Maintain patient on bed rest.

### Rationale

Patients with a myocardial contusion often complain of substernal chest pain that radiates to the neck and shoulder. This type of pain worsens on deep inspiration and increased physical activity. As the pain increases, the patient's level of anxiety increases, and the myocardial oxygen supply is further taxed. Analgesics should be used as indicated. Restricted activity and the use of supplemental oxygen will conserve the myocardial oxygen needs. Because the symptoms are similar to those seen in an acute myocardial infarction, it is imperative to fully evaluate the character of the chest pain. The nurse should continue to observe for subtle ECG changes. Those most frequently seen are nonspecific ST-segment and T-wave changes; however, patients have rapidly progressed into atrial fibrillation, flutter, multiple premature ventricular contractions, or supraventricular tachycardia (3, 4). Also, the nurse should frequently assess the patient's heart sounds, auscultating for diminished sounds, murmurs, or pericardial friction rubs.

## C. Nursing Diagnosis

Anxiety related to lack of knowledge of hospital environment and fear of further injury

### Goal of Care

Decrease anxiety and promote adequate coping mechanisms.

### Nursing Interventions

- Assess patient's level of anxiety.
- Assess patient's knowledge of injury and provide information as needed.
- Provide emotional support and comfort measures.
- Explain all diagnostic tests and treatments.
- Provide opportunities for patient to verbalize questions, fears, and anxieties.

### Rationale

An unplanned admission to the hospital after a motor vehicle accident is likely to cause anxiety or fear in any patient. The anxiety level may be further increased by a diagnosis of myocardial contusion. Many sources state that a cardiac injury is frequently perceived by patients as a direct threat to life (8–10). Anxiety, if not addressed early, can lead to further complications for the patient. Aside from compromising the patient's normal coping mechanisms, anxiety can cause an increase in the myocardial oxygen demand. Therefore, it is important to assess the patient's anxiety level and knowledge of the injury. By providing information to the patient about the injury and proposed hospital course, the nurse may decrease the fear of the unknown. Explanation of all tests and treatments before they occur may further decrease the patient's apprehension and anxiety. Allow the patient opportunities to ask questions and verbalize about the situation. Include family members in this process, as they may also have anxiety about the patient's condition. They can then assist in supporting the patient to cope with a stressful experience.

## ASSOCIATED NURSING DIAGNOSES

A.  Alterations in tissue perfusion
B.  Potential for fluid volume excess
C.  Potential for infection

### REFERENCES

1.  Hammond BB, ed. Cardiac contusion resulting from blunt chest trauma. J Emerg Nurs 1984;10(5):236–238.
2.  Wiener SL, Barrett J. Trauma management for civilian and military physicians. Philadelphia: WB Saunders, 1986:207–213.
3.  Kite JH. Cardiac and great vessel trauma: Assessment, pathophysiology, and intervention. J Emerg Nurs 1987;13(6):346–351.
4.  Cunningham JL. Assessment and care of the patient with myocardial contusion. Crit Care Nurs 1987;7:68–77.
5.  Hart LH. Hidden chest trauma in the heart-injured patient. Crit Care Nurs 1986;6(4):54.
6.  Dunham CM, Cowley RA. Shock trauma/critical care handbook. Rockville, MD: Aspen, 1986:171–174.
7.  Funk M. Preparing the patient for a MUGA study. Crit Care Nurs 1983;3(5):57–60.
8.  Gaglione KM. Assessing and intervening with families of CCU patients. Nurs Clin North Am 1984;19(3):427–433.
9.  Johnson SH. 10 ways to help the family of a critically ill patient. Nursing 1986;16(1):50–53.
10. Rasie SM. Meeting families' needs helps you meet ICU patients' needs. Nursing 1980;10(7):32–35.

# CHAPTER 13

## Ruptured Thoracic Aorta

### Ellen P. Bowers, RN, BSN

## Clinical Presentation

A 20-year-old man was hit by a car while riding his bicycle and thrown 30 feet. On arrival in the emergency department, he was moaning and lethargic (Glasgow Coma Scale score, 12/15), moving all his extremities, and breathing spontaneously.

Further examination revealed tachypnea with dullness to percussion and decreased breath sounds over the left field. He was intubated and placed on 100% oxygen; a left chest tube was inserted, which drained 250 ml of frank blood. Laboratory studies, including blood type and cross-match, were done. A right radial arterial line, a right internal jugular introducer, and a left saphenous introducer were inserted. A Foley catheter and orogastric tubes were placed. Fluid resuscitation with crystalloids and colloids was initiated and continued. Cervical, thoracic, pelvic, and lumbar spine films were negative for fracture. Supine chest x-ray studies demonstrated a widened mediastinum, fractures of left ribs 1 through 5, and a left humeral neck fracture.

After the vital signs stabilized, the patient was transported to the angiography suite, where aortography demonstrated a descending aortic rupture. He was taken directly to the operating room, where a pulmonary artery catheter was placed, and a double-lumen oral endotracheal tube was introduced. Thoracotomy revealed a 95% tear of the descending aorta distal to the left subclavian artery. It was debrided and grafted with tubular Dacron. Neither left heart bypass nor passive aorta-to-aorta shunt was used. Two doses of intravenous mannitol were given during the 35-minute aortic cross-clamping. The estimated blood loss was 3000 ml; the patient was given 7 units of packed red blood cells, 4 units of fresh frozen plasma, 10 units of platelets, and 2000 ml of crystalloids intraoperatively. A diagnostic peritoneal lavage was grossly negative.

On transfer to the intensive care unit, nursing assessment revealed a cold (96°F [35.6°C]), unresponsive patient, now with a single-lumen oral endotracheal tube, with no spontaneous respirations. He was placed on a pressure-cycled ventilator set to deliver a mandatory rate of 16 breaths/minute at a tidal volume of 800 ml, at an $FiO_2$ of 1.0, with 5 cm $H_2O$ of positive end-expiratory pressure (PEEP). Vital signs were as follows: blood pressure, 170/105; heart rate, 96; and respiratory rate, 16. Laboratory studies included assessment of arterial and mixed venous blood gases, and cardiac output was measured. The left chest tube inserted intraoperatively was connected to $-20$ cm $H_2O$ water seal suction, and chest auscultation revealed diminished breath sounds in both bases bilaterally, with rales and rhonchi over the left lung field. Electrocardiogram displayed a normal sinus rhythm, with full pulses and 4-second capillary refill times overall. Intravascular volume support continued with crystalloids; the Foley drained clear yellow urine; and the gastric tube drained bilious contents.

A nitroprusside drip was started when the mean arterial pressure (MAP) remained greater than 85 despite warming. As the patient began to assist the ventilator, the mode was changed to a synchronized mandatory rate of 10 with a pressure support of 20 cm $H_2O$. Later that night, the patient was able to communicate that he was in pain; a morphine sulfate drip was started to titrate for his comfort. Motor-sensory status evaluation revealed that his lower extremities were neurologically intact. The nurse noted that his sputum was blood tinged.

Despite the patient's generally edematous appearance, the nurse was concerned about low flow status and intravascular volume deficit. This concern was based on a cardiac output of 5.5 liters/minute, a decrease in central venous pressure (CVP), urinary output, hemoglobin and hematocrit, and arteriovenous oxygen difference, with increases in heart rate and diastolic blood pressure. Dopamine (5 μg/kg/minute) was administered, and 2 units of packed red blood cells were given. Following this treatment, cardiac output rose but the pulmonary capillary wedge pressure (PCWP) remained unchanged; urinary output, arterial oxygen content, and CVP increased; and MAP decreased to between 85 and 90 mm Hg.

A relative hypoxemia of $PaO_2$ 80 on an $FiO_2$ of 0.4 was treated successfully with chest physiotherapy and suctioning. A heated cascade to the ventilator was used to thin sputum and increase body temperature.

The patient's course was complicated by delayed splenic rupture, adult respiratory distress syndrome, septicemia, and meningitis. He did recover and was eventually discharged home.

## 1. What is the pathophysiological basis for this patient's condition?

According to Greendyke, motor vehicle accident victims thrown or ejected from their vehicles are twice as likely to sustain aortic rupture as those not ejected (1, 2 [p. 177]). In rapid deceleration of the torso, different tissues decelerate at varying velocities, and junctional areas between mobile and more fixed structures are then subjected to great strain. Parmley et al. reported that, for the aorta, the areas most susceptible to rupture are the isthmus (where the thoracic aorta is joined to the arch) and the ascending section connecting the heart and the arch (3). The mobile heart and thoracic sections shear away from the arch, most commonly at the ligamentum arteriosum, just distal to the left subclavian artery (4) (Fig. 13.1).

A majority of these patients will exsanguinate in the field, but 15% may survive to reach the hospital, with the expanding hematoma contained in an aneurysm of the remaining aortic layers and in the posterior mediastinum (3–5). Because the time limit is critical, hospital personnel must be familiar with the physical and radiographic signs that raise suspicion for aortic rupture and dictate the need for aortography (Table 13.1).

Forces of impact will cause the alert patient to complain of chest and back pain; dyspnea may occur if the hematoma compresses the left upper lung and bronchus. Compression of the aorta by the hematoma may result in upper extremity hypertension (2 [p. 183]). Though various signs and symptoms may raise the index of suspicion, aortography remains the definitive diagnostic test (6). If mediastinal widening or loss of the aortic contour is seen on a chest x-ray film, if the mechanism of injury dictates a high index of suspicion, or if the patient cannot have an optimal upright chest x-ray film because of concomitant injuries, then aortography is mandated (3, 7, 8).

During aortography, the femoral artery is cannulated and the tip of the catheter advanced to a point just distal to the aortic valve. Dye is injected and films are taken of the dye dispersal during systole. Risks during and after the procedure include allergic reactions to the dye, neurovascular injury, bleeding, and osmotic diuresis. Appropriate emergency equipment and personnel should accompany the patient to the aortography suite (9).

Aortic rupture repair is undertaken via a left thoracotomy incision, usually in the fourth intercostal space, with the patient in a right dorsal recumbent position. To access the area, a double-lumen endotracheal tube may be used to allow selective deflation of the left lung (2 [p. 195]). Clamps are applied proximal and distal to the tear as well as to the left subclavian artery (Fig. 13.2). Several risks accompany clamping: renal and spinal cord ischemia, left ventricular overload, and cerebral hypertension (10). Fluid overload and hypertension may be minimized by judicious fluid administration, the use of osmotic

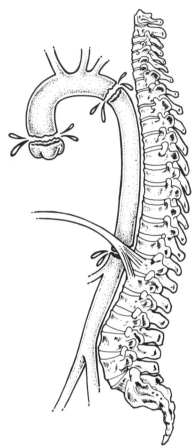

**Figure 13.1.**   Common sites of injury in traumatic rupture of the aorta.

diuretics, and pharmacological vasodilation. Hemodynamic parameters are monitored by a pulmonary artery catheter and right radial arterial line.

Left heart bypass is often contraindicated in the trauma patient because of the risks of total body heparinization in the presence of other injuries. Alternatively, a passive aorta-to-aorta shunt may be used to maintain flow below the distal clamp. Turney found that repair without shunt or bypass is associated with less bleeding, shorter cross-clamp times, and fewer complications (8). When neither shunt nor bypass is used, all efforts are made to complete the procedure within 30 minutes because renal and spinal cord ischemic damage can be caused by longer cross-clamp times (10).

During rupture repair, vagus, phrenic, and left recurrent laryngeal nerves should be identified because they are often in the operative field and at risk for surgical trauma (8). The edges of the tear are debrided, and the gap is often spanned with a tubular Dacron graft (Fig. 13.3). Clamps are released slowly and sequentially to evaluate graft integrity and to monitor for hypertension. The thoracotomy is closed and a left chest tube is left in place.

Postoperative risks include bleeding, atelectasis, hypertension, infection, renal failure, paraplegia, and left laryngeal nerve palsy. Patients may be placed on a short course of

**Table 13.1.** Indications for aortography in patients with multiple injuries[a]

1. History of high-speed deceleration injury
2. Any of the following chest roentgenographic findings:
   a. Superior mediastinal widening
   b. Obscuration of aortic knob shadow
   c. Obliteration of aortic outline
   d. Depression of left main-stem bronchus
   e. Tracheal deviation to the right
   f. Obliteration of aortopulmonary window
   g. Obscuration of medial aspect of left upper lobe
   h. Widening paravertebral stripe
   i. Deviation of esophagus
3. Multiple rib fractures or flail chest or both
4. Fractured first rib or sternum
5. Posteriorly displaced clavicular fracture
6. Unexplained hypotension
7. Massive hemothorax
8. Pulse deficits
9. Upper extremity hypertension
10. Systolic murmur
11. Blood in neck or supraclavicular fossa

[a]*Source*: Kirsh MM, Sloan H. Blunt chest trauma: general principles of management. Boston: Little, Brown, 1977:188–189.

broad-spectrum antibiotics, as seeding of the graft by other septic foci remains a risk. Hypertension is common postoperatively secondary to hypothermia and arch manipulation. Hypothermia, as induced by anesthetic gases and the cooling effect of volume replacement, stimulates sympathetically mediated vasoconstriction. It is thought that baroreceptors on the aortic arch are affected by surgical manipulation in that area and

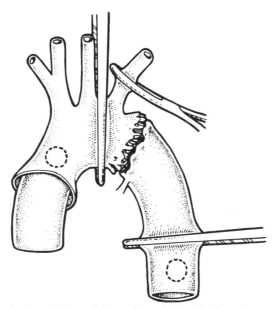

**Figure 13.2.** Positions of clamps in surgical repair of aortic rupture.

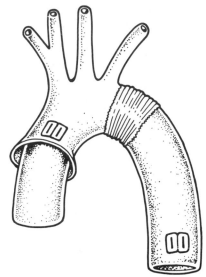

**Figure 13.3.** A Dacron graft in place following aortic rupture repair.

further contribute to the increase in vasomotor tone. Afterload reduction may be necessary to improve cardiac output and protect the graft (2 [p. 200]).

Nursing care priorities are stabilities of cardiovascular dynamics and oxygen delivery; optimization of gas exchange; prevention of infection; and assessment of motor, sensory, and renal status.

## 2. What are the nursing diagnoses of highest priority?

A. Potential for alterations in tissue perfusion
B. Potential for alterations in gas exchange

## 3. What goals of care and nursing interventions are appropriate for the above diagnoses?

### A. Nursing Diagnosis

Potential for alterations in tissue perfusion related to alterations in intravascular volume

### Goals of Care

- Optimize tissue perfusion.
- Prevent cellular hypoxia.

### Nursing Interventions

- Assess color of skin, oral mucous membranes, conjunctivae.
- Monitor capillary refill times, pulse rate, and amplitude.
- Correlate changes in heart rate, blood pressure, and urinary output.
- Assess renal function
  - Input/output (hourly)
  - Specific gravity
  - Creatinine clearance (daily)
- Monitor left and right heart filling pressures.

- Draw samples for arterial blood gases, mixed venous blood gases (MVBG), and cardiac output, and calculate the arteriovenous oxygen difference (a-vDO$_2$) and VO$_2$ index.
- Improve myocardial function by
  - Reducing preload or
  - Increasing preload or
  - Giving inotropes or
  - Reducing afterload or
  - Raising blood pressure to improve venous return or
  - Whatever combination of the above is necessary to create a cardiac output sufficient to provide an oxygen delivery that creates an optimal oxygen consumption
- Provide analgesia and sleep.
- Maintain normothermia.
- Assess for motor-sensory deficits.
- Optimize gas exchange by
  - Maintaining patent airway
  - Adjusting mechanical ventilation parameters

## Rationale

The patient's blood pressure while in the emergency department may vary depending on the amount of bleeding and his or her ability to compensate for it. Aggressive fluid resuscitation may be necessary.

The sympathetically mediated responses to hypovolemia, whether real or relative, attempt to restore circulatory volume and improve venous return to maintain perfusion of vital organs. As mean arterial pressure falls, the baroreceptors in the aortic arch lose their inhibitory effect on the brain-stem medullary vasomotor center, resulting in neuronal outflow that increases vascular tone. The adrenal medulla secretes epinephrine and norepinephrine, and renal arteriolar constriction reduces glomerular filtration rate and urinary output. The adrenal cortex secretes aldosterone, and the pituitary releases antidiuretic hormone, resulting in sodium and water conservation. The total outcome is peripheral venous and arterial constriction that improves venous return; an increase in sodium and water conservation that expands intravascular volume; and an increase in heart rate that, coupled with the improved preload, provides a higher stroke volume and, in the healthy heart, a higher cardiac output (11).

Intraoperatively, the patient may undergo diuresis and vasodilation to reduce left ventricular load during clamping. Limited amounts of fluids may be given.

Postoperatively, therefore, patients may present in a variety of perfusion states. They may be fluid overload in terms of intake and output balances yet also be intravascularly dry as fluid migrates across capillary membranes and into the interstitium, where it is lost to the circulatory process. This shift is referred to as third-space loss (12).

Postoperative nursing care assists in achieving a balance among correcting volume deficits, supporting blood pressure, and protecting the grafted area from the stresses of fluid overload and hypertension (13). The goal is to optimize tissue perfusion and oxygen consumption while providing for graft safety.

Color of skin and nailbeds, temperature, and capillary refill times provide data about peripheral perfusion. Generalized edema will be present if interstitial shifting has occurred. Pulse presence and quality may give clues as to the state of the

**Table 13.2.** Formulas for oxygen delivery and consumption

A. Oxygen Delivery

$(1.34 \times Hbg \times SaO_2) + (0.003 \times PaO_2)$

$= ml\ O_2$ per 100 ml blood (vol%)

$=$ arterial content $(CaO_2)$

where 1.34 is total amount of oxygen that can be carried by 1 gm of hemoglobin

$CaO_2 \times 10 = ml\ O_2$ per liter blood

CO (cardiac output) $=$ liters of blood per min

$(CaO_2 \times 10) \times CO = ml\ O_2$ delivered per min

B. Oxygen Consumption

$(1.34 \times Hgb \times SvO_2) + (0.003 \times PvO_2)$

$= ml\ O_2$ per 100 ml blood (vol%)

$=$ venous content $(CvO_2)$ returning to heart after cellular extraction of oxygen

$CaO_2 - CvO_2 = a\text{-}vDO_2$ (vol%)

$a\text{-}vDO_2 =$ arteriovenous oxygen difference

$=$ difference between what was supplied and what was left over after consumption

$(a\text{-}vDO_2 \times 10) \times CO = ml\ O_2$ consumed per min $(VO_2)$

C. Normal Values (ml/dl $=$ vol%)

$CaO_2 = 16\text{--}18$ ml/dl

$CvO_2 = 14\text{--}16$ ml/dl

$a\text{-}vDO_2 = 2\text{--}4$ ml/dl

Oxygen delivery $= 1000$ ml/min

Oxygen consumption $= 250$ ml/min

compensatory process. Following aortic manipulation and anesthetic gases, the patient may be cold and hypertensive, necessitating warming and pharmacological vascular dilatation to reduce afterload, protect the graft, and prevent dysrhythmias.

Changes in heart rate, blood pressure, urinary output, specific gravity, and intracardiac filling pressures should be correlated frequently to diagnose possible hemodynamic needs and evaluate responses to therapy.

Arterial and mixed venous blood gases, drawn with a hematocrit when cardiac output is measured, allow the calculation of the arteriovenous oxygen difference ($a\text{-}vDO_2$), which is the difference between the arterial oxygen content ($CaO_2$) and the venous oxygen content ($CvO_2$). Arterial content reflects oxygen delivery when combined with cardiac output. Venous content reflects the amount of oxygen returning unused to the right heart after consumption on a cellular level. Therefore, the $a\text{-}vDO_2$ is reflective of the amount of oxygen that was consumed (Table 13.2). The normal range of $a\text{-}vDO_2$ is 4 to 6 vol%. A decrease in the $a\text{-}vDO_2$ may be a process of a fall in arterial oxygen content, necessitating blood transfusion; a fall in flow, dictating volume needs; or a rise in venous oxygen content. A higher venous content results from a decrease in total body oxygen consumption. Because consumption is set by metabolic needs and by delivery, an evaluation of flow and arterial content should follow.

Oxygen consumption is determined by the basal metabolic rate (the oxygen needs of the body) and the number of cells participating in the process. Cells will initially accelerate the rate at which they extract oxygen from the blood when oxygen supply is inadequate. This increased extraction will be reflected in low values for $SvO_2$, $CvO_2$, and $a\text{-}vDO_2$. There is a limit to the amount of oxygen that can be extracted; after that point, anaerobic metabolic processes will ensue, which not only create an oxygen debt but also diminish adenosine triphosphate (ATP) and acidotic end products. Lactic acid, one of the acidic end products, may be measured to quantify the adequacy of oxygen delivery in terms of flow (cardiac output) and carrying capacity (hemoglobin). Persistent failure to provide oxygen will result in cellular hypoxia, multiple organ failure, and death.

Nurses are integrally involved in evaluating and manipulating numerous elements of cardiopulmonary function (e.g., preload, afterload, contractility, cardiac output, $CaO_2$, blood, fluids, drugs, gas exchange), as well as in coordinating care activities in reducing oxygen needs and optimizing consumption (e.g., pain and anxiety relief, sleep, normothermia, asepsis, nourishment).

## B. Nursing Diagnosis

Potential for impaired gas exchange related to alterations in ventilation, secretions, pain, and the effects mechanical ventilation

## Goals of Care

- Re-expand atelectatic lung segments.
- Remove alveolar exudates.
- Prevent respiratory infections.
- Prevent injury.

## Nursing Interventions

- Monitor breath sounds.
- Maintain chest tube patency and function.
- Monitor chest tube output.
- Perform chest physiotherapy.
- Suction secretions as indicated.
- Assess quality and quantity of secretions.
- Monitor pulmonary compliances and peak airway pressures.
- Monitor arterial blood gases.
- Provide analgesia.
- Protect from injury related to mechanical ventilation.
- Integrate chest x-ray findings into assessments and care.

Since the first step in the oxygen delivery process is saturation of hemoglobin with oxygen at the alveolar-capillary interface, pulmonary care is an inherent part of optimizing oxygenation. The patient who has undergone aortic rupture repair is at risk for impaired gas exchange from a number of sources. Intraoperative positioning with the right lung in a dependent position encourages secretion pooling and atelectasis. The deflated left lung receives ventilation at intervals, but the set tidal volumes and lack of sigh volumes may also lead to atelectasis (14). General anesthesia via endotracheal tube is usually delivered without heat or humidity. When coupled with the use of antimuscarinic agents, secretion viscosity may increase, and the mucociliary clearance mechanism may be inhibited to a degree that secretion stasis and atelectasis occur (15).

Pulmonary contusion may result from the same decelerative process that tears the aorta. The resultant alveolar-capillary damage, extravasation of blood and proteinaceous fluids into the interstitium and alveoli, loss of surfactant function, alveolar collapse, and decreased functional residual capacity will alter gas exchange and create intrapulmonary shunting (2). Overhydration can accelerate and exacerbate these pathological changes (14).

The nurse should palpate for tactile fremitus, present over retained secretions, as well as for symmetry of expansion. Decreased breath sounds over atelectatic segments, bibasilar rales in fluid overload or cardiogenic edema secondary to myocardial contusion, unilateral rales over atelectasis, and rhonchi over secretions may be detected on auscultation (15).

The chest tube system should be monitored for air leak as well as quantity and quality of drainage. Intercostal arteries may bleed from surgical trauma; chest tube output that is continually bloody and greater than 200 ml/hr should be reported immediately (16).

Re-expansion of atelectatic segments and clearance of secretions is accomplished by turning to reverse stasis and by chest physiotherapy and suctioning to loosen and remove secretions. Patients on levels of PEEP above 5 cm $H_2O$ are at risk for problems related to decreased venous return and barotrauma. These patients should be assessed frequently for signs and symptoms of decreased cardiac output and for increases in airway pressures necessary to achieve desired volumes. Normal peak inspiratory pressure (PIP) is less than 30 cm $H_2O$ (17); pressures in excess of 30 ml $H_2O$ should be monitored closely.

Maintenance of a patent airway is of utmost importance, and the use of soft wrist restraints in accordance with hospital policy may be needed to prevent self-extubation by the agitated patient. The distance from the teeth to the carina is approximately 27 cm, and the distal end of the tube should rest 1 to 2 cm above it. Periodic monitoring of the endotracheal tube calibration number at the lip or teeth should be incorporated into care. Occlusion of the tube by biting may be prevented by the insertion of a padded tongue blade between the teeth, with less risk of gag and palatal decubitus than with the hard oral airway. Aspiration is prevented by gastric decompression with a gastric tube vented to intermittent suction to remove secretions that are stagnant as a result of postoperative ileus (13).

Adequate cuff seal of the endotracheal tube must be maintained. Cuff pressure should be measured regularly and should not exceed 25 cm $H_2O$ in order to avoid the risk of tracheal ischemia. Serial chest x-ray films verify endotracheal tube placement and identify the need for reposition if necessary.

An additional concern is the loss of sympathetic tone that can result from paraplegia, as a process of the injury itself or because of a long cross-clamp time. Patients may present as paraplegics prior to surgery, possibly because of cord ischemia secondary to intercostal artery compression by the expanding hematoma (4). Nurses should be aware of preoperative motor and sensory status and any period of hypoxia, the intraoperative cross-clamp time, and the use of any shunting or somatosensory monitoring during surgery (18). As soon as possible postoperatively, the patient's motor-sensory status should be documented, as paraplegia not only creates an emotional crisis for the patient and the family but also generates additional concerns for the nurse because of venous pooling and stagnation, which can affect perfusion status.

In addition, cross-clamping suprarenally predisposes the patient to renal dysfunction, with its inherent risks of electrolyte imbalances, fluid retention, and toxicity of renally excreted drugs. Renal function monitoring includes accurate hourly intake and output records, specific gravities, and daily measurement of creatinine clearance.

## ASSOCIATED NURSING DIAGNOSES

A. Potential for infection
B. Alterations in comfort: acute pain
C. Anxiety
D. Fear

E.  Potential for impaired swallowing secondary to left laryngeal nerve damage
F.  Potential for alterations in respiratory function secondary to phrenic nerve damage
G.  Potential sleep pattern disturbance

## REFERENCES

1.  Greendyke RM. Traumatic rupture of the aorta: special reference to automobile accidents. JAMA 1966;195:527.
2.  Kirsh MM, Sloan H. Blunt chest trauma: general principles of management. Boston: Little, Brown, 1977:177.
3.  Parmley LF, Mattingly TM, Manion WC. Nonpenetrating injury to the aorta. Circulation 1958;17:1086–1101.
4.  Beall AC. Surgical treatment of trauma: traumatic rupture of the aorta. Resident Staff Physician 1975;2s–12s.
5.  Knotts FB. Blunt chest trauma. Trauma Q 1987;3(4):23–33.
6.  Cowley RA, Turney SZ. Blunt thoracic injuries: the ruptured aorta. In: Cowley RA, Conn A, Dunham CM, eds. Trauma care. Vol. 1: Surgical management. Philadelphia: JB Lippincott, 1987:172–181.
7.  Mirvis SE. Traumatic disruption of the thoracic aorta: imaging diagnosis. Trauma Q 1988;4(2):49–60.
8.  Turney SZ, Attar S, Ayella RJ, et al. Traumatic rupture of the aorta: a five-year experience. J Thorac Cardiovasc Surg 1976;72:727–734.
9.  Groves MJ. Intrahospital transport of the shock trauma patient. In: Strange JM, ed. Shock trauma care plans. Springhouse, PA: Springhouse, 1977.
10. Piano G, Turney SZ. Traumatic rupture of the thoracic aorta: surgical management. Trauma Q 1988;4(2):61–65.
11. Borg N, Nikas DL, Stark J, Williams SM. Core curriculum for critical care nursing. Philadelphia: WB Saunders, 1981.
12. Folk-Lightly M. Solving the puzzles of patients' fluid imbalances. Nursing '84 1984;14(2):34–41.
13. Dalsing MC, Dilley RS, McCarthy M. Surgery of the aorta. CCQ 1985;8(2):25–37.
14. O'Bryne C. Postoperative care and complications in the thoracotomy patient. CCQ 1985;7(4):53–58.
15. Hughes JM. Postoperative pulmonary care: past, present, and future. CCQ 1983;6(2):67–71.
16. Cardona VD. Trauma reference manual. Bowie, MD: Brady Communications, 1985.
17. Von Rueden KT. Cardiopulmonary assessment of the critically ill trauma patient. Crit Care Nurs Clin North Am 1989;1(1):33–44.
18. Cunningham JN, Lassehinger JC, Merkin HA, et al. Measurement of spinal cord ischemia during operations upon the thoracic aorta: initial clinical experience. Presented at the Annual Meeting of the American Surgical Association, Boston, April 21–23, 1982.

# CHAPTER 14

# Autotransfusion

Deana L. Holler, RN, BSN

## Clinical Presentation

A 24-year-old man was admitted to the emergency department following an attempted robbery. He sustained a gunshot wound to the chest and was transported from the scene within 20 minutes of the assault. Prehospital care providers radioed ahead to report the patient as being tachypneic, hypotensive, and tachycardiac. The patient was placed on oxygen at 15 liters/minute via nonrebreather face mask; one large-gauge intravenous line was started and connected to Ringer's lactate running wide open. Medical antishock trousers (MAST) were put on with leg sections inflated.

On arrival at the hospital the patient presented as follows: conscious, awake, alert, and oriented; sensorimotor intact; labored respirations at 36/minute. The patient was experiencing hemoptysis, and breath sounds were inaudible over the right lung field. Blood pressure was 90/60, heart rate was 122, radial pulses were weak, and conjunctivae were pale.

Inspection revealed an entrance wound immediately below the right scapula and an exit wound in the anterior right seventh intercostal space. Blood was bubbling from the wound, and crepitus was noted in the area surrounding both entrance and exit wounds.

Intravenous lines were started, using a 14-gauge catheter in the right antecubital fossae and a number 7 French introducer in the right groin. Blood samples were obtained and sent to the laboratory for trauma hematology coagulation and chemistry profiles (i.e., HgH, WBC, PT/PTT, platelets, serum electrolytes) and a type and cross-match for six units of packed red blood cells. Rapid infusion of Ringer's lactate followed IV catheter insertion.

A portable supine chest radiograph revealed a moderate hemothorax and pulmonary contusion evidenced by a radiodense area around the wound. A number 38 French chest tube was inserted in the fourth intercostal space in the midaxillary line and connected to an autotransfusion collection system at 20 cm water suction. The initial return was 900 cc of frank blood. This blood was then infused to the patient while a second collection chamber retrieved additional blood. A nasogastric tube and indwelling urinary catheter were inserted, and a tetanus toxoid booster was administered. The patient's chest bleeding tapered off, and a standard chest tube drainage system was employed. The patient did not require surgery and was transferred to the intensive care unit.

## 1. What is the pathophysiological basis for this patient's problem?

The prognostic course of the patient sustaining penetrating chest trauma varies in accordance with weapon, location of injury, and presence or absence of other concomitant injuries. In the patient with an isolated penetrating chest wound secondary to a gunshot would, the severity is generally determined by bullet size, velocity, impact, and anatomy traumatized (1). Injury specifics depend on release of kinetic energy, producing tissue damage in the form of laceration, cavitation, and possibly burns (2). Lacerations or missile tracts are formed as the projectile shears through organs, vessels, and tissue in its path, producing a temporary cavity. The cavitation effect is directly proportional to the amount of kinetic energy transmitted by the bullet to the surrounding tissue (3). Generally, low-velocity missiles produce less cavitation effect but cause the majority of damage from laceration and ricochet. High-velocity missiles usually damage all tissue and structures directly in their path (3). Pulmonary contusion may be produced around the high-velocity projectile tract (3).

An open pneumothorax causes a loss of pressure gradients necessary for gas exchange as atmospheric and intrathoracic pressures equalize. If the chest cavity wound is large, a false passageway is created for gas exchange and the normal route may be bypassed (4). As normal negative intrathoracic pressure is lost, venous return and cardiac output are reduced, leading to hypoxia and metabolic acidosis (3). Clinical signs and symptoms vary, depending on the size of the hemothorax. The patient with a small hemothorax may be asymptomatic. A moderate hemothorax may cause the patient varying degrees of cardiovascular and respiratory distress. The patient with a moderate-to-massive hemothorax will manifest signs of severe hemorrhagic shock and acute respiratory distress. Rapid assessment and immediate intervention are imperative, or death ensues quickly. Bleeding can occur from chest wall vessels, internal mammary or intercostal arteries, accompanying veins, pulmonary parenchyma, diaphragmatic rupture, and mediastinal structure trauma (4). As blood fills the chest cavity, cardiac output is further compromised by a mediastinal shift to the unaffected side. Ventilatory function is compromised as both lungs are compressed (3).

One intravenous line should be inserted below the level of the diaphragm to ensure volume replacement in the event of injury to the superior vena cava. Bleeding from the chest cavity may be systemic, pulmonary, or both. Systemic bleeding usually requires surgical correction, whereas pulmonary bleeding may often be controlled by chest-tube placement and subsequent lung re-expansion. A hole in the bronchus can cause hemoptysis and an air leak (4).

Associated injuries can cause additional complications, such as a cardiopulmonary compression from intrusion of intra-abdominal organs through a ruptured diaphragm or the presence of neurogenic shock secondary to fracture of the vertebrae and trauma to the spinal cord.

## 2. What are the nursing diagnoses of highest priority?

A. Potential for decreased tissue perfusion
B. Potential for impaired gas exchange
C. Potential for infection

## 3. What are the goals of nursing care?

### A. Nursing Diagnosis

Potential for decreased tissue perfusion related to fluid volume deficit secondary to hemorrhage into chest cavity

### Goal of Care

Maintain adequate perfusion by identifying possible sites of hemorrhage.

### Nursing Interventions

- Maintain a high index of suspicion for hemorrhage.
- Assess external chest wall and abdomen for evidence of penetrating trauma, such as entrance and exit wounds.
- Assess for and assist with treatment of resultant and associated injuries:
  - Pulmonary contusion
  - Open pneumothorax
  - Hemorrhagic shock
  - Penetrating intra-abdominal trauma

Other associated injuries secondary to the specific location of the gunshot wound also include:

  − Acute pericardial tamponade
  − Myocardial contusion
  − Spinal cord injury
  − Fractures of the bony thorax
  − Tracheobronchial tree rupture
- Obtain the following information from patient, patient's family, or prehospital providers, if possible:
  − Type of weapon, caliber, and missile type
  − Missile velocity
  − Victim's proximity to weapon
- Assist with diagnostic radiography.

## Rationale

Rapid systematic assessment using the ABCDE approach (airway, breathing, circulation with hemorrhage control, disability:neurological status, exposure:completely undress) is imperative for evaluation of the penetrating chest-injury victim. A complete survey may reveal more than one bullet wound, which may be located on the back, shoulder, or axilla.

By obtaining information regarding type of weapon, missile type, velocity, and victim's distance from the weapon, one can often identify the mechanism and potential severity of the injury as well as associated injuries. Tissue damage from all types of gunshot wounds occurs from direct missile tracking, fragmentation, laceration, and the effect of ricochet. In addition, destruction from kinetic energy release causes cavitation and possibly burns (1).

In any penetrating trauma, the injury's location provides vital clues for determining possible associated injuries. Assess the injury site and assume underlying organ, vessel, and tissue damage until proved otherwise. For example, for any penetrating chest wound:

- Between the midclavicular line on the right and the midaxillary line on the left, assume cardiac involvement
- Above the nipple line, assume cervical involvement
- Below the nipple line, assume intra-abdominal involvement (3)

Radiography helps complete the diagnostic picture by confirming actual and associated injuries. However, radiography may be delayed until patient condition is more stable.

## Goal of Care

Restore and maintain normovolemic state.

## Nursing Interventions

- Monitor the patient for signs of hemorrhagic shock: vital signs every 5 to 15 minutes, electrocardiogram, and neurological status.
- Assist in obtaining venous access with two or more large-bore intravenous catheters.
- Obtain baseline laboratory data and type and cross-match profile.
- Ensure availability of adequate amounts of blood and component therapy solutions.
- Assist with insertion of closed-tube thoracostomy.
- Check function of, and prepare for, operation of autotransfusion equipment. Attach chest tube to autotransfusion collection unit.
- Monitor drainage every 5 to 15 minutes.
- Administer autotransfused blood as ordered.

- Ensure availability of required equipment for possible emergency thoracotomy in the acute resuscitation area.
- Prepare patient for surgery and transfer to operating room (OR) if needed.

## Rationale

Hemorrhagic shock can ensue after damage to lungs, solid organs, and pulmonary and abdominal vasculature. Two injuries commonly associated with gunshot wounds are pulmonary and myocardial contusions. Tissue perfusion may be assessed by following trend analysis of cardiopulmonary and neurological systems and laboratory data. Rapid and aggressive fluid administration with crystalloid, colloid, and blood component therapy can offset the progression of hemorrhagic shock and potentially life-threatening coagulopathies (3).

A number 36 to 40 French chest tube is inserted and connected to an autotransfusion device that provides underwater seal, closed drainage, and suction. Blood from the chest cavity is collected for reinfusion while the system is simultaneously relieving lung compression and allowing re-expansion (5). Autotransfusion uses blood that is warm, safe, readily available, and otherwise wasted (6).

Autotransfusion is a procedure that collects, filters, and reinfuses a patient's own blood for vascular volume replacement. The indications for autotransfusion are:

1. Blunt or penetrating chest or abdominal trauma with acute blood loss
2. Massive/acute blood loss with or without available homologous blood
3. Rare blood type or previous transfusion reactions

There are numerous advantages to autotransfusion in comparison to use of banked blood (see Table 14.1). Most of these advantages are derived from the patient being his or her own donor. The contraindications for autotransfusion are few compared to the advantages and relate primarily to infection control concerns (Table 14.2).

The procedure consists of connecting the underwater seal autotransfusion device to the patient's chest tube. Instill anticoagulants, if ordered, into shed blood collected in autotransfusion device. Infuse shed blood, using micropore blood administration tubing. On completion of the blood collection, connect the chest tube to the stan-

**Table 14.1.** Advantages of autotransfusion in comparison to banked blood[a]

1. Safe for patients who have received previous homologous transfusions and have antigen/antibody problems
2. Eliminates transmission of diseases, such as hepatitis, malaria, syphilis, AIDS, cytomegalovirus
3. Eliminates possible technical errors in type and cross-matching
4. No hemolytic, febrile, allergic, or graft vs. host reactions; no risk of isoimmunization to erythrocyte, leukocyte, platelet, or protein antigen
5. Readily available; no time delay for type and cross-match or for finding a compatible donor blood type
6. Costs significantly less than banked blood
7. Uses blood usually wasted
8. May circumvent religious objections to homologous transfusions
9. Eliminates need to adjust blood to body temperature
10. Provides normal pH, potassium, and ammonia levels
11. Provides normal levels of 2,3-DPG, which promotes tissue/cell oxygenation
12. Contains more viable platelets and red blood cells (RBCs)
13. Contains low hemolysis levels
14. Provides normal clotting factors except fibrinogen (if used within 4 hours)

[a]*Source:* Adapted from Holler DL. Autotransfusion. In: Strange JM, ed. Shock trauma care plans. Springhouse, PA: Springhouse, 1987:334.

**Table 14.2.** Contraindications[a] for autotransfusion[b]

| |
|---|
| Malignancy |
| Infectious process at site or systemic |
| Enteric wound contamination |
| Pre-existing coagulopathy |
| Injury older than 3 hours or wound re-exploration |
| Pre-existing liver or kidney function problems |

[a]Note: The physician may overrule these contraindications in certain circumstances.
[b]Source: Adapted from Holler DL. Autotransfusion. Reprinted with permission from *Shock Trauma Care Plans* copyright 1987, Springhouse Corporation. All rights reserved.

dard underwater seal drainage system. Secure all connections. Potential complications of autotransfusion are listed in Table 14.3.

This patient's autotransfusion used a chest tube thoracostomy collection device.

The larger the chest tube, the less chance of occlusion by blood clots (6). Blood from the thoracic cavity that is collected, filtered, and reinfused may be used alone or in conjunction with blood-component therapy to treat hemorrhagic shock secondary to moderate to massive hemothorax. Nursing interventions accompanying autotransfusion are listed in Table 14.4. An emergency thoracotomy may be performed in the acute resuscitation area if the patient is in, or is about to have, a cardiac arrest. By opening the chest, direct visualization of injury may make it possible to control intrathoracic hemorrhage, release acute pericardial tamponade, and perform internal cardiac massage (3). If emergency thoracotomy is successful, the patient is transferred to the OR for further achievement of hemostasis and the exploration of the abdomen for associated injuries.

The patient who remains stable in the acute resuscitation area without requiring an emergency thoracotomy may require surgical time for wound debridement, irrigation, and exploration.

The patient may lose 800 to 1500 cc of chest-cavity blood and not require a thoracotomy, as treatment with fluid resuscitation, closed tube thoracostomy, and autotransfusion may be adequate (3). Indications for surgery are:

- Loss of >500 cc/hr within 2 hours
- Loss of >200 cc/hr for 3 to 4 hours
- Increasing blood loss over 3 to 5 hours
- Large clotted hemothorax (7)

## B. Nursing Diagnosis

Potential for impaired gas exchange related to interference in ventilation secondary to hemorrhage into chest cavity

## Goal of Care

Maintain patent airway and adequate gas exchange.

**Table 14.3.** Potential complications of autotransfusion[a]

| |
|---|
| Emboli (air or particulate matter) |
| Hemolysis |
| Coagulopathy |
| Citrate toxicity |
| Sepsis |

[a]Source: Adapted from Holler DL. Autotransfusion. Reprinted with permission from *Shock Trauma Care Plans* copyright 1987, Springhouse Corporation. All rights reserved.

**Table 14.4.** Nursing interventions in autotransfusion[a]

1. Monitor vital signs, particularly the cardiovascular and respiratory parameters.
2. Maintain equipment sterility. Monitor and correct breaks in the system.
3. Monitor controlled suction.
4. If anticoagulant is ordered, ensure the proper ratio of anticoagulant to shed blood. (Refer to the manufacturer's guidelines or physician's order.)
5. Monitor laboratory data during and after autotransfusion, particularly hemoglobin/hematocrit levels, coagulation profile, arterial blood gases (ABGs), and calcium levels.
6. Document amount of blood retrieved and reinfused in intake/output.
7. Infuse collected blood within 4 hours of collection.
8. Follow autotransfusion device manufacturer's recommendations on general use of device.

[a]*Sources:* Adapted from:
Davidson SJ. Emergency autotransfusion. Surgery 1984:703–707.
Jurkovich GJ, et al. Autotransfusion in trauma: a pragmatic analysis. Am J Surg 1984;148:782.
Holler DL. Autotransfusion. Reprinted with permission from *Shock Trauma Care Plans* copyright 1987, Springhouse Corporation. All rights reserved.

### Nursing Interventions
- Monitor and report signs of respiratory distress.
- Ensure availability and proper functioning of equipment for humidified oxygen administration, intubation, and mechanical ventilation.
- Monitor vital signs (every 5 to 15 minutes), cardiac rhythm, neurological status, and arterial blood gas results.

### Rationale
The degree of cardiopulmonary compromise is directly related to the size of hemothorax and the presence and degree of associated injuries. This, in turn, dictates the interventions required to provide patent airway and improve gas exchange, such as supplemental oxygen, endotracheal intubation, and mechanical ventilation.

A massive hemothorax is a life-threatening emergency, as the cardiovascular and pulmonary systems are stressed when cardiac output is reduced by blood loss and mediastinal shift. Ventilatory compromise is caused by lung compression on the affected and contralateral side (7). Close monitoring is essential, as progressive hemorrhagic shock or uncorrected hypoxia is fatal.

### C. Nursing Diagnosis
Potential for infection related to introduction of pathogens into the chest cavity secondary to gunshot wound

### Goal of Care
Prevent or minimize infection.

### Nursing Interventions
- Cleanse wound and apply dressing using aseptic technique.
- Obtain medication allergy and tetanus immunization history.
- Administer antibiotics and tetanus prophylaxis as ordered.
- Prepare for possible wound exploration and surgical debridement.

### Rationale
Foreign bodies such as clothing, skin, hair, wadding, and burning and unburnt powder may be propelled into the wound (2). Wound cleansing, debridement, and exploration performed expeditiously may help minimize a potentially infectious process. Dressings provide a mechanical barrier to prevent further introduction of pathogens. The presence of medication allergies may contraindicate use of the antibiotic of choice. Any open wound requires tetanus immunization.

## ASSOCIATED NURSING DIAGNOSES

A. Alteration in cardiac output
B. Alteration in comfort
C. Impaired verbal communication
D. Sleep pattern disturbances
E. Impairment of skin integrity
F. Body image disturbance

**REFERENCES**

1. White KM, DiMaro VJ. Gunshot wounds: medicolegal responsibilities of the ED nurse. J Emerg Nurs (March/April) 1979:29–35.
2. White KM. Evaluating the trauma of gunshot wounds. Am J Nurs (October) 1977;77:1589–1593.
3. Maslyk JE. Respiratory section. In: Strange JM, ed. Shock trauma care plans. Springhouse, PA: Springhouse, 1987:70–83.
4. Hurn PD. Thoracic injuries. In: Cardona VD, Hurn PD, Bastnagel-Mason PJ, et al, eds. Trauma nursing: from resuscitation through rehabilitation. Philadelphia: WB Saunders, 1988.
5. Emminizer S, et al. Autotransfusion: current status. Heart Lung 1981;10:83–87.
6. Jacobs LM, Hirch JW. A clinical review of autotransfusion and its role in trauma. JAMA 1984;251:3283–3287.
7. Dunham CW, Cowley RA. Shock trauma/critical care handbook. Rockville, MD: Aspen, 1986:154–156.

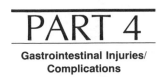

# PART 4

**Gastrointestinal Injuries/
Complications**

# CHAPTER 15

# Liver Trauma

### Kathleen Kwiatowski, RN, BA

## Clinical Presentation

A 24-year-old man was admitted to the emergency department following a 12-foot fall from a ladder while painting his home. The patient landed on a wooden picket fence, sustaining a penetrating injury to the abdomen.

On arrival he was alert and oriented, with a 20-cm portion of the wooden fence protruding from the right upper quadrant of his abdomen. Paramedics at the scene decided to transport the patient with the fence post in place, as hemostasis had taken place and attempts to remove the foreign body may have resulted in a severe loss of blood and probable death. Vital signs on arrival were as follows: blood pressure 80/40, pulse 132, and respirations shallow at 28. Admission laboratory values revealed a hemoglobin and hematocrit of 7.0 gm/dl and 23.5%, respectively. Initial platelet count was 69,000 with a white blood cell count of 21/mm$^3$. Prothrombin (PT) time and partial thromboplastin time (PTT) were elevated.

Because of the patient's clinical presentation, a diagnostic peritoneal lavage and abdominal films were deferred, and he was immediately taken to the operating room for the removal of the foreign body and packing of the liver using large surgical laparotomy packs. Once hemodynamically stable, he was returned to the operating room 24 hours later for a second assessment, removal of the surgical packing, and ligation of any lacerations and obvious bleeders.

Postoperatively, the patient was taken to the intensive care unit (ICU) and mechanically ventilated via a number 8 oral endotracheal tube. His vital signs were stable with blood pressure of 110/60, pulse 100, respirations 20, and temperature 35.5°C (96.6°F). He was arousable to light peripheral pain but had no spontaneous respirations. A Foley catheter was inserted, and an oral gastric tube to low constant suction was placed preoperatively. Packed red cells and fresh frozen plasma were infusing via a left subclavian triple-lumen catheter. A large midline abdominal dressing was in place with a sump tube drain to low intermittent suction extending from the right upper quadrant.

## 1. What is the pathophysiological basis for this patient's problem?

The liver is the largest organ in the body. It is composed of a complex vascular system that contains approximately one-fourth of the body's total blood supply. Because of its location and size, the liver is particularly susceptible to traumatic injury. According to one study of blunt trauma, the liver is second to the spleen in the number of injuries it sustains (1).

The majority of liver injuries are directly related to blunt trauma and are primarily a result of motor vehicle accidents during which the liver is crushed between the ribs and vertebrae.

**103**

**Table 15.1.** Liver injury severity classification[a]

| | |
|---|---|
| Type I | Laceration of Glisson's capsule |
| Type II | Shallow parenchymal lacerations and nonbleeding, nonbursting bullet and stab wounds |
| Type III | Deep lacerations with or without disruption of Glisson's capsule |
| Type IV | Severe bursting injuries |
| Type V | Injuries to the vena cava and/or hepatic veins in addition to parenchymal injury |

[a]*Source*: Olsen W. Late complications of central liver injuries. Surgery 1982;92:733.

Penetrating injuries to the liver are generally due to stab and/or gunshot wounds. The nature of the penetrating object to the abdomen has an effect on morbidity and mortality, in addition to any vascular injury involvement. Stab wounds to the liver produce localized lacerations from which hemorrhage may be easily controlled. However, gunshot wounds may produce diffuse damage to the liver and its surrounding tissue; therefore it may be difficult to isolate hemorrhaging and achieve hemostasis (2).

Injury to the liver is classified by Grades I through V (Table 15.1).

Goals in the management of liver trauma are the control and prevention of bleeding, bile drainage, removal of all severely damaged and nonviable liver tissue, and adequate wound drainage (2). Small liver lacerations may be treated by suturing, with the placement of either Penrose drains or sump drains to ensure adequate drainage and to minimize the risk of intrahepatic hematoma formation. Large liver wounds often require debridement of necrotic tissue and placement of sump drains. If the injury is diffuse, a partial resection (lobectomy) of the nonviable lobe may be necessary to control bleeding (see Fig. 15.1). A 12th rib resection is often required to drain the liver bed effectively.

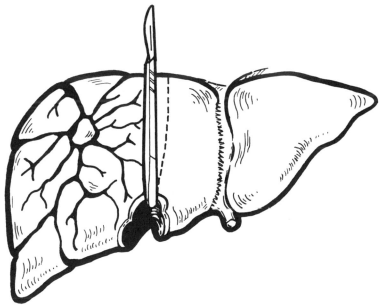

**Figure 15.1.** Typical liver injury requiring hepatic resection. (From McClelland R, Shires T, Poulos E. Hepatic resection for massive trauma. J Trauma 1964;4:282.)

## 2. What are the nursing diagnoses of highest priority?

A. Potential for decreased cardiac output
B. Potential for injury
C. Potential for infection

## 3. What are the goals of nursing care?

### A. *Nursing Diagnosis*

Potential for decreased cardiac output related to massive blood loss, uncontrolled bleeding from undetected liver lacerations, and coagulopathy occurring from liver injury

### *Goal of Care*

Maintain hemodynamic stability.

### *Nursing Interventions*

- Monitor vital signs frequently and observe for signs of shock.
- Monitor hemoglobin, hematocrit, platelet counts, and coagulation profiles.
- Monitor and record drainage from sump drains.
- Assess abdomen and abdominal dressings frequently for abdominal distension.

### *Rationale*

Hemorrhage is the major cause of death in patients sustaining a traumatic liver injury; therefore, it is important to ensure immediate hemodynamic stability in the care and management of these critically ill patients. Patients should be observed closely for 48 to 72 hours, as a number of patients who present with blunt abdominal trauma may not initially develop symptoms of liver injury.

Blood pressure, heart rate, urine output, and central venous pressure (CVP) should be monitored hourly to assess cardiovascular stability and to maintain adequate perfusion. Hemoglobin, hematocrit, platelet counts, and coagulation studies must be obtained at regular intervals several times daily in the initial postoperative phase. A decrease in any of the above values suggests a continued loss of volume, and a fluid replacement regimen of packed red blood cells, fresh frozen plasma, and platelets should be initiated to maintain vascular volume (3, 4).

Nursing observation of the abdomen is emphasized in the physical assessment of the patient. Monitor for increased abdominal distension, guarding to the right upper quadrant of the abdomen, or an increase in pain. The frequency of the need for dressing changes is an important observation, especially if Penrose drains are in place for drainage of the liver bed. Note the color, clarity, and consistency of the drainage. Included in the care of the abdominal wound is the care and maintenance of the drainage sites. Record the amount of drainage from the sump sites and note the color, clarity, and consistency of the drainage. The need for frequent dressing changes with a marked increase in serosanguinous or sanguinous material from the liver is a sign of impending or active hemorrhaging.

### B. *Nursing Diagnoses*

Potential for injury secondary to coagulation disorders related to traumatic injury to the liver, shock, or massive transfusions

### *Goal of Care*

Prevent or minimize further bleeding.

### *Nursing Interventions*

- Monitor coagulation profiles.
- Avoid needlesticks.

- Provide gentle mouth care with a soft brush.
- Prevent skin breakdown.
- Maintain adequate safety measures to prevent injury.

## Rationale

The liver is the site for the production of clotting factors. In addition, it stores vitamin K, which plays a major role in the formation of several of the clotting factors. Therefore, the patient with a traumatic liver injury is susceptible to the development of a coagulopathy.

PT, PTT, and platelet determinations must be obtained at regular intervals daily in the immediate postoperative stage. Replacement therapy consisting of fresh frozen plasma and platelets will begin, based on elevated PT and PTT times. Vitamin K supplements may be necessary to assist the formation of clotting factors.

Nursing care of the patient with a coagulopathy resulting from a liver injury is primarily directed toward the use of appropriate safety measures to minimize the risk of bleeding and to prevent the formation of hematomas and areas of ecchymosis to the skin.

Small-gauge needles are used for injections or for drawing blood. Prolonged pressure to the venipuncture sites may be necessary. Intravenous line sites may leak or ooze blood; therefore, dressings to those sites should be changed as needed. Intramuscular injections should be avoided if possible.

Mouth care is completed with a soft pliable brush or sponge apparatus to alleviate gum irritation and bleeding. Shaving is achieved by the use of either a double-edge razor, or preferably, an electric razor.

The condition of the skin must be included in the complete physical assessment. Inspect areas of petechiae, ecchymosis, and hematoma formation. Establish nursing care standards to maintain skin integrity by turning the patient every 2 hours and administering proper skin care with proper massage techniques. Pad bony prominences with protective foam devices. Additional safety measures include padding the bed rails with pillows or linen to reduce the risk of further trauma of the skin.

## C. Nursing Diagnosis

Potential for infection related to abscess formation in the liver bed

## Goal of Care

Reduce the risk of infection/sepsis.

## Nursing Interventions

- Monitor for signs and symptoms of infection.
- Maintain patency of drainage sumps.
- Maintain strict sterile technique with dressing changes.

## Rationale

An intrahepatic abscess may develop from blood, bile, and foreign body debris remaining in the liver bed. This localized infectious process may rupture and lead to peritonitis, the formation of fistula tracts, bacteremia, and septicemia (2, 5). The potential for these problems necessitates close monitoring for early signs of infection including fever, an increased white blood cell count, and right upper quadrant abdominal pain.

Patency of the sump drains is important to avoid fluid collection at the surgical site. Note the color, clarity, and consistency of the drainage, as well as the presence of a foul-smelling odor. A marked decrease in drainage from the sump site may indicate an occlusion secondary to tissue or exudate, and manual irrigation of the sump by the surgical team may be necessary (6).

Sump drains provide immediate access to the liver bed. Sterile technique is performed with all dressing changes to reduce the risk of bacterial contamination. Dressings should be changed as needed to keep the wound clean and dry, as moisture from blood and body fluids is an excellent medium for bacterial growth and will cause irritation to the surrounding skin edges, resulting in breakdown.

As drainage decreases and the patient improves clinically, drains are advanced and removed, usually in 5 to 7 days. Wound care may include the applications of wet-to-dry, saline-soaked dressings to drainage sites to facilitate closure (2, 7).

## ASSOCIATED NURSING DIAGNOSES

A. Potential for impaired gas exchange
B. Potential for fluid volume deficit
C. Alterations in fluids and electrolytes
D. Potential for nutritional deficits
E. Alterations in comfort

**REFERENCES**

1. Strange JM. Abdominal trauma. In: Cardona VD, ed. Trauma nursing. Oradell, NJ: Medical Economics Books, 1985.
2. Bastnagel-Mason PJ. Abdominal trauma. In: Cardona VD, Hurn PD, Bastnagel-Mason PJ, et al, eds. Trauma nursing from resuscitation through rehabilitation. Philadelphia: WB Saunders, 1988:507.
3. Dunham CM, Cowley RA. Shock trauma/critical care handbook. Rockville, MD: Aspen, 1986.
4. Shires GT. Care of the trauma patient. 2nd ed. New York: McGraw-Hill, 1986.
5. Cox EF, Flancbaum L, Dauterive AH, Paulson PL. Blunt trauma to the liver: Analysis of management and mortality in 323 consecutive patients. Ann Surg 1988;207(2):126–134.
6. Hanna SS, Gorman PR, Harrison AW, Taylor C, Miller HA, Pagliarelo G. Blunt liver trauma at Sunnybrook Medical Center. J Trauma 1987;27(9):965–969.
7. Lowry K Jr., Waltney AD, Branton FS Jr., Strader LD Jr. Treatment of a complex hepatic injury. J Tenn Med Assoc 1987;80(3):138.

# CHAPTER 16

## Blunt Abdominal Trauma with Splenic Rupture and Pancreatic Injury Complicated by Pancreatitis

### Dianne L. Mackert, RN, BSN, CCRN
### Kathleen Kwiatowski, RN, BA

## Clinical Presentation

A 26-year-old man presented in the emergency department after sustaining an assault to the upper abdomen with a lead pipe. He complained of severe generalized abdominal pain that radiated to his back; he was noted to have upper abdominal ecchymosis, slight abdominal distension, and tenderness to palpation over the mid-abdomen. Bowel sounds were absent in all quadrants. Other physical findings were unremarkable except for a few superficial abrasions and contusions over his upper extremities. Vital signs on admission were as follows: blood pressure 80/50, pulse 120 with a respiratory rate of 36. Laboratory profiles on admission revealed a white blood cell count of 20,000/mm$^3$, with a hemoglobin and hematocrit of 7.0 gm/dl and 26.0%, respectively. Chest films showed fractures to the left ninth and tenth ribs without evidence of a hemothorax or pneumothorax. Abdominal films showed signs of an increase in splenic shadowing with a loss of normal outline of the spleen and left kidney.

A diagnostic peritoneal lavage returned bloody fluid; the amylase was 575 Somogyi units. An exploratory laparotomy was performed, during which mesenteric tears were identified and repaired. A hematoma and a complete transection of the pancreas were also found. The proximal pancreas was oversewn, and a distal pancreatectomy was performed. A ruptured spleen was also found, and a splenectomy was performed.

The patient arrived in the intensive care unit (ICU) on a mechanical ventilator with a triple-lumen intravenous catheter, an arterial line, a Foley catheter, a sump nasogastric tube to low continuous wall suction, and two abdominal sump drains to wall suction. Blood pressure was 110/60, pluse 100, temperature 36°C (97°F), central venous pressure (CVP) 6 mm Hg.

Within 36 hours the patient was weaned from the ventilator and extubated, and total parenteral nutrition was begun. Recovery was uneventful initially. The nasogastric tube was discontinued on the sixth postoperative day, and clear liquids were begun on the seventh postoperative day. Within 24 hours after ingesting oral fluids the patient began complaining of nausea and increased abdominal pain, and soon began vomiting. Blood work revealed an amylase of 780 Somogyi units and a white blood count of 17,000. A nasogastric sump tube was reinserted and attached to low wall suction, and total parenteral nutrition was continued.

Within 2 weeks the patient's laboratory values were within normal limits, and the pain had subsided. Oral intake was tolerated without nausea or vomiting. The patient was ultimately discharged to home.

## 1. What is the pathophysiological basis for this patient's problem?

The spleen is an elongated and highly vascular organ situated in the left upper quadrant of the abdomen. It rests near the left kidney and the distal portion of the pancreas. Its close proximity to ribs 7 through 10 on the left makes it susceptible to trauma if these ribs are fractured (see Fig. 16.1).

**108**

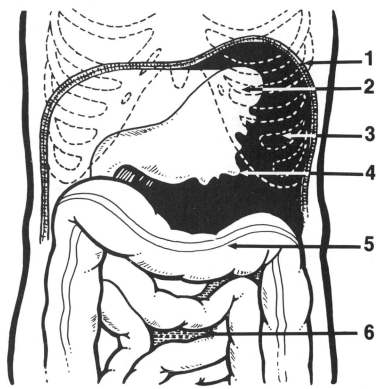

**Figure 16.1.** Radiographic signs of (delayed) rupture of the spleen: 1. left diaphragm raised; 2. stomach dilated; 3. opacity in the left hypochondrium; 4. indentation of the stomach; 5. transverse colon displaced downward; 6. fluid between the coils of intestine. (After V. E. Siler.) (Adapted from Dudley HAF. Abdominal trauma. In: Dudley HAF, ed. Hamilton Bailey's emergency surgery. London: John Wrights & Sons, 1986:399.)

Strange reports that in a study completed by the Maryland Institute for Emergency Medical Service Systems, more than 40% of the patients admitted sustained splenic injuries. Their study reinforced the fact that the spleen remains the most frequently injured organ in blunt abdominal trauma cases (1).

According to Bastnagel-Mason, isolated splenic trauma accounts for less than 20% of all splenic trauma and is associated with very low mortality (2). Cause of death in patients with splenic injuries is generally due to overwhelming postsplenectomy infection or delayed rupture and uncontrolled hemorrhage.

Patients with splenic rupture will exhibit signs of profound hypovolemic shock but may not present in shock for several days, as trauma to the spleen may cause localized encapsulated bleeding. As this subcapsular hematoma builds in size, the pressure exerted causes the splenic capsule to rupture. Injuries to the spleen have been classified by Grades I through V (Table 16.1) (3).

Goals in the management of splenic injury include the control of bleeding and the removal of all nonviable tissue.

If the splenic trauma constitutes an isolated laceration or a capsular tear, then a splenorrhaphy is performed to repair the injury. Splenectomy is indicated in the presence of a

**Table 16.1.** Splenic injury grading system[a]

| | |
|---|---|
| Grade I | Capsular tear or minor parenchymal laceration |
| | Minor suture or splenectomy |
| Grade II | Capsular avulsion |
| | Minor suture and topical hemostatic agent or splenectomy |
| Grade III | Major parenchymal fracture or laceration through gunshot or stab wound |
| | Major suture or splenectomy |
| Grade IV | Severe parenchymal stellate fracture, crush, or bisection or hilar injury |
| | Partial splenic debridement with major suture or splenectomy |
| Grade V | Shattered spleen or multiply injured patient |
| | Splenectomy |

[a]*Source*: Feliciano D, Bitondo C, Mattox K, et al. A four-year experience with splenectomy versus splenorrhaphy. Ann Surg 1985;201:568–575.

splenic rupture, patient instability, and/or uncontrolled hemorrhaging. Drains are not used in isolated splenic involvement or splenorrhaphy; if there has been manipulation or disruption of the pancreatic tail, a soft silastic sump or a bulb suction apparatus is used.

The pancreas curves around the spinal column, making it susceptible to a crush injury between the bony vertebral column and the force of a blow against the abdominal wall (4). Isolated pancreatic injuries are rarely seen; rather, blunt pancreatic trauma is usually discovered in conjunction with other abdominal injuries during surgical exploration (1). This patient's mid-abdomen received the brunt of the blow, injuring the body of the pancreas along with a portion of the mesentery. When the patient's left side receives the force of impact, the tail of the pancreas is most likely injured, whereas the head of the pancreas and the duodenum are at risk of injury when the right abdomen receives a forceful blow (4). Combined pancreatic and duodenal injury increases the risk of sepsis and is perhaps the most lethal of the nonvascular injuries encountered in the management of abdominal trauma (1, 5).

Evaluating blunt abdominal trauma and pancreatic injury is difficult because of the retroperitoneal location of the pancreas. Symptoms of trauma to other organs may delay the detection of pancreatic injury; however, such delays in diagnosis may lead to a significant morbidity and mortality in blunt abdominal trauma (6). In addition, a ruptured pancreatic duct may result in pancreatitis and pancreatic obstruction proximal to the area of injury, with development of a pancreatic fistula, a pseudocyst, or an abscess (4). Table 16.2 lists the complications seen in 150 patients following pancreatic trauma.

**Table 16.2.** Complications of pancreatic trauma in 150 patients[a]

| | Patients | |
|---|---|---|
| Complication | No. | Percent of Total |
| Pancreatic fistula | 20 | 13 |
| Pancreatic abscess | 10 | 7 |
| Hemorrhage | 2 | 1.3 |
| Pancreatitis | 14 | 9 |
| Pancreatic insufficiency | 3 | 2 |
| Diabetes | 1 | 1 |

[a]*Source*: Nance FC. Management of injuries to the stomach, duodenum, and pancreas. In: Worth MH, ed. Principles and practice of trauma care. Baltimore: Williams & Wilkins, 1982:170.

**Table 16.3.** Factors adversely influencing survival in acute pancreatitis[a]

I. Risk factors identifiable on admission to hospital
  A. Increased age
  B. Hypotension
  C. Abnormal pulmonary findings
  D. Abdominal mass
  E. Hemorrhagic or discolored peritoneal fluid
  F. Increased serum LDH levels
  G. Leukocytosis
  H. Hyperglycemia
  I. First attack of pancreatitis
II. Risk factors identifiable during initial 48 hours of hospitalization
  A. Fall in hematocrit less than 10 percent with hydration and/or hematocrit less than 30 percent
  B. Necessity for massive fluid and colloid replacement
  C. Hypocalcemia
  D. Hypoxemia with or without ARDS
  E. Hypoalbuminemia
  F. Azotemia

[a]*Source*: Greenberger NJ, Toskes PP. Approach to the patient with pancreatic disease. In: Braunwald E, Isselbacher KJ, Adams RD, et al, eds. Harrison's principles of internal medicine. New York: McGraw-Hill, 1987:1374.

In addition to these complications, the problem of increased mortality rate has been seen when three or more risk factors are present, either at the time of admission or during the initial 48 hours of hospitalization (see Table 16.3) (7).

Although peritoneal lavage is not especially useful in retroperitoneal injuries, many patients have associated injuries that produce a positive lavage and lead to exploratory laparotomy, which may reveal pancreatic trauma (8). The value of the serum amylase in diagnosing pancreatic injury is controversial because an elevated amylase does not always indicate pancreatic trauma, and a normal serum amylase may occur even in complete pancreatic transection (9). An abdominal computerized tomography (CT) scan may be useful in diagnosing pancreatic injury, since it can reveal collections of fluid around the pancreas (4) (see Fig. 16.1).

The development of pancreatitis is a rare, though potentially lethal, complication occurring in from 1 to 9% of patients after traumatic injuries to the pancreas (6, 10). The medical diagnosis of pancreatitis is generally made when the serum amylase levels remain greater than twice the upper limit of normal (80 to 150 Somogyi units); when there is a history of an etiology known to lead to pancreatitis; and when certain recognized clinical manifestations such as abdominal pain, fever, tachycardia, nausea, and vomiting are present (11, 12). Causes of pancreatitis other than trauma include alcoholism; biliary tract disease; medications such as salicylates, corticosteroids, and thiazides; and metabolic imbalances (12).

Abdominal pain is the foremost symptom of acute pancreatitis, with decreased or absent peristalsis, nausea and vomiting, and moderate abdominal muscle rigidity usually present (11). Hypotension and hyperglycemia occur in 40 to 50% of patients with pancreatitis, and 25% will develop hypocalcemia (11). In addition, pancreatitis may produce other fluid and electrolyte disturbances.

Autodigestion of the pancreas by its own enzymes is one pathogenetic theory (13), yet why the enzymes become activated while in the pancreas rather than waiting to become activated after secretion into the gastrointestinal tract is not understood (14).

Acute pancreatitis may be classified into two types. Edematous pancreatitis involves erosion by enzymes into peripancreatic tissues with an accompanying leakage of fluid into the pancreas, the surrounding tissues, and the peritoneal cavity (14). This type of pancreatitis is generally self-limiting and resolves after 2 to 3 days (13). The more serious type of acute pancreatitis, hemorrhagic, results in more extensive tissue destruction as vascular involvement leads to necrosis (13).

## 2. What are the nursing diagnoses of highest priority?

A. Fluid volume deficit
B. Alteration in comfort
C. Potential for infection

## 3. What are the goals of nursing care?

### A. Nursing Diagnosis

Fluid volume deficit related to extravasation of fluid and electrolytes into the retroperitoneal space

### Goal of Care

Satisfactory fluid and electrolyte balance

### Nursing Interventions

- Monitor intake and output hourly and report urine output less than 30 cc/hr.
- Monitor heart rate, central venous pressure, urinary output, and blood pressure for signs of hypovolemia.
- Monitor serum electrolytes every 6 to 8 hours.
- Check for pressence of Chvostek's sign or Trousseau's sign.
- Check urine-specific gravity every shift.
- Assess basilar breath sounds often for possible rales if fluid challenges are being given.

### Rationale

Hypotension occurs in pancreatitis patients, secondary to hypovolemia, related to extravasation of blood and plasma proteins into the retroperitoneal area (11). An increase in the release of kinin peptides produces vasodilatation, increased vascular and capillary permeability, and decreased myocardial contractility, which may lead to hypovolemia (11). As much as 5 to 6 liters of fluid may be lost into the interstitium (14). Tachycardia, hypotension, decreased central venous pressure, and decreased urine output are indications of insufficient vascular volume and should be reported immediately. A high urine-specific gravity and increased hematocrit provide additional indications of dehydration.

Frequent electrolyte determinations are required to assist in replacing fluids and maintaining values within normal limits. Serum calcium levels are particularly important, as hypocalcemia may develop with pancreatitis. The mechanism for hypocalcemia is thought to involve calcium being bound to areas of fat necrosis within the peritoneum (15). Clinical evidence of hypocalcemia may be demonstrated by assessing the patient for a positive Chvostek's sign, facial twitching in response to tapping over the facial nerve (12). A positive Trousseau's sign, another indicator of low serum calcium, is carpopedal spasm or a curving inwardly of the hand in response to constriction of the upper arm with a blood pressure cuff (12).

Calcium supplementation may be needed to prevent tetany and avoid dysrhythmias, but calcium chloride or calcium gluconate should be given at a rate no greater than 0.7 to 1.5 mEq/minute (14). The severity of the pancreatitis tends to correlate with the degree of hypocalcemia present; a persistent hypocalcemia often indicates a poor prognosis (13, 14).

Approximately half of the calcium in the serum is bound with albumin, so albumin levels should be simultaneously monitored (14). Hypoalbuminemia may account for the low calcium, and the patient may need albumin replacement before normal calcium levels can be achieved (14). Albumin and plasma replacement may be required to help exert colloidal osmotic pressure and attempt to maintain sufficient vascular volume as well (14).

Other potential electrolyte abnormalities must be evaluated in the patient with pancreatitis. Magnesium, sodium, chloride, and potassium losses may be considerable secondary to vomiting or gastric suction, as well as through extravasation, and must be replaced as deemed necessary, based on laboratory determinations (15).

Both hypoglycemia and hyperglycemia may occur, depending on which pancreatic cells are damaged (15). Frequent glucose measurements are a necessity. Total parenteral nutrition may aggravate hyperglycemia; therefore, an infusion pump must be used and insulin administered as required.

These patients are at risk for both metabolic acidosis and alkalosis. Excessive tissue necrosis may result in hyperkalemia and acidosis, and anaerobic metabolism secondary to hypotension may cause lactic acidosis (13, 14). Gastric acid and chloride losses from vomiting or suction may cause metabolic alkalosis (15).

## B. Nursing Diagnosis
Alteration in comfort related to acute pain secondary to pancreatitis

### Goal of Care
Satisfactory pain control

### Nursing Interventions
- Evaluate the patient's pain, noting the location, intensity, and radiation.
- Give Demerol for pain relief.
- Assist the patient to assume comfortable positions.
- Maintain patency of nasogastric tube.
- Offer emotional support.
- Promote rest.
- Restrict oral intake.
- Provide good oral hygiene.
- Assess abdomen for presence of bowel sounds, distension, and tenderness.

### Rationale
Pain is a significant manifestation of pancreatitis, with numerous possible causes. The pain is generally believed to be related to a chemical peritonitis and extravasation of exudate, blood, and enzymes retroperitoneally (11). Distension of pancreatic ducts and the pancreatic capsule, secondary to edema of the inflamed organ, may cause pain, and the swelling may actually lead to obstruction of the duodenum and the pancreatic and biliary ducts (11).

The pain may vary from mild to severe in intensity and generally occurs in the mid-epigastrium and periumbilical areas, though it may radiate to the back because of the retroperitoneal location of the pancreas (11). The pain tends to be worse with the patient in a supine position (11). Assisting the patient to sit up or to assume a position with the thighs and spine flexed may bring some degree of pain relief (11). Pain may radiate to the chest or shoulder areas because of diaphragmatic irritation (14).

Emotional support is a necessary part of care because an individual's pain perception is influenced by his or her mental state at a given time. Anxiety, fear, and depression all increase one's psychological perception of pain as well as increasing the secretion of pancreatic enzymes (12, 15). Encourage the patient to verbalize pain or worries. Be aware that a person's prior experience with pain and the extent of past achievement of pain control determine his or her reaction to discomfort (15). Prompt administration of pain medication when needed fosters trust between patient and nurse. Distraction through music or talking with the patient may be a useful adjunct to achieving pain relief. Observe for nonverbal cues that patients in pain may exhibit, such as clenched teeth or hands, diaphoresing, restlessness, or moaning.

Fatigue may intensify one's perception of pain; therefore, it is a good idea to promote rest whenever possible (16). This can be accomplished by providing nursing care in blocks of time and allowing rest periods to prevent sleep deprivation.

Morphine and codeine are contraindicated for pain relief in pancreatitis because they cause spasm of the sphincter of Oddi, which can interfere with drainage of pancreatic secretions into the duodenum, thus further aggravating the autodigestive process (14). Document the effectiveness of any pain medications administered (usually Demerol), and observe for signs of central nervous system depression so the optimum dosage may be ascertained.

Nausea and vomiting are clinical manifestations of pancreatitis. They result primarily from a combination of gastric and intestinal hypomotility and chemical peritonitis (11). Abdominal distension occurs as a result of paralytic ileus and extravasation of fluid within the peritoneum (11).

Gastric decompression is one of the most important nursing interventions in reducing pancreatic stress. Decompression prevents or severely limits acid flow from the stomach to the small intestines, decreasing the exocrine pancreatic stimulation and allowing the pancreas to rest (14, 16, 17). Decompression is maintained by eliminating oral intake and by the placement of a gastric tube to facilitate the removal of hydrochloric acid from the stomach that may stimulate the release of pancreatic enzymes. Gastric decompression will ultimately provide comfort and effectively reduce pain. Pain management may be achieved by an anticholinergic (Atropine) and a selective analgesic regimen of meperidine hydrochloride (Demerol) and hydroxyzine pamoate (Vistaril) every 3 to 4 hours as needed. Patient activity is limited and bed rest is ordered to minimize pancreatic activity and metabolic demands.

Total parenteral nutrition (TPN) is initiated as soon as possible via a large-bore central catheter in order to meet the patient's nutritional needs and to bypass gastric stimulation of the pancreas caused by oral intake. Nutritional support by TPN may be necessary from 5 days to several weeks. As the serum amylase and the remaining pancreatic enzymes return to normal levels, TPN will be gradually discontinued as normal oral intake is slowly resumed.

## C. Nursing Diagnosis

Potential for infection related to loss of immune support from spleen; development of peritonitis; and abscess formation in the splenic bed

### Goal of Care

Reduce the risk of infection.

### Nursing Interventions

- Monitor for signs of infection.
- Administer polyvalent pneumococcal vaccine (Pneumovax).
- Use sterile technique for dressings and procedures.
- Maintain patency of drainage apparatus.

## Rationale

The most important function of the spleen is primarily that of immune support. Because of the loss of antibody formation postoperatively following a splenectomy, the patient is at greater risk of developing overwhelming postsplenectomy infection. Overwhelming postsplenectomy infection is usually caused by encapsulated organisms, primarily the pneumococcus or hemophilus bacteria, and is characterized by the rapid occurrence of high fever, mental confusion leading to coma, disseminated intravascular coagulation, and hypoglycemia with a toxic, often fatal course (18).

Pneumovax must be given in the immediate postoperative stage, and the administration of broad-spectrum antibiotics at the onset of infection is recommended. Strict sterile technique is maintained during all invasive procedures and dressing changes.

Care and maintenance of the sump drain is essential to facilitate drainage of the pancreatic and splenic bed, thus reducing the risk of abscess formation and peritonitis.

## ASSOCIATED NURSING DIAGNOSES

A. Potential for anxiety
B. Potential for ineffective airway clearance
C. Potential for ineffective breathing patterns
D. Potential for sleep pattern disturbance
E. Potential for impaired skin integrity

### REFERENCES

1. Strange JM. Abdominal trauma. In: Cardona VD, ed. Trauma nursing. Oradell, NJ: Medical Economics Books, 1985:87–97.
2. Bastnagel-Mason PJ. Abdominal trauma. In: Cardona VD, Hurn PD, Bastnagel-Mason PJ, et al, eds. Trauma nursing: from resuscitation through rehabilitation. Philadelphia: WB Saunders, 1988:509–520.
3. Feliciano D, Bitondo C, Mattox K, et al. A four-year experience with splenectomy versus splenorrhaphy. Ann Surg 1985;201:568–575.
4. Frey CF. Injuries to the diaphragm, pancreas, and duodenum. Hosp Physician 1988;24:55–70.
5. Smego DR, Richardson JD, Flint LM. Determinants of outcome in pancreatic trauma. J Trauma 1985;25:771–775.
6. Nance FC. Management of injuries to the stomach, duodenum, and pancreas. In: Worth MH, ed. Principles and practice of trauma care. Baltimore: Williams & Wilkins, 1982:158–171.
7. Greenberger NJ, Toskes PP. Approach to the patient with pancreatic disease. In: Braunwald E, Isselbacher KJ, Adams RD, et al, eds. Harrison's principles of internal medicine. New York: McGraw-Hill, 1987:1374.
8. Feliciano D, Moore EE, Pachter HL, Mucha P. Pancreaticoduodenal trauma. Contemp Surg 1986;29:107–128.
9. Jones RC. Management of pancreatic trauma. Am J Surg 1985;150:698–704.
10. Jordan GL Jr. Pancreatic trauma. Contemp Surg 1985;26:11–17.
11. Greenberger NJ. Gastrointestinal disorders: a pathophysiological approach. 3rd ed. Chicago: Year Book Medical Publishers, 1986:251–255.
12. Fain JA, Amato-Vealey E. Acute pancreatitis: a gastrointestinal emergency. Crit Care Nurse 1988;8:47–60.
13. McConnell EA. Gastrointestinal bleeding and pancreatitis. In: Urosevich PR, ed. Nursing critically ill patients confidently. 2nd ed. Springhouse, PA: Springhouse, 1984:144–145.
14. Roberts SL. Physiological concepts and the critically ill patient. Englewood Cliffs, NJ: Prentice-Hall, 1985:312–335.
15. Orr ME. Acute pancreatic and hepatic dysfunction. New York: Wiley, 1981:26–93.
16. Roberts SL. Nursing diagnosis and the critically ill patient. Norwalk, CT: Appleton & Lange, 1987:100–103.
17. Dunham CM, Cowley RA. Shock trauma/critical care handbook. Rockville, MD: Aspen, 1986.
18. Shatton GW. Injuries to the liver and spleen. In: Worth MH, ed. Principles and practice of trauma care. Baltimore, MD: Williams & Wilkins 1982:183–189.

# CHAPTER 17

## Penetrating Abdominal Trauma: Stab Wound

Joanne M. Walker, RN, MSN, CETN

## Clinical Presentation

At 8 AM a 16-year-old male was brought to the hospital emergency department (ED) via ambulance, accompanied by his mother. His mother stated that when she returned home from working the 11 PM to 7 AM shift she found her son lying unconscious and "covered with blood" in the entry hall of their apartment building. She said that after supper the evening before, her son had gone to basketball practice; he usually returned home between 11 and 11:30 PM. She called him from work every night at about midnight to check on him; when he did not answer the previous night, she assumed he was showering. She was too busy at work to try again later. A policeman who arrived at the ED shortly after the ambulance stated that a bloody butcher knife with an 8-inch blade was found near the boy's body.

The patient was unresponsive, except to painful stimuli. His blood pressure (BP) was 70/40, pulse 130, and respirations 36 and shallow. He had multiple lacerations on his hands and forearms and four distinct open wounds on his abdomen. There was a glistening piece of pink tissue protruding from one of the wounds (1). His abdomen was distended and hard. There were no bowel sounds, and percussion produced dull sounds in all quadrants. He moaned and moved his head from side to side when his abdomen was palpated. A nasogastric tube was placed and returned some undigested food particles and 300 cc of fluid, which was guaiac negative. A Foley catheter was inserted, and it immediately drained 400 cc of clear yellow urine. Rectal exam revealed bright red blood in the rectum. Laboratory tests showed a white blood cell count (WBC) of 18,200 mm$^3$ and a hematocrit of 21%.

Based on the clinical findings a colon injury was suspected. The patient was given intravenous (IV) antibiotics and transported to the operating room for immediate abdominal exploratory laparotomy and double-lumen colostomy formation.

Postoperatively the patient was admitted to the intensive care unit. He arrived with a number 8 oral endotracheal tube, breathing spontaneously. His vital signs were temperature 39°C (102.2°F), pulse 110, respirations 24, and BP 100/60. He responded slowly but appropriately to verbal stimuli. In addition to a Foley catheter, two central line IVs and an arterial line were in place. A unit of packed red blood cells (RBC) was infusing through the right subclavian central line.

The patient had a large abdominal dressing covering an open midline wound, which was packed with sterile saline-soaked gauze. He had a red stoma protruding ½ inch into a colostomy bag on his left upper quadrant and a mucous fistula in his left lower quadrant that was clamped and covered with petroleum gauze and a dressing. His nasogastric tube was draining a minimal amount of clear fluid. The lacerations on his arms were sutured and covered with dry sterile dressings.

### 1. What are the pathophysiological bases for this patient's problems?

Nearly one-third of all stab wounds to the abdomen do not penetrate the peritoneal lining, and patients who show no evidence that the peritoneum has been entered may be admitted for observation for 24 to 48 hours and released without surgical intervention (1). The size of the penetrating object helps to determine the possible extent of the injuries and

**Table 17.1.** Indications for immediate surgical exploration[a]

1. Physical signs of intraperitoneal injury (i.e., hard distended abdomen)
2. Unexplained shock
3. Loss of bowel sounds
4. Evisceration of a viscus (this patient had a piece of omentum protruding from one wound)
5. Blood in the stomach, bladder, or rectum
6. Radiographic evidence of visceral injury, such as pneumoperitoneum.

[a]*Sources*:
Mason PJ. Abdominal trauma. In: Cardona VD, Hurn PD, Bastnagel-Mason PJ, et al, eds. Trauma nursing: from resuscitation through rehabilitation. Philadelphia: WB Saunders, 1988:499–515.
Fulenwider J. Blunt and penetrating abdominal trauma. In: Broadwell D, Jackson B, eds. Principles of ostomy care. St Louis: CV Mosby, 1982:171–182.

potential care requirements. Table 17.1 lists the indications for immediate surgical exploration.

Injuries to the colon may result in bacterial and chemical peritonitis from intraperitoneal fecal spillage and are among the most lethal of abdominal injuries, with a mortality rate nearing 10%. The number of wounds and the delay in treatment are other factors contributing to increased morbidity and mortality (1, 2). A "dirty" or contaminated surgical wound must be left open, disrupting the body's first line of defense against further infection. As the wound heals, dehiscence is always a danger, caused by the increased pressure of swollen tissue, infection, and the stress of increased patient activity.

In colon injuries that have been contaminated for a long time (becuase of treatment delay), and particularly those occurring in the left colon (which is subject to higher luminal pressures and heavy bacterial colonization), primary anastomosis is not possible (2). In this patient's case, a double-barrel descending colostomy was performed (see Fig. 17.1) to achieve total fecal diversion until any abdominal abscess, peritonitis, and sepsis could resolve.

## 2. What are the nursing diagnoses of highest priority?

A. Potential for infection
B. Alteration in self-concept
C. Alteration in bowel elimination
D. Fear

## 3. What are the goals of nursing care?

### A. Nursing Diagnosis

Potential for infection related to disruption of skin integrity, delayed treatment, delayed closing of surgical incision, previous contamination from fecal spillage, and possibility of additional fecal contamination from the colostomy (2, 3)

### Goal of Care

Prevent further infection.

### Nursing Interventions

- Monitor vital signs and laboratory values for signs of infection or alteration in wound healing; report temperature and WBC increases.
- Report swelling of surrounding tissue, discoloration of the wounds, increase in wound drainage, change in the character of the drainage, or onset of a foul smell from the wound.

### Rationale

Incisions made into the abdomen in the presence of fecal contamination are more commonly associated with postoperative wound infections, bacteremia, and sepsis.

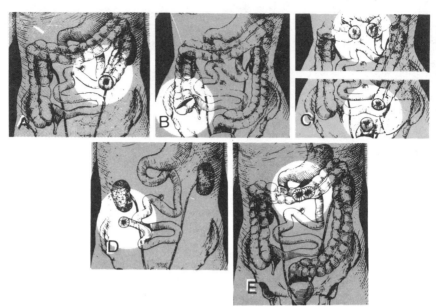

**Figure 17.1.** Types of intestinal diversions. **A** End colostomy. **B** Cecostomy. **C** Double-barrel colostomy. **D** Iliostomy. **E** Transverse loop colostomy. (Reprinted with permission from Pfizer Hospital Products Group, Inc, Largo, FL.)

Successful treatment of colonic injuries includes measures to restore the integrity of the bowel wall and to control fecal spillage at the time of injury and in the future (3). Copious irrigation of the abdominal wound during surgery and postoperative broad-spectrum antibiotic coverage are necessary to prevent these complications. Early detection of signs of infection may enable the health care team to alter the treatment plan, such as changing the dressing type or frequency of changes, before a second operation is necessary. Wounds are not able to heal in the presence of necrotic tissue. If mechanical debridement is ineffective, surgical intervention may again be required (4).

Peritonitis is always a risk in the presence of wound contamination, and the nurse must monitor for this serious complication. Signs and symptoms of peritonitis include acute increase in WBC count; high temperature elevations 39°C (>102°F) with chills; rigid abdomen with guarding and rebound tenderness; absent bowel sounds; severe abdominal pain and distension; nausea and vomiting; shallow, rapid respirations due to abdominal pain; and symptoms of shock (1).

## Goal of Care

Maintenance of skin integrity

## Nursing Interventions

- Do not change the colostomy pouch more often than once every 3 days.
- Change the pouch at first sign of leakage.
- Clean the skin thoroughly with soap and water, rinse, and dry with each pouch change.
- Observe for signs of skin breakdown and treat with powders and/or skin barriers as needed.

- Clean the skin around all other wounds during dressing changes, and keep the skin free from exudate.

## Rationale

Enzymes present in the stool are damaging to the skin. Intact skin is necessary for maintaining a tight seal on an appliance and thus protecting the skin. Too-frequent pouch changes cause mechanical destruction and removal of the skin. If frequent changes are necessary, re-evaluate the pouching system. A durable pouch-anchoring device may be necessary to protect the skin. Yeast infections are common, particularly if the pouch is improperly fitted, allowing exposure of too much skin surrounding the stoma. Ideally, less than ¼ inch of skin should be exposed.

## B. Nursing Diagnosis

Disturbance in self-concept related to alteration in bowel elimination pattern secondary to colostomy formation

## Goal of Care

Independence of the patient in the realm of bowel elimination

## Nursing Interventions

- Develop a teaching plan for the patient that includes his family and proceeds in a slow, step-wise fashion (5, 6).
- Perform colostomy care in a direct manner, including the patient by describing what you are doing, and eventually asking him to help.
- Control facial expression and verbal behavior during stoma care so as not to communicate distaste to the patient.
- Supplement explanations of the colostomy's structure and function that were given by the physician.
- Encourage ventilation of feelings by keeping the teaching sessions uninterrupted and unhurried.

## Rationale

The patient has had a major assault to his self-concept; he is recovering from a frightening attack, a major operation, and a disruption in his concept of his body and its functioning. For a teenage boy, the idea of having bowel movements from a opening in his abdomen may seem like a scene from a horror movie. At a time when peer pressure is especially crucial, this alteration is devastating. He will take cues concerning his peers' acceptance of him from the nurses' response in the hospital. Showing distaste for the stoma may cause irrevocable damage to him. He has to make major adjustments, and his anger and fear may prevent him from learning and from healthy adaptation.

## C. Nursing Diagnosis

Alteration in bowel elimination related to surgical manipulation and resultant ileus formation

## Goal of Care

Adequate elimination of body waste

## Nursing Interventions

- Monitor intake and output.
- Maintain patency of nasogastric tube.
- Maintain adequate fluid intake.
- Use narcotics judiciously for pain control.
- Increase mobility.

### Rationale

Surgical manipulation or traumatic injury to the bowel, sepsis, retroperitoneal hematoma, gastric distension, and overuse of narcotic analgesia may result in postoperative ileus (1). Prolonged ileus may necessitate the use of parenteral alimentation and all its inherent risks; may cause continued gastric suction with associated fluid and electrolyte disturbances and patient discomfort; and may contribute to delayed wound healing and possibly dehiscence from abdominal distension.

Metoclopramide (Reglan) may be useful in relieving nausea and vomiting associated with ileus. Reglan acts by stimulating motility of the upper GI tract without stimulating gastric, biliary, or pancreatic secretions. It increases the tone of gastric contractions, relaxes pyloric sphincter and duodenal bulb, and increases duodenal and jejunal peristalsis, with resultant acceleration of gastric emptying and intestinal transit. It has no effect on gallbladder or colon motility (7, 8).

## D. Nursing Diagnosis

Fear related to hsopitalization, the presence of strangers, separation anxiety, uncertainty about the future, real or imagined loss of love and approval of others, threats to personal integrity, loss of control of developmentally achieved functions, and recall of traumatic events (retaliation of the assailant) (5, 9)

### Goal of Care

Alleviate fear.

### Nursing Interventions

- Identify threat and cause.
- Reduce or eliminate contributing factors.
- Clarify and explain the injury and expected outcomes.
- Explain all procedures in understandable terms.
- Develop a care routine that results from a mutually derived plan.
- Give information as to progress.
- Talk about the future.
- Limit and/or screen visitors.
- Communicate to other involved health care workers the nature of his fears and what behaviors he exhibits that demonstrate those fears (5).

### Rationale

The patient is a teenage boy with no previous hospital experience and very little knowledge about medical procedures. He has been through a terrifying assault and is now surrounded by strangers. He feels that he has lost control; the assault continues, and he is powerless to stop it. Calm reassurance given frequently and a care routine that incorporates the patient in the plan helps him regain some control of his environment (10).

## ASSOCIATED NURSING DIAGNOSES

A. Alterations in comfort related to postoperative pain and delayed wound healing
B. Fluid volume deficit related to blood loss at the time of injury and to intraoperative evaporation
C. Altered growth and development related to loss of achieved mastery of bowel control
D. Knowledge deficit related to colostomy and wound care
E. Alterations in nutrition: less than body requirements

## REFERENCES

1. Mason PJ. Abdominal trauma. In: Cardona VD, Hurn PD, Bastnagel-Mason PJ, et al, eds. Trauma nursing: from resuscitation through rehabilitation. Philadelphia: WB Saunders, 1988:499–515.
2. Fulenwider J. Blunt and penetrating abdominal trauma. In: Broadwell D, Jackson B, eds. Principles of ostomy care. St Louis: CV Mosby, 1982:171–182.
3. Nance FC. Injuries to the colon and rectum. In: Mattox KL, Moore EE, Feliciano DV, eds. Trauma. Norwalk, CT: Appleton & Lange, 1988:495–504.
4. Martin M. Wound management and infection control after trauma: implications for the intensive care setting. CCQ 1988;11:43.
5. Edwards J, Krouse S. Helping the emergency colostomy patient through reality shock. Nursing 87, 1987;17:63–64.
6. Pinnyei M. Management of gunshot injuries. Dimensions Crit Care Nurs 1983;2:350–351.
7. Scherer VC. Nurses' drug manual. Philadelphia: JB Lippincott, 1985:705.
8. Physician's desk reference. 43nd ed. Oradell, NJ: Medical Economics Books, 1988.
9. Craig M, Copes W, Champion H. Psychosocial considerations in trauma care. CCQ 1988; 11:52.
10. Cihlar C. Mental status assessment for the E.T. nurse: psychological impact of physical trauma. J Enterostomal Ther 1986;13:49–53.

# PART 5

**Genitourinary Injuries/Complications**

# CHAPTER 18

## Rhabdomyolysis with Associated Myoglobinuria Resulting in Acute Renal Failure Necessitating Peritoneal Dialysis

Kathy A. Shane, RN, BSN, CCRN, CNRN

## Clinical Presentation

D.H. was a 28-year-old male involved in a single vehicle accident. He was driving while intoxicated and ran his car off the road over an embankment. After being trapped in the car, he was discovered and extricated after approximately 12 hours. He was flown by helicopter to the regional trauma center, where all initial diagnostic studies, such as diagnostic peritoneal lavage, multiple x-rays, and laboratory tests, were found to be negative, and his vital signs were stable. The patient was admitted to the step-down intensive care unit (ICU) with electrocardiogram (ECG) and intake and output monitoring only.

Shortly after admission, the patient became agitated and verbally abusive, and complained of back pain. Spinal x-rays were repeated but again were found to be negative; therefore, in view of his stated history of alcohol abuse, symptoms were attributed to acute alcohol withdrawal. It was later noted that the patient had not voided in 8 hours and he was catheterized for only 100 ml of reddish-brown urine. Laboratory values revealed creatinine of 2.3; blood urea nitrogen (BUN) of 48; Na of 149; potassium of 5.6; glucose of 289; Ca of 6.0; bilirubin of 1.9; serum glutamic oxaloacetic transaminase (SGOT) of 1762; lactic dehydrogenase (LDH) of 1957; creatine phosphokinase (CPK) of 89, 280 with MB of 62; hematocrit of 54; hemoglobin of 16.1; and white blood cell (WBC) count of 16,000. Arterial blood gases on room air were 7.29, $PaO$ of 78, $PaCO_2$ of 30, $HCO_3$ of 15, and $O_2$ saturation of 97%. His vital signs were temperature 38.5°C (101°F), pulse 108, respirations 30, and blood pressure 108/70. The patient had been receiving intravenous (IV) fluids of $D_5$ ½ NS with 20 mEq KC/L at 125 ml/hr since admission 18 hours earlier. The patient was transferred to the ICU with the diagnosis of rhabdomyolysis secondary to pressure necrosis with resultant acute tubular necrosis (ATN) from myoglobinuria.

The patient was started on a drip of $D_5W$ with 25 gm of mannitol and 100 mEq of $NaHCO_3$/ liter at 150 cc/hr and dopamine at 3 μg/kg/minute for renal perfusion. A pulmonary artery catheter was inserted with initial pressure readings of 28/10, mean pulmonary artery pressure (PAP) of 18, pulmonary capillary wedge pressure (PCWP) of 10, and central venous pressure (CVP) of 5. The patient was also given regular insulin 5 units IV and calcium gluconate 1 amp slowly IV. His respiratory status rapidly deteriorated, necessitating intubation and mechanical ventilation on $FiO_2$ 0.45, tidal volume 900, and synchronized intermittent mandatory ventilation (SIMV) 12. Attempts at improving renal function failed; a peritoneal dialysis catheter was inserted, and peritoneal dialysis was begun 28 hours after admission to the ICU. At no time did he exhibit any sign of visible injury, such as ecchymosis or jaundice. The CPK on day 2 was 69,800 and remained elevated for 8 days before returning to normal. The patient was extubated 8 days later, and peritoneal dialysis was continued for 5 weeks with complete recovery of renal function.

## 1. What is the pathophysiological basis for this patient's problem?

Gabin (1982) defined rhabdomyolysis as any condition in which serum creatine kinase (CK) activity is more than five times normal in the absence of brain or heart disease; however, mild rises (~250 IU/ml) have rare clinical significance (1, 2). Rhabdomyolysis is caused by any process that disrupts the integrity of muscle cell membranes, resulting in the release of myoglobin and other components of muscle: SGOT, LDH, CPK, glucose, and potassium. Myoglobin is a heme-containing pigment in muscle cells, necessary for oxygen binding and transport to the site of oxidative metabolism in muscle. It has a greater affinity for oxygen than hemoglobin, and therefore does not release oxygen until oxygen tension is very low (3, 4). Myoglobin stains only the urine, whereas after hemolysis, hemoglobin stains the serum and urine (5). Lysis of as little as 100 gm of skeletal muscle may result in myoglobinuria (6). Myoglobinuria is frequently seen following acute myocardial infarction, but rarely assumes clinical significance (2). Normally, 1 to 2% of skeletal muscle is myoglobin; in patients in chronic malnourished states, such as alcoholism, myoglobin makes up to 3 to 5%, resulting in a redder hue to muscle (3). There are several methods for detecting the presence of myoglobin in urine and blood. Specialized scanning techniques are available to quantitate roughly the amount of muscle damage; however, the diagnosis of rhabdomyolysis is made based on clinical findings and biochemical abnormalities. Visible pigmentation from myoglobin may be transient, lasting only 1 to 2 days, and may have passed by the time other symptoms develop and diagnosis of rhabdomyolysis is made. Patients who are at risk for developing myoglobinuria should have urine myoglobin sent and be treated prophylactically until definitive diagnosis is made. (Table 18.1) The patient may have vague complaints of malaise, myalgia, and weakness. Physical exam reveals decreased deep tendon reflexes, a "doughy" feeling of involved muscles, and hemorrhagic discoloration of skin over injured muscles.

Muscle, by weight, is the largest organ in the body, constituting as much as 40% of body weight (6). Lysis of muscle can release large quantities of the enzyme CPK.

Skeletal muscle contains the MM isoenzyme, and cardiac muscle contains the MB isoenzyme. CPK activity in excess of 100,000 IU/ml is common following muscle injury, but in patients with alcoholic malnutrition, only modest elevations may occur because the CPK content of muscle is decreased. CPK levels should peak in 24 to 36 hours and decrease by half within 48 to 72 hours. If levels remain elevated or rise, this is indicative of further muscle damage (7). The rise of SGOT and LDH is less significant in noncardiac muscle damage.

The three principal consequences of rhabdomyolysis and myoglobinuria are respiratory distress due to muscle weakness, fluid and electrolyte imbalances, and most important, renal failure. Other complications of rhabdomyolysis include compartment syndrome and disseminated intravascular coagulation (DIC) (see case studies regarding these topics).

## 2. What are the nursing diagnoses of highest priority?

A. Alteration in renal tissue perfusion
B. Potential for fluid volume deficit
C. Impaired tissue integrity

## 3. What are the goals of nursing care?

### A. Nursing Diagnosis

Alteration in renal perfusion with resultant renal failure as a result of myoglobinuria

**Table 18.1.** Partial etiologic classification of rhabdomyolysis[a]

---

I. Hereditary (not elaborated)
II. Not Hereditary
  A. Traumatic
    1. Direct
      a. Crush syndrome
        (1) Trauma including surgery
        (2) Compression
      b. Ischemic necrosis
        (1) Arterial occlusion
        (2) Carbon monoxide poisoning
        (3) Coagulopathy or DIC
        (4) Ligation of vena cava
        (5) Air embolism
    2. Indirect
      a. Unusual strenuous exercise (postexertional)
      b. Convulsions (prolonged myoclonus)
      c. Electrical injuries
  B. Nontraumatic
    1. Metabolic disorders
      a. Diabetic ketoacidosis
      b. Hypokalemia
      c. Hypophosphatemia
      d. Hypomagnesemia
      e. Hypo- or hyperthyroidism
      f. Hypo- or hypernatremia
      g. Nonketotic hyperosmolar coma
    2. Inflammatory and degenerative muscle disease
    3. Infection
      a. Viral
        (1) Influenza A and B

    3. Infection—(*continued*)
      a. Viral—(*continued*)
        (2) Herpes simplex
        (3) Mononucleosis
        (4) Coxsackie
        (5) Legionnaires'
        (6) Hepatitis
      b. Bacterial
        (1) *E. Coli* sepsis
        (2) Salmonellosis
        (3) Shigellosis
        (4) Tetanus
        (5) Gas gangrene
        (6) Toxic shock syndrome
      c. Rickettsial
    4. Abnormal body temperature
      a. Hypothermia—exposure or hypothyroidism
      b. Fever
        (1) Tetanus toxin
        (2) Heat injury or heat stroke
        (3) Malignant hyperthermia
    5. Drugs and toxins
      a. Alcohol
      b. Snake or spider venom
      c. Amphotericin B
      d. Amphetamines
      e. Barbiturates
      f. Aminocaproic acid (ischemia)
      g. Tricyclic antidepressants
      h. Steroids

---

[a]*Sources:* Adapted from:
Rowland L. Myoglobinuria. Can J Neurol Sci 1984;I:1–13.
Knochel J. Rhabdomyolysis and myoglobinuria. Ann Rev Med 1982;33:435–443.
Ron D, Teitelman U, Michaelson M, et al. Prevention of acute renal failure in traumatic rhabdomyolysis. Arch Intern Med 1984;2:277–280.
Farmer J, Civette J, Taylor R, Kirby R. Rhabdomyolysis. Critical care. Philadelphia: JB Lippincott, 1988:1569–1573.

## Goal of Care

Prevention of deterioration in renal function

## Nursing Interventions

- Maintain urine output ≥ 100 ml/hr by hydration, loop diuretics, mannitol infusion.
- Check urine pH with every voiding or every 2 to 4 hours if indwelling catheter; maintain pH >7.
- Follow renal function studies (i.e., BUN, creatinine, creatinine clearance) every 12 to 24 hours.
- Send urine myoglobins every day until negative and no further signs of tissue breakdown.
- Prevent crystallization of mannitol infusion.

## Rationale

The exact mechanism by which renal failure occurs following rhabdomyolysis has not been proved. It is postulated that tubular deposition of pigment obstructs the renal tubules with resultant dilatation of the nephrons, leading to compression of afferent arterioles and shunting of blood flow away from affected areas, causing acute tubular necrosis (ATN) (8, 9). Another theory is that vasoactive kinins released from damaged skeletal muscle directly damage the kidney (5, 10). Hemoglobin, also released with muscle damage, has a vasoconstricting effect on renal arteries as well. Whatever the theory, most authorities concur that myoglobinuria seems more likely to cause renal failure if associated with hypotension, dehydration, acidosis, or hypoxia (2, 11). Large amounts of fluid may be sequestered as edema (third-space loss) in damaged muscle, presenting a prerenal factor in the development of acute renal failure (ARF) (6). This hypovolemia or dehydration decreases renal blood flow and increases the concentration of nephrotoxic pigments. Adequate fluid resuscitation is therefore paramount.

Continuous infusion of mannitol and $NaHCO_3$ is controversial, but those who advocate this regimen feel it is beneficial for diuresis and urine alkalinization. Proponents rationalize its use on the fact that low urine pH has two harmful effects: First, it can potentiate the nephrotoxicity of myoglobin, and second, in patients with muscle injury, uric acid is commonly overproduced, and in the presence of acid urine, uric acid precipitation is favored. Opponents feel that rehydration alone is sufficient to improve urine output and "flush" the kidney of nephrotoxic substances (12). They advocate the use of loop diuretics as indicated. They argue that $NaHCO_3$ infusion can exceed the absorptive capacity of the proximal tubules, increasing distal delivery of $HCO_3$ anions and resulting in alkalemia and increased potassium excretion (6). Acetazolamide (Diamox) can be administered concurrently with mannitol and $NaHCO_3$ drip to prevent this alkalemia. The diuretic effect of acetazolamide is due to hydration of carbon dioxide and dehydration of carbonic acid, resulting in renal loss of sodium, water, and potassium, thus promoting urine alkalization and diuresis (13).

It mannitol is used, it must be added just prior to administration and never refrigerated, to prevent crystallization. If crystals are present in the vial, place in warm water until they disappear and preferably draw up mannitol with a filter needle before injection into the IV bag. In-line filters are effective in preventing infusion of crystals that may form during IV administration.

## B. Nursing Diagnosis

Potential for fluid volume deficit or excess with associated electrolyte disturbances secondary to rhabdomyolysis, acute renal failure, and peritoneal dialysis

## Goal of Care

Prevention of abnormal fluid volume and electrolyte disturbances

## Nursing Interventions

- Monitor strictly the intake and output.
- Monitor serum electrolytes, glucose, and osmolality.
- Monitor specific gravity every shift.
- Monitor BUN and creatinine.
- Observe and prevent complications of peritoneal dialysis.
- Maintain aseptic technique.
- Test urine for glucose, blood, and protein every 6 hours.

**Table 18.2.** Fluid and electrolyte imbalances associated with renal failure[a]

| Condition | Possible Etiologies | Signs and Symptoms | Management |
|---|---|---|---|
| Hyponatremia | Sodium loss associated with diuretic therapy, vomiting, diarrhea Reduced intake of sodium—dietary or intravenous Excessive fluid intake in relation to output | Abdominal cramps, nausea and vomiting, twitching, seizures, confusion, weakness, apprehension, fatigue | Control nausea, vomiting, diarrhea. Restrict fluids to prevent further dilutional hyponatremia. Increase dietary or intravenous sodium intake. Monitor serum sodium levels closely. Seizure precautions. |
| Hypernatremia | Excessive intake of dietary or intravenous sodium Increased aldosterone output | Increased deep tendon reflexes, lethargy, restlessness, weakness, dry skin, dry mucous membranes, increased temperature, flushed skin, thirst | Restrict intravenous and dietary sodium. Maximize fluid intake as tolerated. Monitor effects of diuretics. Monitor efficacy of hypotonic solution administration. |
| Hypokalemia | Potassium loss associated with vomiting, diarrhea, or diuretics Decreased potassium intake | Muscle weakness, muscle cramping, irregular pulse, parasthesias, hypoactive or absent bowel sounds, drowsiness, ECG changes (T-wave inversion, ST depression, U-waves) Faint heart sounds, decreased blood pressure, fatigue, vomiting, shortness of breath, weak pulse | Control vomiting, diarrhea. Increase dietary intake of foods high in potassium—tomatoes, oranges, bananas, raisins, figs, dates, apricots, potatoes. Administer potassium supplements, oral and/or intravenous. Administer potassium-sparing diuretics (i.e., Aldactone). |
| Hyperkalemia | Excessive intake of dietary or intravenous potassium Decreased ability of kidney to excrete potassium Increased cellular release of potassium related to metabolic acidosis and hemolysis due to high levels of nitrogenous wastes | Parasthesias; ECG changes (peaked T-wave, prolonged P-R interval, widened QRS); slow, irregular pulse, hyperactive bowel sounds; diarrhea; muscle weakness; muscle flaccidity; nausea; dizziness; muscle cramps; polydipsia | Monitor serum potassium levels closely. Restrict dietary and intravenous potassium intake. Treat metabolic acidosis. Loop diuretics to increase renal excretion of potassium (i.e. Lasix). Reduce body protein catabolism, which releases potassium from tissues. Increase carbohydrate intake (good energy source) to reduce catabolism protein. Decrease activity to reduce energy requirements. Decrease accumulation of nitrogenous wastes, |

| Condition | Cause | Signs and Symptoms | Interventions |
|---|---|---|---|
| Hyperkalemia *(continued)* | | | which decrease lifespan of red blood cells, resulting in hemolysis. If blood transfusion is necessary obtain fresh rather than stored blood. Potassium content of stored blood is higher, and stored blood is more apt to be hemolyzed. Hemolysis of red blood cells results in release of potassium. Administer cation exchange resins. Kayexalate ioncreases intestinal potassium excretion by exchanging sodium for potassium. Administer insulin and hypertonic glucose solutions intravenously to cause shift of extracellular potassium into cells. Prepare for dialysis if above measures fail. |
| Hyperphosphatemia | Decreased ability of kidneys to excrete phosphorus | Seizures, muscle cramps, hyperreflexia, paresthesias | Restrict dietary intake of foods rich in phosphorus (e.g., poultry, milk, cheese, peanuts, peas). Administer phosphorus-binding antacids, such as Amphojel, Basaljel. |
| Hypophosphatemia (rare) | Overuse of phosphorus-binding antacids | | Decrease dosage of phosphorus-binding antacids. |
| Hypermagnesemia | Excessive intake of magnesium-containing antacids and laxatives Decreased ability of kidneys to excrete magnesium | Flushed, warm skin; nausea and vomiting; hypotension; depressed respirations; decreased level of consciousness; hypoactive deep tendon reflexes; bradycardia | Limit use of magnesium-containing antacids and laxatives (Maalox, Mylanta, Riopan, Gelusil, Milk of Magnesia, Mag Citrate). Restrict dietary intake of foods rich in magnesium (milk, legumes, whole-grain breads and cereals, nuts). |
| Hypomagnesemia (rare) | Overuse of magnesium-binding antacids Increased excretion of magnesium by kidneys | Mental status change, numbness and tingling in extremities, positive Chevostek's and Trousseau's signs, tachycardia, neuromuscular irritability, tremors, premature ventricular contractions | Administer MgSO$_4$. Change to magnesium containing antacids. |

*(continues)*

**Table 18.2.** Fluid and electrolyte imbalances associated with renal failure[a] *(continued)*

| Condition | Possible Etiologies | Signs and Symptoms | Management |
|---|---|---|---|
| Hypocalcemia | Rapid correction of acidosis. As pH increases, calcium ionization decreases<br><br>Decreased absorption of calcium associated with kidneys' inability to metabolize vitamin D, which stimulates calcium absorption from the intestines<br><br>Increased phosphorus retention—inverse relationship between phosphorus and calcium | Cardiac arrhythmias; muscle cramps; tetany; seizures; changes in mental status; positive Chevostek's and Trousseau's signs; numbness and tingling of fingers, toes, and circumoral area; abdominal cramps; laryngeal stridor; prolonged QT interval | Increase dietary intake of calcium (dairy products). Avoid too-aggressive treatment of acidosis to prevent reduction in calcium ionization. Avoid stored blood transfusions—citrate binds calcium. Administer activated vitamin D and calcium supplement. Treat hyperphosphatemia. Seizure precautions. |
| Hypercalcemia | Increased dietary or intravenous intake of calcium<br><br>Excessive intake of calcium-containing antacids<br><br>Increased intestinal absorption of calcium associated with vitamin D therapy.<br><br>Increased release of calcium from bone associated with hyperparathyroidism—parathyroids secrete increased amounts of parathyroid hormone in attempt to maintain adequate calcium levels | Cardiac arrhythmias, muscle weakness, muscle flaccidity, nausea and vomiting, anorexia, constipation, mental status change, decreased gastrointestinal (GI) motility, deep bone pain, flank pain, abdominal pains, paralytic ileus, shortening of QT interval, hypertension | Restrict calcium in diet. Avoid calcium-containing antacids (Tums, Rolaids, calcium carbonate, Titralac). Administer corticosteroids to promote urinary calcium excretion, inhibit reabsorption of calcium from bone, and decrease absorption of calcium from intestines. Mobilize patient to reduce calcium loss from bones. Administer calcitonin or mithramycin to inhibit osteoclastic bone resorption and increase renal clearance of calcium. Loop diuretics to increase urinary calcium excretion. Prepare for dialysis to reduce calcium levels. Parathyroidectomy. |

| | | | |
|---|---|---|---|
| Metabolic acidosis | Hyponatremia<br>Hyperkalemia causes hydrogen ions to shift into vascular space<br>Excessive loss of bicarbonate associated with diarrhea and a decreased ability of kidneys to reabsorb bicarbonate<br>Decreased ability of kidneys to excrete hydrogen ions, phosphates, sulfates, and the end products of protein metabolism | Anion gap > 15 mEq/liter, vomiting, headache, nausea, rapid shallow respirations, stupor, disorientation | Treat hyponatremia and hyperkalemia. Control diarrhea. Maintain adequate nutritional status to decrease release of acid end products associated with catabolism of body protein. Administer $NaHCO_3$. Prepare for dialysis to remove excess phosphates and sulfates. |
| Fluid volume deficit | Anorexia, nausea<br>Inability of hypertrophied nephrons to concentrate urine and decreased ability of renal tubules to reabsorb electrolytes<br>Decreased glomerular filtration rate<br>Increased aldosterone output associated with diminished renal blood flow, which causes increased output of renin. This is converted to angiotensin, which then stimulates aldosterone output | Poor skin turgor; thirst; dry mucous membranes; weight loss > 0.5 kg/day; low BP or orthostatic decrease by 15 mm Hg and concurrent rise in pulse; weak, rapid pulse; dyspnea; edema; increased CVP; JVD (jugular vein distension) | Encourage P.O. intake, or administer IV fluids. Prevent vomiting. Control diarrhea. Improve renal blood flow. Prepare for dialysis. |

[a]*Sources*: Adapted from:
Johanson B, Dungga C, Hoffmeister D, Wells S. Standards of critical care. St Louis: CV Mosby, 1981:378–388.
Ulrich S, Canale S, Wendell S. Nursing care planning guide: A nursing diagnosis approach. Philadelphia: WB Saunders, 1986:404–408.
Ellerbe S. Fluid and blood component therapy in the critically ill and injured. New York: Churchill Livingstone, 1981:3–16.
Millar S, Sampson L, Soukup S. AACN procedure manual for critical care. Philadelphia: WB Saunders, 1985:319.

## Rationale

Metabolic features attributable to crush injury are due to the release of intracellular muscle constituents (3). The profound hypocalcemia, hyperglycemia, and hyperuricemia are believed to be secondary to the release of a large endogenous phosphate load with subsequent calcium binding and deposition of calcium salts in soft tissue, glycogen release, and breakdown and release of uric acid. Other factors contributing to hypocalcemia are hyperphosphatemia and skeletal resistance to vitamin D, which leaks from injured muscle cells. As the patient's condition improves, these calcium deposits can be released back in the circulation with resultant hypercalcemia. To prevent metastatic calcification, administration of calcium salts should, therefore, be reserved for symptomatic cases only (5). In addition, indiscriminate use of calcium may potentiate muscle cell injury. Hyperkalemia is due to the release of intracellular potassium from necrotic muscle.

Skeletal muscle breakdown results in the release of creatine, the storage compound of high-energy phosphate. Creatinine is the metabolic waste product of creatine degeneration and is filtered by the glomeruli, not reabsorbed. In rhabdomyolysis, creatinine formation exceeds the filtration rate; therefore, measured creatinine is characteristically out of proportion to BUN, which is typically low with these patients (10).

Treatments for myoglobinuria may also produce fluid and electrolyte and acid-base derangements. These include hypokalemia, metabolic alkalosis, and hypovolemia, and must be monitored and treated accordingly.

If renal failure should develop, a multitude of fluid and electrolyte imbalances may occur depending on which phase of renal failure the patient is in, high output or oliguric (Table 18.2).

Treatment of acute renal failure may be by hemodialysis (see Chapter 22 on acute renal failure) or by peritoneal dialysis. Peritoneal dialysis is superior to hemodialysis in that it is simpler (it may be performed by patient or family after discharge), may be performed immediately after insertion of a trocar, is less costly, affords patient mobility, and results in more gradual physiological changes. The drawbacks of peritoneal dialysis versus hemodialysis are that there is an increased risk of infection, pulmonary and peritoneal; it is less useful for the removal of toxins; it cannot be used if the peritoneal membrane is not intact; it is associated with increased albumin loss; and there is increased patient discomfort (14) (Table 18.3).

Glucose in the dialysate increases osmotic pressure, drawing extracellular fluid from the patient across a semipermeable membrane (peritoneum), and also increases urea clearance and electrolyte removal. The more concentrated the glucose solution, the greater the pull. Potassium is added to the solution to replace losses in the effluent. Urea clearance is maximized and body heat loss minimized when the dialysate is near body temperature (14, 15).

Keep in mind that dosages of drugs, particularly antibiotics, must be adjusted with renal failure, and some drugs are dialyzable (16).

## C. Nursing Diagnosis

Impaired tissue integrity secondary to pressure and/or ischemia

## Goal of Care

Prevention of further tissue breakdown

## Nursing Interventions

- Turn patient every 2 hours.
- Avoid positioning on affected side.

**Table 18.3.** Problems associated with peritoneal dialysis[a]

| Problem | Possible Etiologies |
| --- | --- |
| Bowel or bladder perforation | Traumatic insertion of trocar or later erosion of trocar |
| Skin excoriation | Leakage at catheter insertion site |
| Ileus | Inflammation from dialysate or infection |
| Peritonitis | Poor aseptic technique, contaminated dialysate |
| Air in system (patient will complain of shoulder pain) | Loose connections, too rapid infusion rate (knee chest or Trendelenburg positioning will help remove air from peritoneum) |
| Pulmonary insufficiency | Elevated diaphragm from enlarged abdomen during dwell phase |
| Hypotension | Too-rapid removal of intravascular volume, vena cava compression |
| Hypertension | Anxiety, pain during "dwell phase," hypervolemia |
| Arrhythmias—premature beats | Dialysate too cold |
| Bradyarrhythmias | Overdistension |
| Catheter obstruction | Clots, fibrin, adhesions, tubing kink |
| Malnutrition | Protein loss, decreased calcium and iron absorption |

[a]*Sources:* Adapted from:
Physicians' desk reference. 43rd ed. Oradell, NJ: Medical Economics Books, 1989:1116.
Fleming L, Kane V. Step-by-step guide to safe peritoneal dialysis. RN (Feb) 1984:44–47.

- Monitor CPK, SGOT, and LDH levels.
- Monitor perfusion, particularly in affected extremities every 2 to 4 hours.
  - Check distal pulses
  - Check color
  - Check warmth
  - Check movement
  - Check sensation

There have been reports of patients found unconscious for unknown periods of time, who are admitted with ARF due to rhabdomyolysis from pressure necrosis (3). Additional muscle damage from either pressure or ischemia from edema is an important goal of treatment. Any increase in CPK, SGOT, and LDH is indicative of further muscle breakdown. Any decreases in sensation, movement, changes in color (pallor or mottling), and change in temperature should be reported immediately, as loss of distal pulses is a late symptom.

Turning the patient will help prevent further tissue compromise. If unable to turn the patient because of injuries or unstable condition, a low air loss bed may be useful.

Alcohol has a direct toxic effect on muscle. In addition, the alcoholic patient is often malnourished, with associated metabolic abnormalities, such as hypokalemia, hypophosphatemia, and hypomagnesemia, all of which may intensify skeletal muscle injury and complicate its treatment. It is, therefore, important to obtain information regarding alcohol use from patient or family.

Fortunately, after recovery there is no residual muscle atrophy. If rhabdomyolysis is caused by excess exercise, resumption of the same exercises do not cause reappearance of symptoms, which may suggest that adaptive changes have occurred in the muscle, making it more tolerant to exertion (5).

## ASSOCIATED NURSING DIAGNOSES

A. Ineffective breathing pattern
B. Impaired gas exchange
C. Alteration in comfort
D. Potential for infection
E. Alteration in nutrition
F. Impaired physical mobility

**REFERENCES**

1. Gabow PA, Kaehny WD, Kerleher SP. The spectrum of rhabdomyolysis. Medicine 1982;6:141–152.
2. Rowland L. Myoglobinuria. Can J Neurol Sci 1984;I:1–13.
3. Knochel J. Rhabdomyolysis and myoglobinuria. Ann Rev Med 1982;33:435–443.
4. Ron D, Teitelman U, Michaelson M, et al. Prevention of acute renal failure in traumatic rhabdomyolysis. Arch Intern Med 1984;2:277–280.
5. Farmer J, Civette J, Taylor R, Kirby R. Rhabdomyolysis. Critical care. Philadelphia: JB Lippincott, 1988:1569–1573.
6. Ratcliffe P, Berman P, Griffith R. Pressure-induced rhabdomyolysis complicating an undiscovered fall. Age Ageing 1983;12:245–248.
7. Dunham M, Cowley R. Shock trauma/critical care handbook. Rockville, MD: Aspen, 1986:501.
8. Reid W, McQueen A. Acute rhabdomyolysis in a marathon runner. Br J Sports Med 1987;21:49.
9. Hart PM, Ferrfeld DA, Briscoe AM, et al. The effect of renal failure and hemodialysis on serum and urine myoglobin. Clin Nephrol 1982;18:144–143.
10. Schrier R. Acute renal failure: pathogenesis, diagnosis, and management. Hosp Pract (Mar) 1981:93–112.
11. Zuidema GD, Rutherford RB, Ballingen WF, et al. The management of trauma. 4th ed. Philadelphia: WB Saunders, 1985.
12. Guechot J, Cynuber L, Lioretin N, et al. Rhabdomyolysis and acute renal failure in a patient with thermal injury. Intensive Care Med 1986;12:159–150.
13. Physicians' desk reference. 43rd ed. Oradell, NJ: Medical Economics Books, 1989:1116.
14. Hadak C, Coallo B, Lohr T. Critical care nursing. Philadelphia: JB Lippincott, 1986:377–390.
15. Johanson B, Dungga C, Hoffmeister D, Wells S. Standards of critical care. St Louis: CV Mosby, 1981:378–388.
16. Eisenberg M, Furukawa C, Ray G. Manual of antimicrobial therapy and infectious diseases. Philadelphia: WB Saunders, 1980:240–244.

# CHAPTER 19

## Ruptured Bladder

### Denise Cost, RN, CCRN

## Clinical Presentation

A 51-year-old woman was admitted to the emergency department after being struck by a car as a pedestrian. At the scene, she was alert and talking, and the smell of alcohol was on her breath. The patient's prehospital blood pressure was 86/60, and medical antishock trousers (MAST) were applied. On admission to the emergency department, she complained of shortness of breath and hip pain. Her Glasgow Coma Scale score was 14/15. Her blood pressure was 116/80; pulse was 96; and respiratory rate was 18 breaths/minute. Her pupils were equal and reactive to light. Further examination revealed distended neck veins, and rales were heard on auscultation. Normal heart sounds were present. Hypoactive bowel sounds were present, and her abdomen was nontender. Further palpation revealed an unstable pelvis with motion on lateral pressure and right hip crepitation with external rotation. No gross blood was detected by rectal examination, and no masses were palpated. Chest x-ray films showed bilateral pulmonary edema. Arterial blood gases (ABGs) were $PaO_2$, 70; pH, 7.33; $PaCO_2$, 35; and $HCO_3^-$, 18. Pelvic x-ray films demonstrated pubic rami fracture with pelvic ring disruption. An intravenous pyelogram (IVP) was negative. Cystogram revealed a large intraperitoneal bladder disruption with dye extravasation. During this exam, the patient experienced tachypnea and required intubation and mechanical ventilation. She received furosemide (Lasix) for pulmonary congestion. She also received 5 units of packed red blood cells, 10 units of fresh frozen plasma, and 3500 ml of lactated Ringer's solution during resuscitation. After stabilization she was taken to the operating room for an exploratory laparotomy. Surgical exploration revealed a 3-cm anterior intraperitoneal bladder rupture, which was debrided and repaired. Serosal tears of the terminal ileum and colon were also repaired. A drain was placed above the bladder, and a pelvic Hoffman device was applied. Preoperatively, her neurovascular status to both lower extremities was normal. The patient was transported to the intensive care unit in stable condition with arterial and venous lines in place, a Foley catheter for drainage, and an orogastric tube for drainage and was intubated on mechanical ventilation.

### 1. What is the pathophysiological basis for this patient's problem?

Blunt injuries to the lower abdomen or pelvis, such as those sustained in motor vehicle crashes, are the most common cause of bladder injury (contusions or rupture). Crush injuries result in penetration and rupture of the bladder by fractured bone. Penetrating injuries are also caused by stabbings, gunshot blasts, or foregin objects or are iatrogenic (induced by pelvic operations or endoscopic instrumentation).

An empty bladder is extremely resistant to most types of trauma (1). A distended bladder is more likely to be ruptured by blunt trauma, to be torn by fragments of bone from pelvic fractures, or to present a bigger target for penetrating missiles. It extends higher up into the abdomen, becoming more prone to both penetrating and blunt trauma.

There are two major types of injury to the bladder: contusion and rupture. Signs and symptoms of bladder injury are listed in Table 19.1.

A simple bladder contusion is an injury to and hemorrhage in one or more layers of

**133**

**Table 19.1.** Signs and symptoms of bladder injury

Gross hematuria
Inability to void
Severe lower abdominal pain and tenderness to palpation, although pain may be minimal in some patients
Dullness to percussion due to hematoma formation or distended bladder
Signs of peritonitis can be present with intraperitoneal bladder rupture.
Enlarging pelvic mass on rectal or vaginal exam

the vesical wall, with the wall remaining intact and no extravasation of urine. Hematuria is usually the only symptom.

Rupture of the bladder is the most common bladder injury and can result in intraperitoneal or extraperitoneal extravasation of urine. Intraperitoneal ruptures occur most commonly following trauma to the lower abdomen in patients with bladder distension (2 [p. 1398]). The dome of the distended bladder, the part covered by peritoneum, is the weakest, most unprotected area of the bladder wall and thus is prone to rupture, causing leakage of the urine into the peritoneal space. Extraperitoneal rupture is usually associated with fracture of the bony pelvis (3), leading to extravasation of urine into the extraperitoneal spaces (2 [p. 1399]). Extraperitoneal ruptures are the most common rupture of the bladder (4). Isolated bladder rupture (i.e., rupture of the bladder without other associated injury) is rare.

Bladder rupture is diagnosed by cystography, which will reveal the presence or absence of extravasation of contrast medium and intraperitoneal or extraperitoneal rupture. Bladder perforations are treated with surgical debridement, repair with absorbable sutures, and decompression of the bladder. Penrose drains are used to drain the perivesical space (5). Decompression is accomplished with a Foley catheter or suprapubic cystotomy. The bladder is allowed to decompress, and catheters are left in place for 7 to 14 days (6). If intraperitoneal ruptures remain untreated, peritonitis may develop in 24 to 48 hours because of urinary drainage into the peritoneal cavity (7).

Complications of appropriately treated bladder rupture are few due largely to the organ's considerable recovery potential (8). Mortality rates in patients with bladder rupture have been reported as high as 22%; death is usually related to the severity of the associated injuries and sepsis rather than to the bladder injury (9).

## 2. What are the nursing diagnoses of highest priority?

A. Potential for infection
B. Alteration in comfort

## 3. What are the goals of nursing care?

### A. Nursing Diagnosis

Potential for infection related to disruption of skin and genitourinary tract

### Goals of Care

- Decrease risk of infection.
- Identify signs of infection.

### Nursing Interventions

- Monitor patient for signs and symptoms of infection: temperature, white blood cell (WBC) count, wound drainage, appearance of catheter insertion sites, appearance of suture lines, urine cultures and urinalysis results, and skin integrity.
- Change dressing routinely every 12 to 24 hours or as ordered.

- Perform routine Foley catheter care using iodine-based antiseptic solution for cleansing of catheter site.
- Perform cystotomy catheter site care and dressing change once daily and as needed.
- Assess abdomen, perineum, and thighs for tenderness, swelling, and/or redness.

## Rationale

The treatment of ruptured bladder is decompression of the bladder with catheters to allow the suture line to heal without undue pressure. Attention must be paid to the care and maintenance of the Foley catheter and the cystotomy catheter to prevent bladder and urinary tract infection and sepsis. Catheter insertion sites should be cleansed gently but thoroughly. In the case of unrecognized urinary extravasation due to undetected bladder rupture, abscess formation with dissection along the fascial planes can occur in the retroperitoneum up the anterior abdominal wall and down into the perineum, resulting in extensive necrosis (7). Symptoms may include swelling, redness, flank tenderness, or tenderness of the lower abdomen, perineum, or penis.

## B. Nursing Diagnosis

Alteration in comfort related to presence of invasive catheters and surgical incisions

## Goal of Care

Alleviate pain.

## Nursing Interventions

- Stabilize catheters.
- Administer pain medication.

## Rationale

Stabilization of catheters and tubes is necessary to prevent pressure on the bladder and urethra and prevent dislodgment. Proper stabilization of catheters contributes to the patient's comfort. In males, Foley catheters should be stabilized on the abdomen; this straightens the urethral curve and reduces the chance of pressure necrosis within the urethra. In females, the catheter should be taped to the inner thigh with enough length to allow mobility of the lower extremity without pulling the catheter balloon down on the bladder neck.

# ASSOCIATED NURSING DIAGNOSES

A. Anxiety
B. Disturbances in self-concept
C. Alteration in patterns of urinary elimination

**REFERENCES**

1. Shoemaker WC, Thompson WL, Holbrook PR. The Society of Critical Care Medicine textbook of critical care. Philadelphia: WB Saunders, 1984:903.
2. Schwartz G, Safar P, Stone J, Storey P, Wagner D. Principles and practices of emergency medicine. 2nd ed. Philadelphia: WB Saunders, 1986.
3. Weiskittel P, Sommers MS. The patient with lower urinary tract trauma. Crit Care Nurse 1989;9:54–64.
4. Hayes EE, Sandler SMN, Corriere N. Management of the ruptured bladder secondary to blunt abdominal trauma. J Urol 1983;129:946–947.
5. Cowley RA, Dunham CM. Shock trauma critical care manual: initial assessment and management. Baltimore: University Park Press, 1982:180.
6. Kinney MR, ed. AACN's clinical reference for critical care nurses. New York: McGraw-Hill, 1981:680.
7. Tritschler V. Abdominal-genitourinary injuries. In: Harmon AR, ed. Nursing care of the adult trauma patient. New York: Wiley, 1985:214.
8. McAninch JW. Genitourinary trauma. In: Mattox KL, Moore EE, Feliciano DV, eds. Trauma. Norwalk, CT: Appleton & Lange, 1988:545–547.
9. Montie J. Bladder injuries. Urol Clin North Am 1977;4:59.

# CHAPTER 20

# Renal Trauma

Jocelyn A. Farrar, RN, MS, CCRN

## Clinical Presentation

A 17-year-old student was admitted to a hospital following an injury during a high school football game. The patient had been tackled, receiving a severe blow to the back and right flank. On arrival, the patient was awake and oriented to time, place, and person. He was moving all four extremities but complained of abdominal and right flank pain. His blood pressure was 90/60 mm Hg; pulse was 130; and respirations were 32/minute and shallow. The patient was pale and diaphoretic, with thready rapid pulses. His medical history indicated that he had suffered from glomerulonephritis as a child.

Examination revealed severe costovertebral angle pain on the right and palpable mass in the right flank. A large ecchymotic area was evident over the area of the 11th and 12th ribs and flank on the right.

A radiograph examination of the abdomen revealed fractures of the right 11th and 12th ribs, with an abnormal obliteration of the psoas margin and renal shadow. The KUB (a flat plate radiographic examination of the kidney, ureter, and bladder) showed an abnormal outline of the right kidney.

Based on the mechanism of injury and the clinical presentation of the patient, blunt renal trauma was suspected, and a urology consult was obtained. A urinary catheter was passed, which revealed gross hematuria. Urethrogram and cystogram revealed a normal urethra and bladder. An intravenous pyelogram (IVP) was then done, which revealed an abnormal right kidney, with dye extravasation into the right retroperitoneal cavity. The left kidney was normal. A renal arteriogram indicated an intact renal vascular pedicle but major laceration of the renal parenchyma, extending through the renal capsule and the collecting system with major extravasation of contrast material.

The patient was transported to the operating room, where an exploratory laparotomy was performed. A major laceration of the right kidney was found, which extended through the renal capsule into the collecting system. The renal parenchyma was repaired, and nonviable tissue was debrided. A large retroperitoneal mass of blood and extravasated urine was evacuated. Following repair of the collecting system, a temporary nephrostomy tube was inserted. A Penrose drain was placed and exited through the flank.

On admission to the intensive care unit, the patient was mechanically ventilated through a number 8 endotracheal tube. His blood pressure was 120/70 mm Hg; pulse was 90; respirations were 20/minute; and temperature was 98.8°F (37.0°C). A nephrostomy tube and indwelling Foley catheter were present, both of which were draining grossly bloody urine. A pulmonary artery catheter was in his right subclavian vein, and an arterial line was in his right radial artery. The patient was receiving transfusions of packed red blood cells. A nasogastric tube was draining green fluid. The midline laparotomy incision and the right flank nephrostomy and Penrose drain sites were covered with dry sterile dressings.

## 1. What is the pathophysiological basis for this patient's problem?

The kidneys lie within the upper retroperitoneal space at the level of the 12th thoracic and the first three lumbar vertebrae. The left kidney is protected anteriorly by the spleen, pancreatic tail, descending colon, and chest wall. The right kidney, positioned

1 to 2 cm lower than the left, is protected by the liver, duodenum, and diaphragm (1). The psoas and quadrats lumborum muscles protect the kidneys posteriorly, with the ribs providing further protection posteriorly and laterally (2).

The renal parenchyma is surrounded by a strong fibrous renal capsule. A layer of perinephric fat surrounds the kidney and is confined by Gerota's fascia. When not damaged, this fascia is capable of providing a tamponade for renal hemorrhage (2). The kidney is a mobile organ attached to the aorta by the renal artery and to the vena cava by the renal vein. A ureter provides the connection to the urinary bladder. This mobility can become a disadvantage when sufficient force is applied to the kidney to cause disruption of this renal vascular pedicle (2).

Renal trauma may be classified as either blunt or penetrating (3). Blunt renal injuries are associated with motor vehicle accidents, falls, or sports injuries and are often the result of a direct blow to the back, flank, or abdomen. This blow may cause the kidney to set into a rapid acceleration/deceleration motion on the vascular pedicle. This type of renal trauma, known as a contrecoup injury, results when sufficient force is applied to cause stretching and tearing of the renal pedicle vasculature. The result may be a renal pedicle avulsion with hemorrhage or excessive stretching of the renal artery with laceration of the intima. This laceration is followed by the formation of a renal artery thrombosis at the site of the tear (4, 5).

Blunt trauma may produce a crushing injury to the kidney. Crush injuries may result from the patient being caught between two objects or from a strong blow causing an inward rotation of the 12th rib. This rib may then compress the kidney into the lumbar spine (3). A fracture of a rib or of the lumbar transverse process may result in a parenchymal laceration (2).

Penetrating renal trauma is generally the result of a gunshot or stab wound. Penetrating injuries are relatively rare: 8% of all patients with penetrating injury incur a renal injury (3).

The incidence of renal trauma is high among patients who have diseased or congenitally deformed kidneys. Consequently, patients should be assessed for renal abnormalities such as polycystic, pelvic, or horseshoe kidneys; glomerulonephritis; hydronephrosis; or renal tumor. Major renal injury caused by minor trauma may indicate that renal disease existed prior to the injury (1, 5).

Often, renal trauma is masked by a more acute injury to another organ system. Therefore, a high index of suspicion must be maintained for patients experiencing blunt trauma to the torso, pelvis, back, or flank; or lower thoracic or upper spine injury or when ecchymosis is present over the flank (Grey-Turner's sign), indicating a retroperitoneal hematoma (1, 3, 6).

Both blunt and penetrating renal injuries may be classified according to severity. Minor injuries include contusions, simple parenchymal lacerations, and small subcapsular hematomas (Fig. 20.1). There is usually no urinary extravasation. Major renal injuries include renal rupture, parenchymal lacerations with arterial occlusion, tears of the renal vasculature, laceration or avulsion of the renal artery or vein, parenchymal lacerations with enlarging perirenal hematomas, and parenchymal fractures that extend into the collecting ducts with extravasation of urine and hematoma formation (5) (Fig. 20.2).

Minor renal trauma is usually treated conservatively. The patient with microscopic hematuria and no other associated injuries may be placed on partial bed rest with increased hydration. A repeat IVP may be obtained to monitor the healing process. Patients experiencing gross hematuria may be placed on strict bed rest with trend analysis of vital signs, hematuria, urinary output, serum and urine creatinine, blood urea nitrogen, creatinine clearance, hemoglobin, and hematocrit. If the patient's condition deteriorates, surgery may be indicated (1, 5).

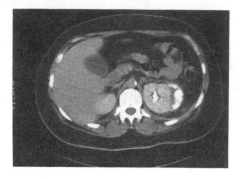

**Figure 20.1.** Minor renal injuries. Simple laceration and subcapsular hematoma. (From Peters PC, Bright TC. Management of trauma to the urinary tract. Adv Surg 1976;10:197–244.)

Major renal trauma involving avulsion injuries, early renal artery thrombosis, urinary extravasation, an expanding retroperitoneal hematoma, or unstable cardiovascular status should be explored surgically (1, 5, 6). Goals of surgical intervention include control of vascular pedicle bleeding, identification of injury, debridement of nonviable parenchyma, hemostasis, closure of the collecting ducts, repair of viable parenchyma, and extraperitoneal drainage (5, 6).

Complications following renal trauma include delayed bleeding, abscess formation, urinary fistula formation, renal atrophy (from renal artery thrombosis), renovascular hypertension, arteriovenous fistula formation, hydronephrosis, and renal failure (2, 6).

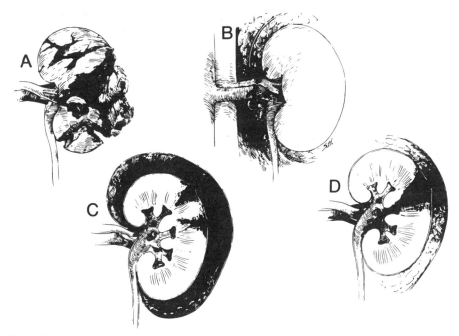

**Figure 20.2.** Major renal injuries. **A** Renal rupture. **B** Laceration of renal artery and vein. **C** Perirenal hematoma. **D** Laceration through collecting system. (From Peters PC, Bright TC. Management of trauma to the urinary tract. Adv Surg 1976;10:197–244.)

## 2. What are the nursing diagnoses of highest priority?

A. Potential for fluid volume deficit
B. Potential for infection

## 3. What goals of care and nursing interventions are appropriate for the above diagnoses?

### A. *Nursing Diagnosis*

Potential for fluid volume deficit related to hemorrhage secondary to renal trauma

### *Goal of Care*

Maintain normovolemic state.

### *Nursing Interventions*

- Monitor vital signs and pulmonary artery pressures and report signs of hemorrhagic shock.
- Monitor serial hemoglobin, hematocrit, coagulation profile, and urine hematest results.
- Assess flank mass size and note trends.
- Observe surgical site for bleeding.
- Monitor intake and output measurements and urine specific gravity.
- Note trends in blood urea nitrogen, serum creatinine, urinalysis, urine creatinine clearance, and electrolytes.

### *Rationale*

The patient experiencing renal trauma is at risk for massive hemorrhage. Gerota's fascia, when intact, is capable of providing a tamponade for bleeding following minor renal trauma. Damage to this fascia limits its tamponade effect, with the potential for a massive bleed into the large retroperitoneal space (1, 2). Vital signs must be monitored hourly (more often during cardiovascular instability), and trends that could indicate hemorrhage must be noted and reported (7). Fluid volume status must be assessed, and trends in intake, output, and pulmonary artery pressures must be monitored (1).

The presence of an expanding flank mass could indicate continued bleeding into the retroperitoneal space. The size of the mass should be monitored by measuring abdominal girth or by cautious palpation of the mass. Although abdominal girth measurement is a less exact method of assessing flank mass size, it is potentially safer because palpation of this mass may disrupt clots and cause further bleeding (1).

Patients with major renal trauma may experience severe hemorrhage and require massive blood and fluid resuscitation. Consequently, trend analysis of serial hemoglobin, hematocrit, and coagulation profile is essential (1, 7).

During hemorrhage, decreased cardiac output produces a selective shunting of blood to vital organs, with a subsequent decrease in the perfusion of the renal capillaries. Because the kidneys have a high rate of metabolism, renal tissues are especially susceptible to damage from ischemia and hypoxia. Ultimately, tubular necrosis and complete renal shutdown may occur (8). Therefore, renal function must be assessed carefully. Hourly intake and output measurements and urine-specific gravity must be documented and trends noted. Serum values of blood urea nitrogen, creatinine, and urine creatinine clearance must be assessed daily. In addition, serial urinalysis parameters will give useful information regarding kidney function (1, 8, 9).

## B. Nursing Diagnosis

Potential for infection related to disruption of skin integrity, presence of invasive lines and drains, and presence of extravasated blood and urine in the retroperitoneal space

### Goals of Care

● Decrease risk of infection.
● Patient will experience no undetected signs of infection.

### Nursing Interventions

● Clean operative and line and drain insertion sites according to institutional policy.
● Ensure strict aseptic technique during line and drain care.
● Monitor temperature, vital signs, and white blood cell count.
● Maintain patency of drainage systems.
● Monitor suture lines and invasive sites for redness, warmth, swelling, drainage, and odor.
● Assess urine for odor, color, and sediment, and monitor culture results.

### Rationale

Critically ill trauma patients are predisposed to infection. Risk factors such as hypovolemia, shock, tissue ischemia, and hematoma formation can alter the inflammatory response, potentiate tissue necrosis, and create an environment in which microorganisms thrive (10). The renal trauma patient, experiencing one or all of the above risk factors, will be predisposed to infection.

Postoperatively, the renal trauma patient has numerous invasive monitoring lines and drainage tubes. These may include Foley catheters, suprapubic catheters, nephrostomy tubes, Penrose drains, and sumps. Each is a potential avenue for infection. It is essential that strict aseptic technique be maintained during line and drain care (1, 10).

Foley catheter care is essential in preventing infection. Foley care with a povidone–iodine-based solution should be administered at least every 8 hours (1). The drainage system should remain closed and patent, with the tubing free of kinks and the drainage bag below the level of the patient at all times (1, 8, 10). Other line and drain sites should be cleaned according to institution policy.

Urine and blood extravasation into the retroperitoneal cavity may create a medium for bacterial growth (7). Consequently, the patient must be monitored for signs and symptoms of infection. Trends in white blood cell count, temperature, and vital signs must be noted. The surgical site and invasive line and drain sites must be assessed for redness, warmth, pain, swelling, drainage, and odor.

In addition, the urine must be assessed for color, odor, and evidence of sediment, and the results of urine cultures must be documented.

## ASSOCIATED NURSING DIAGNOSES

A. Knowledge deficit
B. Alterations in patterns of urinary elimination
C. Alterations in comfort
D. Ineffective airway clearance
E. Sleep pattern disturbance
F. Impaired tissue integrity
G. Anxiety

## REFERENCES

1. Cook LS. Genitourinary trauma. In: Cardona VD, Hurn PD, Bastnagel-Mason PJ, et al, eds. Trauma nursing: from resuscitation through rehabilitation. Philadelphia: WB Saunders, 1988:620–626.
2. Anonymous. G.U. trauma inside and out: The kidneys. Emerg Med 1985;17:25–27, 31–33, 35, 38–39.
3. Knezevich BA. Trauma nursing: Principles and practice. Norwalk, CT: Appleton-Century-Crofts, 1986:113–139.
4. Paulson DF. Genitourinary trauma. In: Moylan JA, ed. Trauma surgery. Philadelphia: JB Lippincott, 1987:309–316.
5. Frentz GD, Erich KL. Trauma to the urinary tract. In: McSwain NE Jr, Kerstein MD, eds. Evaluation and management of trauma. Norwalk, CT: Appleton-Century-Crofts, 1987:195–231.
6. Dunham CM, Cowley RA. Shock trauma/critical care handbook. Rockville, MD: Aspen, 1986:253–265.
7. Strange JM. Shock trauma care plans. Springhouse, PA: Springhouse, 1987:120–122.
8. Luckman J, Sorensen KC. Medical-surgical nursing: a psychophysiologic approach. Philadelphia: WB Saunders, 1987:227, 243–235, 1216–1218.
9. Cook LS. Renal trauma: a challenging assessment, a cause for cautious care. RN 1983:46, 58–63.
10. Hoyt NJ. Infection and infection control. In: Cardona VD, Hurn PD, Bastnagel-Mason PJ, et al, eds. Trauma nursing: from resuscitation through rehabilitation. Philadelphia: WB Saunders, 1988:229–232, 251–252.

# CHAPTER 21

## Acute Tubular Necrosis Requiring Hemodialysis

Shirley Roth, RN, MS, CCRN

## Clinical Presentation

A 24-year-old man was admitted to the hospital after falling while cliff climbing. His medical diagnoses included fractured pelvis, bilateral fractured femurs, ruptured spleen, multiple lacerations, contusions of the small bowel, and pulmonary contusion.

He was admitted with a blood pressure of 60 palpable and a pulse of 140. After successful fluid resuscitation, he was taken to surgery and underwent splenectomy, repair of small bowel lacerations, and pinning of bilateral fractured femurs.

On admission to the intensive care unit, hemodynamic parameters were monitored continuously via a left radial arterial line and subclavian pulmonary artery catheter. An infusion of $D_5$ ½ normal saline with KCl was administered through a peripheral intravenous catheter in his right forearm. An indwelling Foley catheter was in place. He was intubated and mechanically ventilated on $FiO_2$ of 0.4, tidal volume of 800 ml, and synchronized intermittent mechanical ventilation (SIMV) of 12 breaths/minute. Antibiotics and antacids were given over the next 5 days, during which his hospital course was unstable. He experienced several episodes of hypotension requiring fluid resuscitation as well as temperature elevations greater than 102°F (39°C) requiring sepsis evaluation. Additional complications were progressive hypoxemia with $PaO_2$ of 50 and declining renal functioning with a urinary output less than 30 ml/hr, blood urea nitrogen (BUN) of 100, and creatinine of 6.8 mg/dl.

His acute renal failure was thought to be related to acute tubular necrosis (ATN). After conservative treatment, including fluid replacement to improve hydration and renal perfusion and diuretics to increase urinary output, proved unsuccessful, hemodialysis was initiated.

### 1. What is the pathophysiological basis for this patient's problem?

Acute renal failure (ARF) is defined as a sudden deterioration in renal function which may occur over hours, days, or even weeks. ARF is usually, but not always, associated with oliguria (400 ml or less of urine in 24 hours). Common causes of ARF are ischemic, toxic, or obstructive injury to the kidney. These etiologies are categorized as prerenal, intrarenal, or postrenal. Prerenal factors are related to hypoperfusion states such as hypovolemia (large third-space loss, dehydration, hemorrhage), cardiovascular insufficiency (congestive heart failure, sepsis, shock), or bilateral renal artery occlusion. Intrarenal causes lead to renal parenchymal damage such as occurs in glomerular diseases, vasculitis, acute interstitial diseases, nephrotoxins, crush injuries, and hepatorenal syndrome. Postrenal factors are related to complete or incomplete obstruction of the urinary tract, such as occurs from renal calculi, tumors, prostatic hypertrophy, and surgical accidents (1, 2).

Seventy-five percent of all cases of ARF are related to ATN (2). Ischemia and exposure to nephrotoxic drugs are the major causes. Although the pathophysiology of ARF is not well understood, a number of hypotheses suggest that oliguria may result from

- Decreased glomerular filtration rate
- Increased renal vasoconstriction

- Intratubular obstruction due to fibrin, necrotic cells, pigments, and so on
- Back leak of glomerular filtrate into the interstitium and/or vasculature
- Renal cellular edema and no vascular reflow

ARF associated with nonoliguria (1000 ml of urine per day) may be related to an inability of the renal tubules to reabsorb glomerular filtrate.

There are three phases of acute renal failure: the oliguric phase, the diuretic phase, and the recovery phase. The oliguric phase occurs when the urinary output falls below 400 ml/day. Hyperkalemia, acidosis, hypocalcemia, hyperuricemia, hypermagnesemia, and edema occur during this phase. Anemia may also develop. Plasma creatinine usually rises 0.5 mg/day, and BUN rises 10 to 20 mg/day. Oliguria usually begins within hours of the insult and may last 1 to 4 weeks. The diuretic phase begins with a steadily increasing urinary volume, indicating tubular regeneration; but renal function remains impaired, as evidenced by continually elevated creatinine and BUN levels. Diagnosis of ARF is based on clinical findings of poor urine output in response to fluid challenge or diuretics in the oliguric phase and ineffective concentrating ability in the high output phase, as evidenced by urine Na <20 mEq/liter and specific gravity <1.010 (2). During the last phase, the recovery phase, the urine is concentrated, which indicates returning tubular function. The blood creatinine and BUN levels return to normal. Renal function continues to improve over the next 3 to 12 months or longer (2, 3).

Recovery from ARF is related to several factors, including the patient's preinjury health, age, underlying disease processes, timing of interventions, and the patient's response to these interventions. The principal cause of death is related to sepsis and the illness or injury that precipitated the renal failure (1).

Patient management includes diagnosing and correcting the underlying cause, reestablishing normal urine flow, optimizing intravascular volume and cardiac output, and maintaining electrolyte as well as acid-base balances (3, 4). If these care strategies are ineffective, dialysis may be required. This approach may include hemodialysis, peritoneal dialysis, or continuous arterial/venous hemofiltration (CAVH).

Dialysis is the diffusion of dissolved particles through a semipermeable membrane separating two solutions. The solutes removed are the end products of metabolism (1, 5).

Dialysis is indicated in patients with ATN when uremia progresses to a point where it can no longer be controlled by conservative medical measures. Uremic symptoms include neurological impairment, uremic pericarditis, fluid overload, hyperkalemia, and/or severe metabolic acidosis (Table 21.1.).

Hemodialysis rapidly shifts the patient's plasma levels toward normal by quickly removing unwanted solutes and fluid. One hemodialysis treatment usually lasts 3 to 4 hours. When the patient has severe fluid overload and/or a hypercatabolic state, the treatments are done daily. If the patient is stable, then treatments are performed less frequently. Hemodialysis provides rapid removal of solutes and is therefore the treatment of choice in emergency situations, including poisoning, pulmonary edema, and hyperkalemia (1).

Hemodialysis is also indicated when peritoneal dialysis is contraindicated, such as in patients who are unable to accept a peritoneal catheter because of multiple abdominal adhesions, abdominal infections, diaphragmatic leaks, or damaged peritoneal membrane.

**Table 21.1.** Patient problems associated with increased nitrogenous wastes—creatinine, urea, organic acid[a]

Metallic taste
Stimulation of chemoreceptor trigger zone, leading to nausea and vomiting
Vagal or sympathetic stimulation due to irritation of gastric mucosa by nitrogenous waste
Muscle cramps due to nerve irritation
Paresthesias related to peripheral neuropathies
Stomatitis—excessive salivary urea converted to ammonia by the enzyme urease, which is
    present in bacteria on teeth; ammonia irritates mucosa
Dry skin and pruritus due to atrophy of sweat glands, subcutaneous precipitation of calcium
    phosphate crystals, and presence of urate crystals on skin (uremic frost)
Depressed immune response
Decreased number of effective platelets and clotting, factors III and VIII
Dysrhythmias
Pericarditis associated with irritation of pericardium from accumulated nitrogenous wastes
Impotence

[a]*Source*: Adapted from Ulrich S, Canale S, Wendell S. Nursing care planning guides: a nursing diagnosis approach. Philadelphia: WB Saunders, 1986:402–429.

## 2. What are the nursing diagnoses of highest priority?

A. Alterations in fluid volume: deficit or excess
B. Alterations in thought processes
C. Potential for infection
D. Alterations in cardiac output

## 3. What goals of care and nursing interventions are appropriate for the above diagnoses?

### A. Nursing Diagnosis

Alterations in fluid volume: deficit or excess related to the effects of ultrafiltration during hemodialysis and the inability of the kidneys to remove excess fluid

### Goal of Care

Fluid volume within normal limits

### Nursing Interventions

- Assess cardiovascular status including weight, blood pressure, central venous pressure/pulmonary artery wedge pressure (CVP/PAWP), heart sounds, quality of peripheral pulses, breath sounds, peripheral edema, intake and output, and current medication.
- Be prepared to treat potentially unstable blood pressures that may occur while large amounts of fluids are removed during ultrafiltration.
- Monitor for signs and symptoms of hypovolemia during dialysis, including hypotension, tachycardia, decreased CVP/PAWP, and altered level of consciousness.
- Be prepared for early treatment, including
    Trendelenburg positioning
    – Fluid replacement
    – Intravenous administration of osmotic agents such as mannitol or albumin
    – Administration of inotropic drugs

### Rationale

The patient with ATN requiring hemodialysis will experience increasing fluid volumes between dialysis treatments. Problems associated with hemodialysis are listed in Table 21.2. The need to remove this excess fluid during dialysis predisposes the patient to episodes of hypotension. Water is first removed from the plasma, after which the water shifts from interstitial spaces and cells into the plasma. If the rate of ultrafiltration from

**Table 21.2.** Problems associated with hemodialysis[a]

| Problem | Possible Etiologies |
|---|---|
| Anemia due to hemolysis | Dialysate bath too hot or cold, inadequate heparinization, improper dialysate concentration, turbulent flow, blood reaction |
| Air embolus | Loose tubing connections, improper priming of filter, air detector malfunction |
| Shunt failure | Infection, clotting, kinking, aneurysm formation, vessel sclerosing, vessels are too small or do not dilate |
| Congestive heart failure | Hypervolemia between treatments |
| Angina | Hypotension due to too-rapid filtration, anxiety |
| Arrhythmias | Rapid potassium shifts, hypotension |
| Hemorrhage | Accidental disconnection, inadvertent systemic overheparinization |
| Hypertension | Fluid overload, anxiety, disequilibrium syndrome |
| Disequilibrium syndrome | Disorientation caused by cerebral edema, rapid dialysis |
| Poor flow | Vessel spasm, immature vessel or small vessels, improper needle positioning, too-small needle size |
| Hypotension | Diversion of 300 ml of blood initially into machine, antihypertensives block sympathetic vasoconstriction, kinked tubing, filter damage with blood leak |
| Infection | Poor aseptic technique, contamination of dialyzer |
| Seizures | Disequilibrium syndrome, hypotension |

[a]*Sources*: Adapted from:
Johanson B, Dungga C, Hoffmeister D, Well S. Standards of critical care. St Louis: CV Mosby, 1981:378–388.
Ulrich S, Canale S, Wendell S. Nursing care planning guides: a nursing diagnosis approach. Philadelphia: WB Saunders, 1986:402–429.
Cairoli O, Voyce P. Memory bank for hemodialysis. Pacific Palisades, CA: Nurseco, 1982:50–89.
Millar S, Sampson L, Soukop M. AACN procedure manual for critical care. Philadelphia: WB Saunders, 1985:319.

the vascular space is greater than the refill rate from the interstitium and cells, then hypovolemic hypotension will occur (1). An osmotic agent such as mannitol or albumin can facilitate the movement of fluid from the extravascular space to the plasma. If hypotension is prolonged or severe, normal saline can be administered to restore volume. If hypotension fails to respond to IV fluids, an inotropic drug may be necessary to maintain blood pressure during dialysis.

If blood pressure support cannot be maintained during dialysis, treatment must be discontinued and attempted again at a later time.

## B. Nursing Diagnosis

Alteration in neurological status related to cerebral edema

### Goal of Care

Decrease risk of neurological disequilibrium.

### Nursing Interventions

- Perform a baseline neurological assessment.
- Monitor for signs of increased intracranial pressure during the dialysis treatments and for several hours thereafter.
  - If patient is awake, instruct him or her to report headache and/or nausea during the treatment.
  - If patient is disoriented, uncooperative, or confused, closely monitor for signs of decreasing cerebral functioning.

– If patient is comatose, monitor for signs of increased intracranial pressure, including hypertension, bradycardia, and widening pulse pressure.
• Be prepared for early treatment of neurological disequilibrium, including
  – Intravenous administration of osmotic agents such as mannitol or albumin
  – Administration of anticonvulsant drugs
  – Decreasing dialysis treatment times

## Rationale

The patient with ATN requiring hemodialysis is predisposed to dialysis disequilibrium syndome; cerebral edema is thought to be the major cause. Urea is cleared more slowly from cerebrospinal fluid than from plasma, resulting in acidic cerebrospinal fluid. This altered pH may impair mentation. Intracellular acidosis of brain tissue increases osmolarity, resulting in cerebral edema and further alteration in neurological function (4).

Disequilibrium syndrome may occur in highly uremic patients toward the end of dialysis or after cessation of treatment. The patient may exhibit symptoms of increased intracranial pressures, including headache, nausea and vomiting, restlessness, disorientation, changes in sensorium, twitching, and/or seizures. Untreated symptoms may lead to coma or death (1, 5).

The effects of disequilibrium syndromes may be diminished or prevented by initiating dialysis before severe biochemical disturbances occur. If correction of plasma urea is too rapid, osmotic agents such as mannitol, albumin, and hypertonic saline may be administered (6).

Shorter, more frequent dialysis treatments are the preferred method for prevention of disequilibrium syndrome; if this approach is not feasible, anticonvulsant drugs may be effective as a preventive measure. Phenytoin is used as a preventive and treatment modality, whereas intravenous diazepam is used for the suppression of acute seizure activity.

## C. Nursing Diagnosis

Potential for infection related to immune system compromise

## Goal of Care

Decrease risk of infection.

## Nursing Interventions

• Monitor patient for signs and symptoms of infection, including fever, increased white blood cell count, a change in wound appearance or drainage, or a change in the chest x-ray film.
• Invasive monitoring lines should be removed as soon as they are no longer needed, or the sites should be rotated every 3 to 4 days according to institution policy.
• Meticulous care should be given to all invasive line sites and wounds.

## Rationale

Infection is the most common cause of death in ARF. Nitrogeous end products of protein metabolism, i.e., urea, uric acid, decrease the phagocytic and chemotactic activities of the neutrophils. These alterations in the body's normal defense mechanisms result in an increased susceptibility to infections as well as a decreased ability to fight them (3).

Steps should be taken to prevent infections. This includes the avoidance of invasive procedures whenever possible. For example, once renal failure has been diagnosed and it is no longer necessary to monitor hourly urinary output, the indwelling catheter may be discontinued and intermittent catheterizations employed (4, 7).

## D. Nursing Diagnosis

Alterations in cardiac output related to uremic or dialysis-related pericarditis, pericardial effusion, or pericardial tamponade

### Goal of Care

Restore or maintain adequate cardiac output.

### Nursing Interventions

- Monitor for signs and symptoms of uremic pericarditis, including
  - Fever or leukocytosis
  - Sternal chest pain sometimes radiating to the neck and shoulders (this pain is aggravated by deep breathing or laying flat)
  - Friction rub, best heard at the left midsternal area during systole
- Monitor for signs and symptoms of pericardial effusion, including
- - Paradoxical pulse greater than 10 mm Hg
  - Unexplainable hypotension
  - Increased central venous pressures with increased jugular vein distension
  - Weakened peripheral pulses
  - Narrowed pulse pressure
- In the event of cardiac tamponade, be prepared for emergency pericardiocentesis.

### Rationale

Pericarditis occurs in approximately 5% of the ARF population. If left untreated, it may lead to hemorrhagic pericardial effusion and cardiac tamponade.

In renal failure, the pericardial sac may become inflamed by nitrogeous end products of protein metabolism, bacteria, or viruses, causing the pericardial layers to rub together during contraction rather than gliding over each other. Often the inflammatory process of pericarditis will precipitate effusion of fluid and blood into the pericardial space (1, 5).

## ASSOCIATED NURSING DIAGNOSES

A. Alterations in comfort
B. Alterations in bowel elimination
C. Alterations in nutrition
D. Impaired gas exchange
E. Fear
F. Knowledge deficit

**REFERENCES**

1. Schoengrund L. Renal problems in critical care. New York: Wiley Medical Publications, 1984.
2. Johanson B, Dungga C, Hoffmeister D, Well S. Standards of critical care. St Louis: CV Mosby, 1981:378–388.
3. Kinney M, Dear C, Packa D, Voorman D. AACN's clinical reference for critical care nursing. New York: McGraw-Hill, 1981.
4. Ulrich S, Canale S, Wendell S. Nursing care planning guides: a nursing diagnosis approach. Philadelphia: WB Saunders, 1986:402–429.
5. Nurses Clinical Library. Nursing 84 Books. Renal and urologic disorders. Springhouse, PA: Springhouse, 1984:67.
6. Blagg C. Acute complications associated with hemodialysis. In: Drukker W, ed. Replacement of renal function by dialysis. Lancaster: Martinus Nijhoff Publishers, 1986:612.
7. Brennan DT. Standards of clinical practice for nephrology nursing. Pitman, NJ: Anthony J Jannette, 1988:67.

# CHAPTER 22

## Acute Renal Failure Treated with Continuous Arteriovenous Hemofiltration

Nancy L. Palmer, RN, CCRN

## Clinical Presentation

A 71-year-old man was transported via air to the hospital following a motor vehicle accident. Details of the accident were unknown. The patient was trapped in the vehicle for 1 to 2 hours prior to extrication.

The patient was awake and lethargic but could be aroused by painful stimuli. He was intubated immediately, secondary to cyanosis, shallow respirations, and a palpable blood pressure of 80.

Admission laboratory studies showed a $PaO_2$ of 76 mm Hg, pH of 7.37, $PaCO_2$ of 30 mm Hg, $O_2$ saturation of 95%, $FiO_2$ of 1.0, and positive end-expiratory pressure (PEEP) of 5 cm. Hemoglobin and hematocrit were 8.7 and 28.6, respectively. Sodium was 138, potassium 4.4, serum osmolality 290, blood sugar 183, blood urea nitrogen (BUN) 14, and creatinine 1.7. Chest x-ray showed clear lungs bilaterally.

The patient sustained massive crush injuries with degloving of the left lateral thigh and calf, and bilateral open fracture dislocation of the ankles. Diagnostic tests included head and abnominal computerized tomography (CT) scans, x-rays of cervical, thoracic, lumbar spine, and both lower extremities; an angiogram of the thoracic aorta; and an arteriogram of both lower extremities.

After initial resuscitation, evaluation, and stabilization the patient was taken to the operating room for exploration and debridement of his leg wounds. External fixation devices were applied to stabilize both ankles. The left wrist was splinted and the scalp laceration was sutured.

A pulmonary artery catheter was inserted in the operating room and showed a pulmonary artery mean of 28, a pulmonary capillary wedge pressure (PCWP) of 11, a central venous pressure (CVP) of 8, and a cardiac output of 4.1 liters/minute. The patient's blood pressure ranged from 90/50 to 120/60. His heart rate was 55 beats/minute, with regular sinus bradycardia. Dopamine infusion was started at 6 μg/kg/minute, along with dobutamine at 12 μg/kg/minute. Blood pressure increased to 135/70, heart rate increased to 80 beats/minute, and cardiac output increased to 6.3 liters/minute.

Fluid resuscitation in the emergency department and operating room included 2000 cc normal saline, 3000 cc Ringer's lactate, 500 cc Plasmanate, 7 units of packed cells, and 6 units of fresh frozen plasma. Estimated blood loss was 3000 cc. Urine output was 2430 cc. Total fluid intake was 8870 cc and total output was 5430 cc, yielding a positive fluid balance of 3440 cc.

Ten hours after admission the patient was admitted to the intensive care unit (ICU). Despite initial postoperative hypothermia, the patient spiked a temperature of 38.5° C (102.6° F) in the first 24 hours after admission. Cultures of the patient's blood, sputum, urine, and leg wounds were sent to the laboratory. Antibiotic coverage with Keflex 2 gm/day IV had been initiated in the operating room to treat tissue contamination from the bilateral open ankle fractures and was continued for 48 hours. The patient's fever was treated with acetaminophen 650 mg per rectum and a cooling blanket.

Over the next 3 days the patient's hemodynamic status deteriorated, with clinical and laboratory findings indicative of sepsis (see Chapter 31). The patient continued to require additional ventilatory support on a volume-cycled ventilator. Renal function deteriorated as evidenced by the patient's urinary creatinine clearance, which significantly dropped each day. Urine output ranged from 10 to 40 cc/hr on the fourth day after admission. An above-the-knee amputation of the left leg was performed in an aggressive attempt to eliminate a septic foci. Postoperatively, vascular access lines were placed to begin hemofiltration to treat the impending renal failure.

## 1. What is the pathophysiological basis for this patient's problem?

Many trauma patients survive their initial injuries only to succumb to overwhelming septicemia in the posttraumatic phase. Reasons for increased risk of infection posttrauma include the following (1):

- Shock states alter the immune response, so normally nonpathogenic organisms may have a pathogenic effect.
- Hospital-acquired organisms may be of a highly resistant nature.
- Invasive procedures compromise body defenses by providing ports of entry for bacteria.
- While treating one organism, antibiotic therapy may allow another organism to proliferate.
- Bloody or serous wound drainage provides an excellent medium for bacterial growth.

The source of this patient's septic state was most likely the left leg degloving injury. The initial hypovolemia from trauma and vasodilation in septic shock led to tissue hypoperfusion, which is a frequent cause of renal failure. In addition, crush and degloving injuries release myoglobin and hemoglobin from damaged muscle, which can precipitate in the renal tubules, causing tubular necrosis (see Chapter 18). Acute renal failure occurs commonly in the settings of surgery, trauma, sepsis, and hypotension; two or more of these problems may exist concomitantly as they do in this patient (2).

Acute renal failure describes any abrupt deterioration of renal function (2). The various causes of acute renal failure are classified as prerenal, intrarenal, and postrenal; examples of clinical conditions associated with these etiologies are listed in Table 22.1. The overall mortality rate of acute renal failure is 50%, but in selected settings, such as ruptured abdominal aortic aneurysm, it may be 90% or greater (3).

Prerenal failure is caused by factors outside the kidney that decrease renal blood flow either by vasoconstriction or by reduction in blood pressure. This decreased blood flow reduces glomerular perfusion and can be caused by hypovolemia associated with hemorrhage, burns, cardiac insufficiency, and septic shock, or by renal artery obstruction by a thrombus or an embolus.

Postrenal failure is caused by obstruction of the urinary tract flow at any point along its course. Blockage can be from calculi, tumors, or trauma. Urine backs up into the renal pelvis and parenchyma, resulting in anuria.

The etiology of intrarenal failure include diseases such as acute glomerulonephritis and acute pyelonephritis, and systemic diseases such as disseminated lupus erythematous. In the trauma patient, intrarenal failure may be due to myoglobinuria, hemoglobinuria, or aninoglycosides. There is damage to the renal parenchymal tissue itself, resulting in malfunctioning of the nephrons. This problem leads to a condition commonly known as acute tubular necrosis (ATN). ATN can follow major surgery, crush lesions, major trauma, incompatible blood transfusions, and septicemia.

Pathophysiological changes that occur in ATN vary with the cause. For example,

**Table 22.1.** Common etiologies of acute renal failure[a]

| Classification | Examples of Clinical Conditions |
|---|---|
| **Prerenal** | |
| Hypovolemia | Vascular loss—hemorrhage |
| | Gastrointestinal loss—vomiting, diarrhea |
| | Renal loss—diuretic abuse, osmotic diuresis associated with diabetes |
| | Integumentary loss—burns, diaphoresis |
| Cardiovascular failure | Myocardial infarction |
| | Tamponade |
| | Vascular pooling—sepsis |
| | Vascular occlusion—thrombosis, embolism |
| **Postrenal** | |
| Obstruction | Ureteral—fibrosis, calculi, crystals, clots, accidental ligation |
| | Bladder—neoplasms |
| | Urethral—stricture, prostatic hypertrophy |
| **Parenchymal** | |
| Glomerulonephritis | Acute poststreptococcal, systemic lupus erythematosus, Goodpasture's syndrome, bacterial endocarditis |
| Vasculitis | Periarteritis, hypersensitivity angiitis |
| Interstitial nephritis | Acute pyelonephritis, allergic nephritis, hypercalcemia, uric acid nephropathy, myeloma of the kidney |
| Renal vascular disease | Renal artery occlusion, renal vein thrombosis |
| Acute tubular necrosis | |
| Postischemia | Hypovolemia, cardiogenic shock, endotoxic shock |
| Nephrotoxins | Heavy metals, organic solvents, glycols, antibiotics, anesthetics, radiographic contrast media |
| Pigments | |
| Hemoglobin | Intravascular hemolysis—transfusion reactions, toxic hemolysis |
| Myoglobin | Rhabdomyolysis—trauma, muscle disease, seizures, severe exercise, prolonged coma |

[a]*Source*: Baer CL. Acute renal failure. Newport Beach, CA: American Association of Critical Care Nurses, 1989:408.

during renal ischemia the tubular cells are damaged from lack of oxygen and slough off, plugging the tubules.

As tubular cells are damaged, there are changes in renal functioning. These changes are most often reflected in a decrease in urine output. Urine output less than 400 ml in 24 hours is oliguria; anuria is urine output less than 50 ml in 24 hours. The accumulation of nitrogenous wastes (azotemia) is reflected in the elevation of BUN and creatinine. Azotemia may begin even before urinary output decreases.

Renal failure will usually be detected prior to oliguria if a daily urine creatinine clearance is performed. Creatinine clearance primarily reflects glomerular function. During the first 3 to 5 days postinjury, a low creatinine clearance implies inadequate cardiac output or renal parenchymal damage from the initial shock state. A fall in creatinine clearance after the first 3 to 5 days is likely to reflect inadequate cardiac output, sepsis, or nephrotoxicity from drugs (4).

Acute renal failure may be reversible with successful treatment, resulting in minimal residual dysfunction. Great care should be devoted to minimizing sepsis in patients with acute renal failure, since sepsis is the major cause of death in these patients. The first clinical phase of renal failure, the oliguric phase, lasts from 1 to 4 weeks. Following this phase there is a period of diuresis, during which urine gradually increases. Renal function is still abnormal, but the glomerular filtration rate starts to recover. The period of recovery begins as renal function gradually improves, and it may last from 3 to 12 months. There is usually a permanent, partial loss of some glomerular filtration rate and concentrating ability.

In the critical care setting the treatment of renal failure may be hemodialysis, peritoneal dialysis, or continuous arteriovenous hemofiltration (CAVH). The choice will depend on the patient's injuries and the stability of his or her hemodynamic status.

## 2. What are the nursing diagnoses of highest priority?
A. Potential for infection
B. Fluid volume excess

## 3. What are the goals of nursing care?

### A. Nursing Diagnosis
Potential for infection related to alteration of skin integrity

### Goal of Care
Recognize early signs of infection.

### Nursing Interventions
● Nursing interventions are described fully in Chapter 31, Septic Shock in the Trauma Patient.

### B. Nursing Diagnosis
Fluid volume excess related to overhydration

### Goal of Care
Restore and maintain normovolemic state.

### Nursing Interventions
● Insert indwelling Foley catheter on physician order.
● Measure intake and output hourly.
● Obtain baseline laboratory data and repeat as ordered.
● Administer IV diuretics as ordered.
● Initiate and maintain CAVH.
 – Prime hemofiltering device according to manufacturer's instruction.
 – Assist with insertion of vascular lines for hemofiltration.
 – Prepare and infuse replacement therapy.
 – Administer heparin bolus dose and start heparin infusion.
 – Maintain adequate systemic blood pressure—mean arterial pressure (MAP) greater than 60 mm Hg.
 – Position hemofilter securely; maintain visibility at all times.
 – Record hourly filtration rate.
 – Monitor ultrafiltrate for occult blood.
 – Monitor for signs of a clotted filter.
 – Monitor electrolytes and partial thromboplastin time (PPT): every 4 hours × 2, every 8 hours × 3, then every 12 hours during the course of CAVH.
 – Check pulse distal to access line every 4 hours.

### Rationale
CAVH is an extracorporeal technique for use in preventing or alleviating hypervolemia and/or toxic solute accumulation in patients with acute renal failure. This technique uses an extracorporeal circuit that blood enters through an arterial access, flows through a hemofilter, and re-enters the body through a venous acccess line.

**Table 22.2.** Indications, advantages, and disadvantages of CAVH[a]

*Indications*
Pulmonary edema with cardiogenic shock
Oliguria unresponsive to diuretics
Massive fluid overload
Respiratory compromise with acute renal failure (ARF)
Hemodynamic instability making hemodialysis unfeasible
Parenteral nutrition restricted because of hypervolemia
ARF following abdominal surgery making PD unfeasible

*Advantages*
Continuous gradual treatment
Allows flexibility in fluid balance
Less technical training than hemodialysis
More reliable and rapid than PD

*Disadvantages*
Requires two large-bore vascular access sites
Infections
Bleeding problems due to anticoagulation
Requires strict monitoring of patient
Potential blood loss from filter

---

[a]*Source:* Adapted from:
Kaplan AA, Longnecker RE, Fulkert VW. Continuous arteriovenous hemofiltration. Ann Intern Med 1984:358–367.
Golper TA. Continuous arteriovenous hemofiltration in acute renal failure. J Kid Dis 1985;VI(6):373–386.

CAVH removes plasma water and dissolved solutes from the intravascular fluid while allowing conservation of the cellular and protein components of the circulating blood. Net filtration pressure inside the filter causes an ultrafiltrate to form. CAVH removes fluid slowly and continuously over a 24-hour period. It is not effective for the rapid removal of toxic substances such as drug overdoses.

This process is slow, relative to conventional hemodialysis; rapid electrolyte shift does not occur, and there are no wide fluctuations in vital signs. Therefore, critically ill patients may be more hemodynamically stable using CAVH than with other fluid removal strategies. In addition, the extracorporeal circuit can be kept in place for hours or even days. CAVH is a temporizing procedure that can be used until the kidneys resume normal function (5). Certain clinical conditions often seen in the ICU, such as congestive heart failure, pulmonary edema, hepatorenal syndrome, and hypervolemia respond well to CAVH (6, 7). Table 22.2 lists other selected features of CAVH.

The CAVH system relies primarily on the patient's own arteriovenous pressure gradient. A MAP of at least 60 mm Hg and a normal central venous pressure are necessary to maintain blood flow through the system (7). If the patient has a high central venous pressure, indicating high venous resistance, a higher blood pressure may be necessary to maintain this gradient; inotropic support may be necessary to achieve or maintain gradient.

Nursing responsibilities include assisting the physician with insertion of vascular access lines for CAVH and maintenance and monitoring the CAVH system as well as the patient's response to it. The femoral artery and vein are frequently used insertion sites. The femoral site provides easy percutaneous entry and improved filter flow because of the large lumen size. Despite a MAP greater than the recommended 60 mm Hg, an arterial catheter lumen less than 16 gauge does not permit effective system functioning (5). Prior to catheter insertion, the CAVH filter

**Table 22.3.** Signs of filter clotting[a]

A decrease in the hourly ultrafiltration rate
Relative coolness to touch of the venous tubing as compared to the arterial tubing
A decline in the ratio of dialysate to plasma BUN or creatinine. The filter is usually changed
when the ratio decreases to 0.5. (The highest possible ratio is 1.0)
Gravity separation of blood into cells and plasma in the blood tubing (a late sign
necessitating immediate filter change to prevent access clotting)

[a]*Source*: Adapted from Lawyer L. Clinical experience and application of continuous arteriovenous hemodialysis in the intensive care unit. Third International Symposium on Acute Continuous Renal Replacement Therapy, 1987.

should be primed according to the manufacturer's instructions. The patient may be started on a low-dose heparin drip through the arterial side of the system. Anticoagulation improves blood flow and prevents filter clotting, thus prolonging filter life. The goal of the heparin infusion is to prevent clotting of blood within the filter without causing systemic anticoagulation in the patient, with the latter being problematic in multisystem injured patients. Usually a loading dose of heparin ranging from 500 to 2000 units is given prior to starting the heparin infusion (5). The heparin infusion may be titrated according to the patient's coagulation status; 50 units/hr to 100 units/hr is a typical dosage range in the trauma patient (7). Occasionally CAVH will be attempted without heparinization, depending on the patient's clinical status. Using the venous side of the system for administration of replacement IV fluid or hyperalimentation will help maintain the patency of the venous catheter.

Additional nursing responsibilities prior to the initiation of CAVH are documentation of baseline vital signs and hemodynamic parameters. These include heart rate, blood pressure, MAP, cardiac output, PCWP and CVP, and they should be accessed hourly during CAVH. Baseline laboratory data include serum chemistries, liver function, and coagulation studies.

The physician will connect the hemofilter circuit to the arterial and venous access lines. The arterial side is attached first. Blood is allowed to fill the filter before connecting to the venous access to prevent bolusing with priming solution. Allow 5 minutes to lapse after attaching both sides before opening the ultrafiltrate ports, as this pause ensures adequate blood flow (8). Perform IV catheter care according to hospital protocol. Secure the hemofilter to the patient to prevent any tension or kinking of lines. Check all connections for tightness to prevent leaks or accidental disconnections; non-Luer-Lok connections should be taped. Accidental disconnections are a serious complication, as exsanguination will rapidly occur (8).

Ongoing patient assessment continues throughout CAVH treatment. Monitor vital signs closely. Notify the physician immediately for severe hypotension. Replacement fluids are usually ordered and will need regulation on an hourly basis, depending on the rate of ultrafiltration. Record the replacement fluid and ultrafiltrate on the intake and output flow sheet. Monitor electrolytes every 4 hours × 2, every 8 hours × 3, then every 12 hours. Check pulses distal to the access sites every 4 hours to ensure perfusion distally to the limb.

To maintain adequate blood flow the hemofilter must be placed below the level of the heart. The greatest possible vertical distance between filter and ultafiltrate drainage bag should be maintained to increase the "pull" of fluid through the filter. Elevating the bed to the highest level will help achieve this maximum distance.

Always keep the hemofilter visible and never obscured by dressings or bed linen, to facilitate frequent filter monitoring for cell separation and air in the system.

**Table 22.4.** Factors affecting ultrafiltrate rate[a]

| |
| --- |
| Hydrostatic pressure |
| Venous return |
| Serum oncotic pressure |
| Blood viscosity |
| Length and gauge of blood tubing |
| Filter surface area |
| Ultrafiltrate column height |
| Ultrafiltrate suction level |
| Intrinsic filter membrane characteristics |

[a]*Source:* Adapted from Golper TA. Arteriovenous hemofiltration in acute renal failure. Am J Kid Dis 1985;VI(6):373–386.

Hypotensive episodes may precipitate clotting within the filter. A gradual decrease in the rate of ultrafiltrate is the first indication of this problem. Other indications of clotting of the filter are listed in Table 22.3. Factors affecting the ultrafiltration flow rate are delineated in Table 22.4.

At least once every hour, check the ultrafiltrate for occult blood, which would indicate a rupture of fibers in the filter. If blood is present, clamp the ultrafiltrate tubing and notify the physician. Begin priming a new filter. In the interim, to assure patency of the venous and arterial access lines in the event of clotting or fiber rupture, the physician will attach each side to a heparinized saline infusion using a pressurized flush delivery system or an infusion pump. Clamps and access line connections should be readily accessible at the bedside for an emergency situation.

## ASSOCIATED NURSING DIAGNOSES

A. Impaired physical mobility
B. Potential for alterations in cardiac output
C. Anxiety
D. Impairment of skin integrity

**REFERENCES**

1. Childs CS. Vasogenic shock. In: Strange JM, ed. Shock trauma care plans. Springhouse, PA: Springhouse. 1987:22.
2. Oken DE, Wolfert AI, Gehr TWB. The pathosphysiology and differential diagnosis of acute renal failure. In: Shoemaker WC, Ayres S, Grenvik A, et al, eds. Textbook of critical care. Philadelphia: WB Saunders. 1989:712.
3. Beck C. Disordered renal function: diagnosis. In: Civetee JM, Taylor RW, Kirby RR, eds. Critical care. Philadelphia: JB Lippincott. 1988:1315.
4. Dunham CM, Cowley RA. Shock trauma/critical care handbook. Rockville, MD: Aspen. 1986:508.
5. Price CA: Continuous arteriovenous ultrafiltration: A monitoring guide for ICU nurses. Crit Care Nurse 1989;9(1):12–19.
6. Kaplan A. CAVH: An alternative to dialysis in the intensive care setting. VA Practitioner. 1984.
7. Paradiso C. Hemofiltration: An alternative to dialysis. Heart Lung 1989;18(3):282–290.
8. Palmer JC, Koorejian K, London JB, et al. Nursing management of continuous arteriovenous hemofiltration for acute renal failure. Focus Care 1986;13(5):23.

# PART 6

**Musculoskeletal Injuries/
Complications**

# CHAPTER 23

## Compartment Syndrome following Extremity Injury: Muscle Rupture and Femur Fracture

Robbi Lynn Hartsock, RN, MSN, CCRN

## Clinical Presentation

### Case I (1)

While pitching for his softball team, a 30-year-old man noticed a "pop" in his arm that produced intense pain. As the evening progressed, his discomfort worsened, and he presented to the emergency department (ED). Because his x-rays were normal, he was told to elevate the arm in a sling and was sent home. Several hours later, he returned to the ED with increased pain, but again was sent home because of lack of diagnostic findings.

The following day he presented to a second ED with massive swelling in his arm, exquisite pain, and paresthesias with distal neurocirculatory and functional compromise. He was diagnosed as having gas gangrene and was referred to a third facility for hyperbaric oxygen (HBO) therapy. On arrival, he was evaluated and found to have significant swelling, tenseness, and severe pain. Direct measurement of compartment pressures was done and compartment syndrome was diagnosed. Emergency fasciotomy and exploration revealed a ruptured medial head of the triceps muscle. After a short convalescence, the patient made a full recovery without neuromuscular deficit.

### Case II (1)

A 22-year-old man was involved in a single-car motor vehicle accident in which he was ejected from the automobile. He sustained a severe closed head injury (CHI), a closed right femur fracture, and a contusion of the right lower leg. He presented to the resuscitation area with a Glasgow Coma Scale (GCS) score of 4 and was emergently intubated and resuscitated for symptoms of neurogenic shock. X-rays demonstrated a right femur fracture, but were negative for right tibia/fibula fracture. Because of the severity of his head injury and increasing intracranial pressure, operative therapy for the femur fracture was deferred. A tibial pin was inserted, a long-leg cast was applied, and his leg was elevated in cast-roller (Neufeld's) traction. He was transported to the intensive care unit (ICU), where he continued to have massive cerebral swelling with intracranial pressure problems. His GCS remained at 4. Approximately 3 days later, the nurses noted sluggish capillary refill times (CRT) in the right foot and reported this finding to the orthopedic surgeons. The surgeons did not concur with this assessment, and no medical intervention occurred. On day 5, there were obvious delays in the CRT of the right foot as well as an unexplained fever. At that time the cast was removed, compartment syndrome was diagnosed, and immediate fasciotomy was per-

**155**

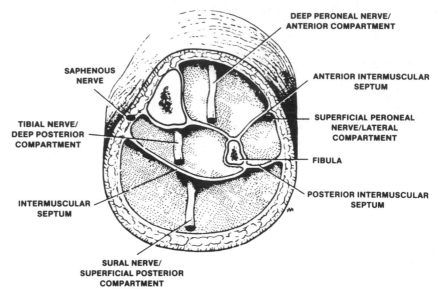

**Figure 23.1.** Cross-section at junction of the middle and distal thirds of the leg, illustrating the four compartments and their respective nerves. (Source: Adapted from Mubarak SJ, Owen CA. Double incision fasciotomy of the leg for decompression in compartment syndromes. J Bone Join Surg 1977;59:184.)

formed. On day 7, however, the leg was determined to be nonviable and was amputated in the operating room.

## 1. What are the pathophysiological bases for these patients' problems?

Muscle groups are surrounded by dense layers of semirigid fascia that form compartments (Fig. 23.1). Contained within the compartments are bones, muscle tissue, and vasculature, as well as nerves. Because the fascia literally surrounds these compartments in a fairly inflexible envelope, increases in pressure within it can compromise vascular and neuromuscular function.

A rise in compartment pressure may be due to an increase in compartment contents or to a decrease in the compartment size. Regardless of the etiology, an unchecked rise in compartment pressure may eventually exceed the microcirculation pressure within the compartment, and muscle tissue ischemia begins. Thus, the term *compartment syndrome* refers to a condition in which neuromuscular and circulatory compromise result from increased compartment pressure and subsequent ischemia due to a variety of etiological factors.

Although any space surrounded by fascia can potentially be at risk for compartment syndrome, the compartments of the forearm and lower leg are most commonly affected (2). Both external and internal predisposing factors are listed in Table 23.1.

Clinical findings vary with the compartment(s) involved, but in general, compartment syndrome almost always involves pain disproportionate to the injury. There is also an increase in the pain on passive stretching of the involved muscle groups. In addition, both light touch and two-point discrimination are diminished early in the course of compartment syndrome (2–6). As illustrated in Case II, however, neither pain nor changes in neurosensory function can be determined in the presence of decreased level

**Table 23.1.** Predisposing factors for the development of compartment syndrome

---

**External**—*Cause: Decrease in compartment size*

Surgical closure of muscle fascia defects
Circumferential dressings or casts
Prolonged, localized external pressure (i.e., extended extrication time, long operative
  procedures)
Prolonged use of medical antishock trousers (MAST)
Crush injury
Open fractures
Circumferential burns
Prolonged compression of a limb during an unconcious state

**Internal**—*Cause: Increase in compartment contents*
Revascularization of injured extremity
Infiltration of an IV catheter
Increased capillary permeability (i.e., burns, intracompartmental hemorrhage)
Soft tissue or muscle edema
Injury of or injection into arterial vessel
Closed fractures
Snake bites
Impaired arterial and venous circulation to an extremity (i.e., prolonged intra-aortic balloon
  pump (IABP) placement)
Arterial embolism
Reduction of long-bone fracture
Vigorous exercise

---

of consciousness. Spinal cord injury or general anesthesia also preclude pain or neuro-sensory assessment.

Palpable tension or firmness of the involved compartment and paresthesias in the involved nerve distribution are common. Muscle weakness, an early sign, progressing to paralysis, may also be encountered if the ischemia remains untreated.

Quality and/or presence of peripheral pulses, however, is *not* a reliable diagnostic sign. Even relatively high intracompartmental pressures are usually not sufficient to compromise arterial perfusion (2–6).

Diagnosis of compartment syndrome is based primarily on the presence of signs and symptoms, since laboratory and radiographic data are nonspecific. Compartment syndrome can occur following both minor and catastrophic injuries. Therefore, a high index of suspicion is an essential diagnostic tool that should be integrated into the nursing assessment of a patient with extremity trauma.

Direct intracompartmental pressure measurement is the only reliable diagnostic modality available. Intermittent monitoring via a central venous pressure water manometer and continuous intracompartmental monitoring using a pressure transducer may both be used. In either option, a sterile needle or IV catheter is inserted directly into the compartment requiring monitoring. Both the water manometer and the pressure transducer

**Table 23.2.** Signs and symptoms of compartment syndrome[a]

---

Disproportional pain
Pain on passive stretch and motor weakness
Hypesthesia (lessened sensibility to touch)
Swelling or tenseness
Compartment hypertension (>30 mm Hg)

---

[a]*Source*: Adapted from Brown OW, LiCalzi L, Kerstien MD. Vascular trauma. In: McSwain NE, Kerstien MD, eds. Evaluation and management of trauma. Norwalk, CT: Appleton-Century-Crofts, 1987:326.

systems are filled with sterile saline and then attached to the needle or catheter to obtain the pressure (2–6).

Normal pressure within a compartment is ≤8 mm HG (2). There appears to be considerable controversy over what pressures constitute a need for fasciotomy, which is the surgical treatment of choice for compartment syndrome. In general, most sources cite an intracompartmental pressure ranging between 30 and 60 mm Hg as an indication for fasciotomy. The threshold varies, though, with the patient's reliability as an information source. The more compromised the level of consciousness, the lower the threshold is for performing a fasciotomy (2–6).

Besides the obvious complication of muscle death and amputation, there are other sequelae of compartment syndrome. Volkmann's ischemic contracture, a condition in which necrotic muscle is replaced by fibrous tissue leading to contracture formation, occurs in 80% of untreated cases of compartment syndrome (2). Renal failure due to myoglobinuria may also occur because of muscle necrosis. Myoglobin is released during muscle death and obstructs the renal tubules. (See Chapter 18 on rhabdomyolysis for further discussion of this problem.) Mannitol and other diuretics may help to decrease tubular necrosis, and the administration of intravenous sodium bicarbonate will alkalinize the urine (2–4, 6).

## 2. What are the nursing diagnoses of highest priority?
A. Alteration in tissue perfusion
B. Potential for injury

## 3. What are the goals of nursing care?

### A. Nursing Diagnosis
Alteration in tissue perfusion related to increase in compartment volume or decrease in compartment size

### Goal of Care
Prevent compartment syndrome or reduce risk for development.

### Nursing Interventions
- Monitor characteristics and trends in patient's pain and discomfort.
- Palpate muscles of affected extremity frequently.
- Perform neurovascular checks to affected extremity hourly.
- Avoid elevation of affected extremity.
- Monitor extremities with circumferential dressings for swelling or neurovascular changes.
- If indicated, monitor and record direct intracompartmental pressures hourly.
- Monitor body temperature and white blood count.
- Notify physician at once of any changes or abnormal findings.

### Rationale
Unrelenting pain out of proportion to the injury is a hallmark finding in compartment syndrome. Commonly, passive muscle stretch increases the discomfort, and palpable firmness/tension of the involved compartment is found.

Necrosis of muscle and neural tissue may occur within 6 hours of the onset of compartment syndrome (6). An early finding, and one that may prevent progression to necrosis, is paresthesias distal to the involved compartment. Capillary refill times may be sluggish, but are not reliable diagnostic aids, nor are elevations in body temperature or white blood counts. The affected extremity may be cooler that the other one, but peripheral pulses may be normal, since occlusion pressure of the microcirculation is reached long before that of arterial diastolic pressue (2–6). Direct measurement of intracompartmental pressures is the most reliable diagnostic tool. Meticulous sterile technique should be maintained with the monitoring system because of infection risks.

Casts and tight-fitting and/or old blood-soaked dressings may indirectly restrict compartment size and interfere with perfusion. Likewise, elevation of the affected extremity may also impede perfusion, since venous return is not facilitated once intracompartmental pressure is excessive (2–4).

## Goal of Care

Promote optimal healing postoperatively *following* fasciotomy.

## Nursing Interventions

- Elevate extremity unless otherwise contraindicated.
- Perform sterile wet-to-wet dressing changes to fasciotomy sites unless otherwise ordered.
- Monitor fasciotomy sites for signs of infection (i.e., inflammation, necrotic tissue, pus, etc.).
- Continue neurovascular checks as before fasciotomy, progressing to decreasing frequency as postopertive edema resolves.
- Begin range-of-motion exercises when ordered.

## Rationale

Elevation of the extremity *following* fasciotomy facilitates venous return and decreases swelling (4). Continuing neurovascular checks will ensure that all involved compartments were incised and will detect abnormal changes due to postoperative swelling.

Moist dressings provide a physiological environment for muscle/wound healing. However, the risk of infection is increased because of a constant moisture state as well as by preoperative hypoperfusion of muscle compartments.

## B. Nursing Diagnosis

Potential for injury related to myoglobinuria secondary to muscle necrosis

## Goals for Care

Decrease risk of renal failure.

## Nursing Interventions

- Monitor urine for presence of myoglobin.
- Monitor urine output hourly and notify physician for declining volume. Administer diuretics as ordered.
- Monitor urinary pH hourly.
- Begin bicarbonate infusion as ordered.

## Rationale

Myonecrosis releases myoglobin into the circulation that may precipitate in the renal tubules, resulting in tubular necrosis (6). Volume expansion or diuretics are used to maintain a urinary output of about 100 cc/hr to prevent myoglobin precipitation. Likewise, large volumes of alkaline urine (pH $\geq$ 7) may lessen tubular necrosis (3).

Early mobilization of the affected extremity helps prevent contracture formation and permanent disability. In addition, optimal functioning of the peripheral vasculature is supported.

# ASSOCIATED NURSING DIAGNOSES

A. Alteration in comfort: Acute pain
B. Potential for infection

C. Impaired physical mobility
D. Impairment of skin integrity

## REFERENCES

1. Bathon GH. September 20, 1988. Personal Communication.
2. Silverhus SW, Amis JA. A practical guide to acute compartment syndrome. J Musculoskeletal Med (Sept) 1988:88–103.
3. Dunham CM, Cowley RA. Shock trauma/critical care handbook. Rockville, MD: Aspen. 1986.
4. Cardona VD, ed. Trauma reference manual. Bowie, MD: Brady Communications Company. 1985.
5. Strange JM, Kelly PM. Musculoskeletal injuries. In: Cardona VD, Hurn PD, Bastnagel-Mason PJ, et al, eds. Trauma nursing: from resuscitation through rehabilitation. Philadelphia: WB Saunders. 1988:525–569.
6. Kelly PM. Compartment syndrome. In: Strange JM ed. Shock trauma care plans. Springhouse: Springhouse, PA: 1987:267–269.

# CHAPTER 24

## Pelvic Fracture Treated with External Fixation

Robert H. Welton, RN, MSN, CCRN
Mary Helen Hoff, RN

## Clinical Presentation

A 76-year-old obese woman was admitted to the emergency department (ED) after a motor vehicle accident in which she was a belted passenger. On arrival in the ED she was awake, alert, and oriented to person and time, but had poor recall of the accident. She was moving all four extremities but complained of pain in her lower back and right hip. Her blood pressure was 90/40, her pulse was 134 and thready, and her respirations were shallow at 36. Medical antishock trousers (MAST) were in place and fully inflated.

A large-bore intravenous cannula was inserted into her left antecubital vein, and Ringer's lactate was infusing at 200 cc/hr. An arterial line was inserted into her right radial artery, measuring a blood pressure of 92/38. She was orally intubated with a number 8 endotracheal tube and placed on a volume-cycled ventilator set at $FiO_2$ of 0.40, tidal volume ($V_T$) of 800 ml, and synchronized intermittent mechanical ventilation (SIMV) at a rate of 8 breaths/ minute. A Foley catheter was inserted into her bladder draining clear yellow urine, which was hemetest negative. Initial examination revealed bony crepitus on palpation over her right iliac crest and ecchymosis over her right hip and lower back. An anterior–posterior pelvic x-ray showed displaced fractures of the right inferior and superior rami, the right sacrum, and the right iliac crest.

After hemodynamic stabilization with infusions of crystalloids, fluids, and blood products, she was transported to the angiography suite for a pelvic arteriogram. Arteriography revealed a bleeding site from the right external iliac artery. The patient was transported to the operating room where she underwent a laparotomy to repair the bleeding vessel and for application of a pelvic Hoffman external fixator device. Postoperatively she was transferred to the intensive care unit (ICU) for postanesthesia recovery and monitoring.

### 1. What is the pathophysiological basis for this patient's problem?

Pelvic fractures may be simple and nondisplaced, or they may be associated with significant hemorrhage and other system injuries, namely to the genitourinary tract, rectum, and sacral and sciatic nerves (1). A number of classification systems have been devised for pelvic fractures; a commonly used one is that developed by Trunkey and his associates (Table 24.1) (2). Pelvic fractures may also be classified as open or closed, with the open type associated with higher mortality and morbidity (1).

Mortality associated with pelvic fractures is directly related to the severity of injury and ranges from 5 to 50% (2–4). The higher percentages within this range represent the mortality associated with open pelvic fractures, which is four times that of closed fractures (5). In a study of 604 patients with pelvic fractures, Rothenberger found that 40% died within 5 hours of admission to the hospital; within 2 days of admission an additional 18% died (6).

Hemorrhage is the leading cause of death from severe pelvic fractures (7), which may cause blood loss up to 15 units of blood (8). This blood loss can occur at the fracture

**161**

**Table 24.1.** Classification of pelvic fractures according to Trunkey[a]

| Type | Category | Characteristics |
|---|---|---|
| I | Comminuted (crush) injuries | • The most severe fractures, involving three or more major components of the pelvis (rami, ilium, acetabulum, sacrum)<br>• Often unstable and accompanied by severe hemorrhage and soft tissue injuries<br>• Associated with the highest morbidity and mortality |
| II | Unstable | • Requires immobilization or traction to reduce hemorrhage or maintain position of weight-bearing portions of the pelvis<br>• Includes displaced and non-displaced diametric fractures,[b] open-book (sprung) pelvis, and acetabular fractures. |
| III | Stable | • Immobilization usually unnecessary except for symptomatic relief<br>• Includes isolated fractures and fractures of the pubic rami |

[a]*Source:* Adapted from Trunkey DD, Chapman MW, Lim RC, et al. Management of pelvic fractures in blunt trauma. J Trauma 1974;14:913.
[b]A diametric fracture is any fracture that extends through the pubic rami and pubic symphysis anteriorly and through the sacrum, the sacroiliac joint, or the ilium posteriorly so there is potential or actual cranial displacement of the hemipelvis.

site, in surrounding soft tissues, or at venous and arterial injury sites. Ecchymosis and swelling in the pelvic region are signs of pelvic fracture (Table 24.2).

The extensive vascular network in the pelvic region is often referred to as the "vascular sink," which receives its arterial blood supply from the hypogastric artery and is drained by a complex venous system (7). In addition, there are multiple interconnected arterial and venous collaterals, and the veins are valveless, rendering them capable of bidirectional flow (1). Early recognition of bleeding sites and intervention are required in patients with pelvic fractures who have massive continuous bleeding.

The priorities of early care of pelvic fracture patients are identical to those applied to any multiply injured patient and emphasize airway management, replacement of intravascular fluid volume deficits, and control of bleeding (9). Control of bleeding is one of the most challenging problems the health care team faces in managing patients with severe pelvic fractures. A number of strategies have been used to control pelvic bleeding from trauma (Table 24.3). Cowley and Dunham propose a plan that uses some of these strategies (1) (Fig. 24.1).

Pelvic angiography may be used for diagnosing as well as treating pelvic arterial bleeding. Immediate surgical intervention may be indicated if a large arterial bleeding site is visualized. Embolization of the bleeding vessel can be performed during angiography if small arterial branches are identified as the source of bleeding. Embolization is achieved by injecting various clotting agents proximal to the bleeding site.

Ligation of the hypogastric artery has been used to control pelvic hemorrhage when conservative therapy has been unsuccessful; however, this strategy is regarded as con-

**Table 24.2.** Signs and symptoms of pelvic fracture[a]

Pain in the region of the pelvis
Instability of the pelvis
Ecchymosis and swelling of the genitalia, perineum, medial thigh, lumbosacrum, or buttocks
Groin and suprapubic swelling
Peripheral neuropathy

[a]*Source:* Adapted from Seibel RE, Flint LM. Pelvic trauma. In: Maull KI, ed. Advances in trauma. Chicago: Year Book Medical Publishers, 1986;1:226.

**Table 24.3.** Strategies to control hemorrhage from pelvic trauma[a]

Transfusion and expectant waiting
Surgery including packing, vascular repair or ligation, hypogastric artery ligation
Angiography and transcatheter embolization
Reduction of pelvic fracture with external skeletal fixation devices
Pneumatic trouser compression with MAST device

[a]*Source:* Adapted from Soderstrom CA. Severe pelvic fractures: problems and possible solutions. Am Surg 1982;48(9):443.

troversial by some (10). The extensive collateral arterial vasculature of the pelvis may account for some of the skepticism over this technique.

Stabilization of pelvic fractures may be helpful in controlling bleeding if fractures are severely displaced or unstable. Methods of stabilization include use of MAST, external fixation, femur traction, pelvic slings, casting, or open reduction with internal fixation.

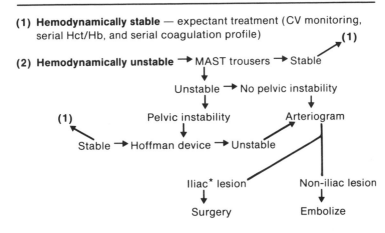

**(1) Hemodynamically stable** — expectant treatment (CV monitoring, serial Hct/Hb, and serial coagulation profile)

**(2) Hemodynamically unstable** → MAST trousers → Stable → **(1)**

Unstable → No pelvic instability

**(1)** ← Pelvic instability → Arteriogram

Stable → Hoffman device → Unstable

Iliac* lesion / Non-iliac lesion

Surgery / Embolize

**(3) (a) Persistent hemodynamic instability** despite **(2)**, or
(b) Patient with **"nonresuscitable shock,"** i.e., cannot control with massive volume infusion — **laparotomy** (rapidly expanding hematoma:
__ Embolize **and** ligate hypogastrics
__ Pack the pelvis
__ Repair major arterial injury
__ Hemipelvectomy

**(4) Pelvic hematoma found at laparotomy**
(a) Nonexpanding or pulsatile — **(1)**
(b) Modest expansion and/or pulsatile — Close the abdomen and perform an arteriogram (embolic tamponade)
(c) If rapidly expanding — **(3)**

*Iliac — common or external

**Figure 24.1.** Flowchart for the management of hemorrhage associated with pelvic fractures. (*Source:* Cowley RA, Dunham CM. Shock trauma/critical care manual. Baltimore: University Park Press, 1982:199.)

**Table 24.4.** Findings suggestive of urologic injury associated with pelvic fractures[a]

| |
|---|
| Hematuria |
| Bloodly urethral meatal discharge |
| Scrotal or perineal fullness and/or ecchymosis |
| Inability to void spontaneously |
| Difficulty passing or poor drainage from a bladder catheter |
| Boggy, "high riding," or absent prostate on rectal exam |
| Abdominal pain |

[a]*Source:* Adapted from Soderstrom CA. Severe pelvic fractures: problems and possible solutions. Am Surg 1982;48(9):443.

MAST, pneumatic compression trousers applied to the legs and lower abdomen, are generally used in the prehospital care phase to assist in managing hypotensive patients. Their use has been associated with a significant increase in survival of such patients; however, use of MAST is limited to the early resuscitative phase of care (11, 12).

External fixation is a treatment method that provides stabilization of a fracture or dislocation by using pins placed percutaneously into the bone and attached to a rigid external frame (13). Although originally intended for open fractures of long bones, these devices have assumed a major role in the management of pelvic fractures. An external fixation apparatus placed across the front of the pelvis will provide stability and may help to control bleeding (9). The control of bleeding is thought to result from minimizing pelvic motion that may loosen clots (14).

Urologic injuries occur in approximately 15% of all pelvic fractures (15). Findings suggestive of urologic injury are listed in Table 24.4. Specific injuries may be identified by pyelography, ureterography, and cystography. It is interesting to note that as many as one-third of patients with pelvic fractures and hematuria do not have renal, bladder, or urethral damage (16). Neurological injuries associated with pelvic fractures are rare; however, sciatic nerve injuries do occur in approximately 16% of hip dislocations (17).

## 2. What are the nursing diagnoses of highest priority?

A. Potential for alterations in tissue perfusion
B. Potential for infection

## 3. What are the goals of nursing care?

### A. Nursing Diagnosis

Potential for alterations in tissue perfusion related to alterations in intravascular volume secondary to bleeding from pelvic trauma

The goals of care and nursing interventions for alterations in tissue perfusion are discussed fully in Chapter 13, Ruptured Thoracic Aorta.

### B. Nursing Diagnosis

Potential for infection related to altered skin integrity due to external fixator pins

### Goal of Care

Decrease risk of infection.

### Nursing Interventions

- Monitor for signs and symptoms of infection of pin sites and suture lines: inflammation, change in character and amount of drainage from pin sites, elevation of white blood cells (WBCs), fever.
- Monitor pin sites to ensure that they are clean without skin or soft tissue tension.

- Perform pin care every 4 hours until drainage decreases, then every 8 to 12 hours as necessary.
- Prevent pressure areas and excoriation of surrounding skin.
- Prevent contact between skin and external frame.
- Maintain integrity of the device by ensuring that it is rigid with all the nuts and components tightened; report loose connections and pins to the orthopedic surgeon.

## Rationale

Unstable pelvic fractures have been treated with bed rest, pelvic slings, skeletal traction, casts, and internal fixation, most of which usually require prolonged hospitalization. In addition, Trunkey et al. have identified a high incidence of pulmonary problems associated with these modes of treatment (2). Open reduction and internal fixation have also been associated with catastrophic bleeding and limited success in fracture stabilization (18).

External fixation stabilizes skeletal injuries with a metal framework outside the skin, attached to bone via pins through the soft tissue. Various devices have been used to provide external fixation of the pelvis, such as the Wagner device, the AO/ASIF tubular system, and the Hoffman apparatus. Several studies have shown that patients with unstable pelvic fractures treated with external fixation have reduced morbidity and fewer nursing demands than those treated with other nonsurgical means (19–21).

External fixation devices are applied in the operating room, using appropriate sterile technique. Skin incisions are made prior to the placement of each pin to avoid tension at the site. Pin dressings should allow for some initial bleeding; however, gentle compression may be applied, if needed, to control it (14).

The most important component of an external fixation system is the interface of the bone, pin, and skin, as failure at these sites may lead to premature removal of the fixator (22). Disadvantages of external fixation relate primarily to the use of percutaneous pins that tend to loosen or become infected before the fracture heals (14). Therefore, meticulous pin care must be maintained while the Hoffman fixator is in place. Pin care is initiated immediately after the operation by gently wiping the sites with sterile applicators or gauze using a half-and-half solution of normal saline and hydrogen peroxide. Keratinaceous growths of skin up the pin may be prevented by pushing downward on the skin around the pin while cleaning. Iodine-containing solutions may react chemically with the stainless steel pins and should not be used (22). Pin sites normally do not require dressings; however, if drainage is excessive or pin site involves a large denuded area, gauze can be wrapped loosely around each pin. Drainage from pin sites should never be obstructed by tight wrapping or by allowing crust formation from dried drainage. The junction of the pin and the skin should be free of tension to avoid skin necrosis. Tension on pin tracks should be avoided and may be treated with surgical extension to prevent skin tearing, which increases the risk of infection and pain to the patient. If excess tension is present, the skin may require incision with a number 11 scalpel blade under local anesthesia (22). This procedure is carried out by the physician. The obese patient may require additional care because excess adipose tissue and skin folds may come in contact with the external frame. This contact may cause pressure ulceration (22). Skin protection can be achieved by applying skin care products, such as Duoderm and Stomadhesive, to skin and tissue folds adjacent to pin sites. Padding these areas with ABD pads or rolled towels prior to turning or position changes will prevent undue pressure from the metal apparatus against skin folds.

After a few days, pin sites usually become fairly comfortable unless problems arise (23). Pain at the pin site may be due to excessive soft tissue tension, to loosening of the pin in the bone, or to infection, which usually begins in the adjacent soft tissues but can spread to bone, especially if the pin is loose or if heat from pin insertion with a power drill has caused local bone necrosis (14). Painful pin sites should be reported to the orthopedist as soon as possible. Pain may be due to pin wound contraction during healing, even if an adequate incision was made initially. Tension from infection and wound contraction are indications for surgical release of tension by incision and local anesthesia as described previously. If there is evidence of cellulitis or purulent drainage, antibiotic treatment based on sensitivity of cultured organism may be ordered to control soft tissue infections. It is important to confirm that pins in infected sites remain secure in the bone. Loose pins should be removed promptly by the physician, as they offer no stability and may contribute to the further risk of bone infection (14).

Routine maintenance of the Hoffman fixator includes cleaning the metal frame to remove drainage or other contaminants. The device should remain rigid with all nuts and connecting rods tight to maintain necessary traction and stability. Close observation of confused patients is necessary to prevent them from tampering or loosening the orthopedic hardware. If a pelvic computerized tomography (CT) scan is required, the dimensions of the opening in the CT scanner should be compared with the patient's pelvis with the Hoffman device in place. The orthopedic surgeon may be required to reposition or reduce the size of the external frame temporarily so the patient and the Hoffman frame will fit into the CT scanner. Once the scan is completed, the modified Hoffman frame may need to be adjusted to its prescan dimensions; the orthopedic surgeon is responsible for these adjustments.

## ASSOCIATED NURSING DIAGNOSES

A. Impaired physical mobility
B. Alterations in comfort
C. Anxiety

### REFERENCES

1. Cowley RA, Dunham CM. Shock trauma/critical care manual. Baltimore: University Park Press. 1982.
2. Trunkey DD, Chapman MW, Lim RC, et al. Management of pelvic fractures in blunt trauma. J Trauma 1974;14:912–923.
3. Mucha P, Farnell M. Analysis of pelvic fracture management. J Trauma 1984;24:379–386.
4. Perry JF. Pelvic open fractures. Clin Orthop 1980;151:41–45.
5. Mucha P. Recognizing and avoiding complications with pelvic fractures. Infect Surg (Jan) 1985:53–62.
6. Rothenberger D, Fisher R, Strate R, et al. The mortality associated with pelvic fractures. J Trauma 1978;84:356–361.
7. Soderstrom CA. Severe pelvic fractures: problems and possible solutions. AM Surg 1982;48(9):441–446.
8. McMurty R, Walton D, Dicherson D, et al. Pelvic disruption in the polytraumatized patient: a management protocol. Clin Orthop 1980;151:22–30.
9. Seibel RE, Flint LM. Pelvic trauma. In Maull KI, ed. Advances in trauma. Chicago: Year Book Medical Publishers. 1986;1:217–243.
10. Patterson FP, Morton KS. The cause of death in fractures of the pelvis, with a note on treatment by ligation of the hypogastric (internal iliac) artery. J Trauma 1973;13:849–856.
11. Flint LM, Brown A, Richardson JD, et al. Definitive control of bleeding from severe pelvic fractures. Ann Surg 1979;189:709–716.
12. Gaffney FA, Thal ER, Taylor WF, et al. Hemodynamic effects of medical anti-shock trousers (MAST garment). J Trauma 1981;21:932.
13. Mears DC. External skeletal fixation. Baltimore: Williams & Wilkins, 1983·1
14. Trafton PG, Herndon JH. External fixators in fracture management. In Maull KI, ed. Advances in trauma. Chicago: Year Book Medical Publishers. 1986;1:245–266.
15. McAninch JW. Trauma to the bladder and urethra. Infections Surg 1983:133–148.
16. Levine JI, Crampton RS. Major abdominal injuries associated with pelvic fractures. Surg Gynecol Obstet 1963;116:223–226.
17. Morton K. Traumatic dislocation of the hip: a follow-up study. Can J Surg 1959;3:67–74.

18. Mears DC, Fu FH. Modern concepts of external skeletal fixation of the pelvis. Clin Orthop 1980;151:65–73.
19. Saucedo T, Matta J. The treatment of unstable pelvic ring injuries [Abstract]. In: Abstracts of the 53rd annual meeting of the American Academy of Orthopaedic Surgeons, New Orleans. 1986:40.
20. Tile M. Fractures of the pelvis and acetabulum. Baltimore: Williams & Wilkins, 1984:4.
21. Wild JJ, Hanson GW, Tullos HS. Unstable fractures of the pelvis treated with external fixation. J Bone Joint Surg 1983;64:1010.
22. Zych GA. Multiple fractures: practical guide and essential checklist. In: Civetta JM, Taylor RW, Kirby RR, eds. Critical care. Philadelphia: JB Lippincott, 1988:645–656.
23. Green SA. Complications of external skeletal fixation. Springfield, IL: Charles C Thomas. 1981:39.

# CHAPTER 25

## Maxillofacial Injury: LeFort III Fracture

### Diana O. Williams, RN, MS, CCRN

## Clinical Presentation

A 32-year-old woman was admitted to the hospital following a head-on collision in which she was the driver. She was not wearing a seat belt. She arrived awake but disoriented, with no history of loss of consciousness. She was moving all of her extremities, denied abdominal pain, had severe lacerations around both eyes, and was expectorating blood from her mouth. Her blood pressure was 130/60 mm Hg; pulse was 90 beats/minute; and respirations were 30/minute and shallow.

Severe maxillofacial bone disruption was suspected, and an emergency tracheostomy was performed for airway management. A computerized tomography (CT) scan of the face showed bilateral LeFort III injury with a fractured mandible. The patient was transported to the operating room, where she underwent open reduction and bone grafting of the fractures.

On admission to the intensive care unit (ICU), she was mechanically ventilated through a number 8 cuffed tracheostomy tube. Her vital signs were as follows: blood pressure, 110/50; pulse, 100 beats/minute; respirations, 20/minute; and temperature, 96.8°F (36°C) rectally. She had no spontaneous respirations and was unresponsive to verbal and tactile stimuli. An indwelling Foley catheter had been placed in her bladder, a double-lumen central venous catheter in her left subclavian vein, an arterial line in her right radial artery, and a peripheral intravenous cannula in her right forearm.

A suture line extended from ear to ear horizontally across the temporal-parietal-frontal region and was covered by a large dressing. Drains were in place at both ends of this coronal incision. Her eyelids were sutured closed, with the suture ties taped upward onto her forehead. Multiple small lacerations on her face were closed with fine sutures. An oral gastric tube was connected to low continuous suction and draining bloody fluid.

### 1. What is the pathophysiological basis for this patient's problem?

Maxillofacial fractures can be grouped according to the LeFort classification proposed in 1901 by the French surgeon Renee LeFort (Figs. 25.1–25.3). The LeFort I fracture separates the maxillary arch from upper facial bones, and the LeFort II fracture involves a separation of the nasomaxillary triangular segment from the zygomatic and orbital facial bones (1). LeFort III fractures, also known as craniofacial dysfunction, separate the midface from the cranium through the orbits. This fracture may extend from the nasofrontal bones down the medial wall of the orbit and lateral maxilla (2). Splits in the hard palate and associated mandibular fractures are not uncommon, and LeFort III fractures frequently present as comminuted lesser LeFort fragments.

Facial muscles, orbital ligaments, and sinus structures are disrupted, and tears in the dura, causing cerebrospinal fluid (CSF) leaks, are seen in LeFort II and LeFort III fractures. CSF leaks through the nose can be clouded by nasal bleeding.

The coronal flap approach to repair involves an incision through the scalp, across the frontal region of the head from ear to ear. The tissues of the face are then peeled away to expose the bony structures, which are repaired or stabilized. This approach eliminates major incisions on the face.

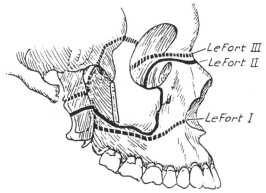

**Figure 25.1.** LeFort fracture lines. (From Worth MH Jr, ed. Principles and practice of trauma care. Baltimore: Williams & Wilkins, 1982:244.)

A ventral approach may be used and involves incisions made within the oral cavity to expose the fracture sites. Fractures are then reduced and wired internally or grafted. Severely damaged or absent bone may be replaced by bone from the patient's rib, skull, or iliac crest (3).

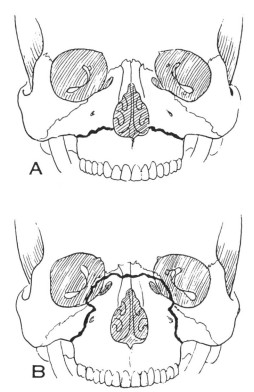

**Figure 25.2.** **A** Low maxillary (LeFort I or Guerin's) fracture. **B** Pyramidal (LeFort II) fracture. (From Worth MH Jr, ed. Principles and practice of trauma care. Baltimore: Williams & Wilkins, 1982:244.)

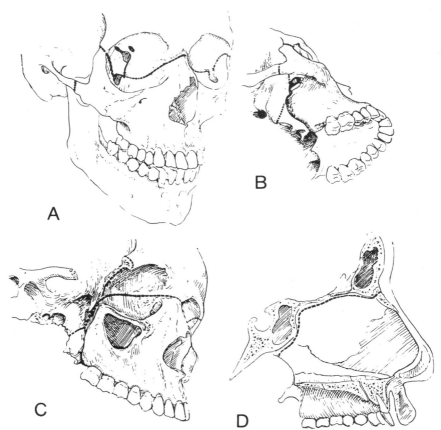

**Figure 25.3.** Lines of fracture in LeFort III fracture. **A** Line of fracture extending through nasofrontal junction to inferior orbital fissure and upward to frontozygomatic junction. **B** Fracture line through zygoma and pterygoid processes. **C** Zygoma has been removed to show more detail. **D** Lines of fracture through septum. (From Worth MH Jr, ed. Principles and practice of trauma care. Baltimore: Williams & Wilkins, 1982:245.)

## 2. What are the nursing diagnoses of highest priority?

A. Potential for ineffective airway clearance
B. Potential for infection
C. Fear

## 3. What goals of care and nursing interventions are appropriate for the above diagnoses?

### A. Nursing Diagnosis

Potential for ineffective airway clearance related to tracheostomy, effects of anesthesia, and decreased level of consciousness

### Goal of Care

Maintain patent airway.

## Nursing Interventions

- Monitor for signs of respiratory distress: cough, increased inspiratory pressures, techypnea, noisy respirations, rhonchi, diminished breath sounds.
- Suction airway and oral cavity as needed.
- Reposition patient every 2 hours.
- Keep wire cutters at bedside of patients with wired jaws.
- Prevent premature self-extubation.
- Maintain patency of and suction to gastric suction tube.
- Begin patient's ambulating early.

## Rationale

The patient with maxillofacial trauma usually requires an artificial airway and mechanical ventilation until facial and neck edema subsides. Facial injuries frequently occur concurrently with neurological injury; depression of neurological function is not uncommon. The patient has undergone a long operative period, frequently under general anesthesia for as long as 16 to 20 hours, and will require postoperative narcotic analgesia and sedation. In addition, chest physiotherapy with postural drainage may be delayed for the first 24 hours and the head of the bed kept elevated in order to decrease facial swelling. For these reasons, patients with facial trauma have difficulty clearing airway secretions effectively. Monitoring airway patency and suctioning are nursing priorities. Tracheal lavage with 1 ml of preservative-free normal saline may stimulate the cough reflex, which mobilizes secretions that can be removed by suctioning (3). Provide adequate hydration to liquefy secretions. Ausculate breath sounds after suctioning to evaluate its effectiveness. Monitoring to ensure appropriate inflation of the tracheostomy or endotracheal tube cuff will prevent aspiration of oral and gastric secretions. In addition, underinflation of the cuff can increase the potential for unintentional extubation (4). Suctioning the oral cavity and positioning the patient in the side-lying position with the head elevated will also decrease the chance of aspiration. Early ambulation will stimulate deep breathing, assist in mobilizing secretions, and facilitate coughing.

Patients with jaws closed by wires or elastic bands should have wire cutters or scissors at the bedside to cut these restraints in the event of hemorrhage or vomiting (4 [p. 150]). Ensuring gastric tube patency and suction provides gastric decompression, which reduces the chance of vomiting and aspirating. Premature self-extubation by the patient may be life threatening because reintubation may be difficult or impossible because of edema (3). A secure tube fixation system is essential. Padded hand restraints, used in compliance with hospital policy, keeping the patient calm through reassurance, and mild sedation also may prevent self-extubation. Use of a "swivel adaptor" along with support to ventilator tubing will prevent excess weight and traction on the artificial airway which may contribute to unintentional extubation (4).

## B. Nursing Diagnosis

Potential for infection related to disruption of integrity of skin and mucous membranes

## Goal of Care

Decrease risk of infection.

## Nursing Interventions

- Cleanse operative sites and wounds at least three times a day.
- Perform oral hygiene with oral lavage at least three to four times a day.

- Monitor amount and odor of nasal and oral drainage.
- Use orogastric tubes instead of nasogastric tubes.

### Rationale

All facial and scalp suture lines must be kept free of dried blood and secretions, which are excellent growth media for bacteria. Cleanse operative sites with cotton-tipped applicators soaked in a 50% solution of normal saline and hydrogen peroxide, using gentle pressure to dislodge encrusted material. Iodine-based products should be avoided because they can damage cells responsible for tissue repair, impeding granulation and antimicrobial defenses, and can contribute to facial scarring (5). Apply a thin layer of non-iodine-based antibiotic ointment over suture lines and abrasions. Special considerations should be given to incisions and wounds around the eyes. Periocular wounds and incisions should be cleansed with normal saline and dressed with an ophthalmic antibiotic ointment. Nonophthalmic ointments should not be applied close to the eyes, as they may be inflammatory to the sclera.

Hair is another excellent medium for bacteria growth. Any blood or road dirt should be washed from the scalp, and the hair should be tied or braided to remove it from suture lines and wounds.

Trauma to the mid-face may disrupt the frontal, ethmoid, and maxillary sinuses. The presence of a tube in the nasal cavity may obstruct sinus drainage and lead to sinusitis; therefore, the use of orogastric tubes instead of nasogastric tubes is recommended (6).

### Goal of Care

Recognize signs of infection.

### Nursing Interventions

- Monitor for signs of infection: fever, elevated white blood cell count, delayed healing, disproportionate swelling, and foul-smelling and/or purulent drainage.

Assess the volume and nature of any drainage from the nasal and oral cavities. Application of a nasal drip pad—a folded gauze pad, which is changed as needed—is a method of collecting and quantifying this drainage. Do not pack, probe, or suction the nares, as doing so may introduce microorganisms and increase intracranial pressure. Nasal and ear drainage may be tested for glucose to distinguish secretions from CSF leaks. CSF leakage down the patient's throat may cause a salty taste (4 [p. 148]). Bloody, purulent, and/or foul-smelling drainage may be an early indication of meningitis or bacteremia and should be reported to the physician immediately. Instruct the patient not to blow his or her nose, as doing so may aggravate bleeding.

### C. Nursing Diagnosis

Potential for fear related to surgery, injury, intubation, and mechanical ventilation

### Goal of Care

Alleviate or diminish fear.

### Nursing Interventions

- Identify source(s) of fear and contributing factors.
- Reduce or eliminate contributing factors.
- Orient and reorient patient to accident, injuries, surgery, and ICU environment.
- Explain plan of care in simple terms.
- Explain all procedures prior to intervening and repeat the explanation each time the task is performed.
- Explain sounds in the ICU (such as alarms or suction).

**Table 25.1.**   Interventions cited by patients as reducing stress[a]

| Stressor | Intervention |
|---|---|
| Suctioning | Reassurance of nurses<br>Holding breath<br>Breathing bag assistance |
| Extubation | Explanation of event<br>Presence of nurses<br>Knowledge that they were breathing spontaneously |
| Inability to communicate | Sign language<br>Miming<br>Writing |
| Mechanical ventilation | Confidence in caregivers<br>Faith<br>Family<br>Being alive |

[a]*Source:* Adapted from Gries ML, Fernsler J. Patient perceptions of the mechanical ventilation experience. Focus Crit Care 1988:15:57.

- Monitor conversation in the presence of the patient.
- Provide a system for communicating.
- Provide a means for the patient to summon help.

## Rationale

The patient's experience following maxillofacial surgery can be extremely frightening. Consider waking up from general anesthesia, not knowing where you are or why you are there. Attempts to open your eyes are unsuccessful because your eyelids have been sutured closed. Attempts at opening your mouth are thwarted because your jaws are wired closed. Air is forced through an opening in your throat, and you feel unable to breathe when secretions obstruct your airway. Attempts to lift your arms to summon help are unsuccessful because your arms are restrained. This scenario is not uncommon for patients following facial trauma.

Many trauma patients are unable to recall their accident as well as the early hours or days of their hospitalization. The general anesthesia required for this long surgery has an amnesic effect, which may contribute to fright and confusion.

The critical care environment is strange and unfamiliar to patients, and it can be frightening and stressful. Sources of stress in the ICU are numerous and include personnel, noise level, equipment, and interactions among the staff and the patient. Strichter studied patients who were mechanically ventilated and found that these patients frequently reported complaints of inability to catch their breath, inability to communicate, confusion, fear of the ventilator, and frequent nightmares (7). Additional research has revealed lack of information as a frequent patient complaint (8, 9). Another study of patient experiences while mechanically ventilated found the inability to recall explanations to be a significant source of stress (10). Interventions cited by these patients as helpful in reducing stress are listed in Table 25.1.

Provisions for emotional support should focus on information and communication. Explanations and reorientations offered in a calm, reassuring approach are essential and should be repeated as often as necessary. Knowing what to expect may help reduce stress, particularly with predictable experiences such as suctioning and its accompanying hyperventilation. The rationale for and temporary nature of hand restraints should be repeated often. The patient should be reassured that the pain and pressure from facial wounds and edema will resolve and be treated with analgesics and sedation. A sign posted over the patient's bed reminding staff that the patient is awake and that bedside conversations should be monitored may prevent the patient from misinterpreting conversations about other patients. Families should be prepared for the drastic change in physical appearance they will encounter on visiting the patient for the first time; families can benefit from the same explanations and orientations given to the patient. Informing family members that the patient's facial edema will resolve over time, and reinforcing this information, may be useful in reducing their fear.

The patient must be provided with an alternate means of communication to replace verbal communication until he or she is able to speak again. If writing with a pad and pencil is not feasible because of the placement of vascular lines or extremity injuries, a system of head nods in response to asking "yes" and "no" type questions may be used, as may an alphabet board. Lip reading may not be effective because of facial and lip edema and mandibular fixation.

Fear may also be reduced by providing some means of summoning help. Call lights are sometimes not provided in the belief that the patient is in constant attendance by the staff; unfortunately, this knowledge reassures only the staff (11). Call lights or some other help-summoning device (bells, buzzers) should be provided.

The management of fear in patients with maxillofacial injuries can present a significant challenge to the nurse. In some patients, such as those with complications due to severe head injury, alcohol intoxication, or substance abuse, the use of drug-induced paralysis with neuromuscular blockade and sedation may be needed to prevent disruption of facial bones, grafts, suture lines as well as artificial airways and drainage tubes.

## ASSOCIATED NURSING DIAGNOSES

A. Potential for fluid volume deficits
B. Alterations in comfort
C. Alterations in oral mucous membranes
D. Sleep pattern disturbances
E. Impairment of skin integrity
F. Disturbances in self-concept/body image

**REFERENCES**

1. Cowley RA, Dunham CM, eds. Shock trauma/critical care manual: initial assessment and management. Baltimore: University Park Press, 1982:93.
2. McCarthy JG, Godrey NV. Facial trauma. In: Worth MH, ed. Principles and practice of trauma care. Baltimore: Williams & Wilkins, 1982:223–254.
3. Deli SL, Bower TC. Maxillofacial and soft tissue injuries. In: Cardona VD, Hurn PD, Bastnagel-Mason PJ, et al, eds. Trauma nursing: from resuscitation through rehabilitation. Philadelphia: WB Saunders, 1988:592.
4. Pesiri AJ, Stewart K, Kobe E, Stewart W. Protocol for the prevention of unintentional extubation. Crit Care Nurs Q 1990;12(4):87–90.
5. Deli SL. Maxillofacial trauma. In: Cardona VD, ed. Trauma nursing. Oradell, NJ: Medical Economics Books, 1985.
6. Holler DL. Maxillofacial injuries. In: Strange JM,

ed. Shock trauma care plans. Springhouse, PA: Springhouse, 1987:202.
7. Dunham CM, Cowley RA. Shock trauma/critical care handbook. Rockville, MD: Aspen, 1986:110.
8. Strichter AR. A description of patient responses during the weaning process after prolonged artificial ventilation. [Master's thesis.] Newark, DE: University of Delaware, 1973.
9. Dodge J. Factors related to patient's perceptions of their cognitive needs. Nurs Res 1969;18:502–513.
10. Wilson-Barnett J. Patients' emotional reactions to hospitalization: an exploratory study. J Adv Nurs 1976;1:351–358.
11. Gries ML, Fernsler J. Patient perceptions of the mechanical ventilation experience. Focus Crit Care 1988;15:52–59.
12. Brown MA, Daly BJ. Care of the patient with respiratory problems. In: Daly BJ, ed. Intensive care nursing. 2nd ed. New York: Medical Examination Publishing Company, 1985:227.

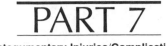

# PART 7

**Integumentary Injuries/Complications**

# CHAPTER 26

# Degloving Injury, Acute Stage

Mary T. deLauney, RN, BSN

## Clinical Presentation

A 26-year-old female fire fighter fell from the right bucket seat of a 15-ton fire truck as it was pulling out of the firehouse. She was trapped and pushed along the road in front of the right rear wheel for 28 feet before being discovered by the other fire fighters. They found her awake, talking, and extremely bloody, with a palpable systolic blood pressure of 50 mm Hg. Seventeen minutes after the accident occurred she was transported by ambulance to the local hospital emergency department.

Her injuries included the following: a degloving injury of the right and left buttocks, both thighs, and right calf, and a rupture of the iliac vein. In addition, she had an evisceration of the bowel with serosal and cecal tears, an open pelvic fracture with right sacroiliac joint separation, a disruption of the symphysis pubis, a fractured pelvic rami, and a comminuted left ileum. She had also dislocated her left knee.

The initial resuscitation process involved the insertion of large-bore catheters for the rapid infusion of fluids, after which an emergency laparotomy and colostomy were performed. The open pelvis was wired, and arterial embolectomy was performed. The wounds were irrigated, debrided, and partially closed in an attempt to achieve hemostasis. Resuscitation fluids included 90 units of packed cells. During this time she experienced a cardiac arrest that responded to drugs and fluids.

Following surgery, she was transferred to the ICU. Surgeons told her family that despite their efforts they believed she would not survive the night. Twenty hours later she was transferred to a trauma center in hypovolemic shock with a systolic blood pressure of 80.

Resuscitation efforts continued. Massive quantities of crystalloids and colloids were infused. During the ensuing surgical procedures, which involved extensive debridement, reembolization of the pelvis, and bilateral fasciectomies of the thighs and calves, a second cardiac arrest occurred. She was again successfully resuscitated, and medical antishock trousers (MAST) were applied to further stabilize the pelvis, tamponade the bleeding, and support circulation.

Achieving wound hemostasis remained a problem. The massive destruction and loss of tissue allowed the unimpeded flow of serum and blood. Dressings soaked with Avitene (a fibrous topical hemostatic agent that attracts platelets and adheres to fibrils) and the application of epinephrine-soaked dressings were partially successful in slowing the rate of fluid loss. Despite this marginal success, within 12 hours she required additional wound debridement. The combination of tissue disruption with circulatory collapse resulted in a continual upward advancement of the line of demarcation between salvageable and necrotic tissue. At this time a nursing decision was made to place the patient on a Stryker frame to facilitate dressing changes. The wounds extended from mid-back down both thighs, the anterior segment of the perineum, and most of the abdomen.

**175**

By the fourth day postinjury this patient had received a total of 173 units of packed red blood cells, 203 units of fresh frozen plasma (FFP), 176 units of platelets, and 26 units of cryoprecipitate. Despite this unprecedented massive blood transfusion, she demonstrated a surprising ability to compensate and stabilize with support.

Expected complications and difficulties began to develop by the second day postinjury. Paramount of these were continued fluid loss with coagulopathy, medullary renal washout, renal polyuria, wound infection, and wound management.

Following the massive transfusion of stored blood, a severe coagulopathy developed, platelets were ineffective, and white blood cells had been depleted. She was placed in protective isolation, platelets were given as needed, and FFP was infused at 200 cc/hr continuously. For the next 17 days an hourly intake of 500 cc/hr was maintained. The amount of FFP was gradually decreased and was eventually discontinued as her coagulation studies improved.

The presence of myoglobin, hemoglobin, and albumin in the urine greatly increased the potential for acute renal failure. The initial fall in urine output, believed to be due to hypovolemia and myoglobinuria, was treated with increased fluid intake, doses of Lasix and mannitol, and urine alkalinization, with intravenous fluids containing sodium bicarbonate. The downward trend in urine output gradually improved with this therapy. When the urine output exceeded 200 cc/hr despite a drop in fluid intake, diabetes insipidus (DI) was suspected. However, based on laboratory results (see Chapter 1) and a test dose of Pitressin, DI was ruled out. Crystalloids and colloids were then used to replace the urine output. An hourly intake of 200 cc/hr, plus the previous hour's urine output, was maintained. At one point intake equaled a total of 675 cc/hr for several hours. Medullary renal washout, renal polyuria, was diagnosed. The inability of the kidneys to concentrate urine necessitated restarting continuous FFP infusion to support fluid loss. Potassium chloride and acetate infusions were needed as well to replace urinary losses. The serum creatinine remained within normal limits despite what appeared to be high output renal failure. Because of the problems posed by the kidney's inability to concentrate the urine, interventions included monitoring and replacing serum electrolytes, especially potassium, and maintaining the volumes of fluids needed to replace the excessive losses. These interventions continued for more than 2 months.

Wound management was another challenge. The initial dressings were Avitene- and epinephrine-soaked gauze covered with Silvadene cream, which were changed by the surgeons in the operating room. By the fourth day postinjury most of the radical debridement had been performed, wound hemostasis had been achieved, and mesh grafts had been applied. The massive loss of fluid and serum from the wounds, which continued to present life-threatening intravascular deficiencies, was treated with intravenous fluids and vasopressor drugs.

The presence of infection and sepsis, as indicated by the cardiovascular profile and serial blood and wound cultures, was treated with the administration of amikacin, vancomycin, and moxalactam. The patient was also placed on protective isolation. Even the Stryker linens were prepackaged and sterilized.

By the seventh day postinjury, whirlpool treatments were initiated. The once-daily treatment lasted 30 minutes; however, the trip to and from the whirlpool tank took 2½ hours. A surgical fellow, two nurses, an attendant, and a respiratory therapist were required for the trip. The patient remained relatively unstable, requiring an average of 500 cc/hr of fluids to maintain hemodynamic stability. She was on a Stryker frame, was orally intubated, and had an arterial line, a Swan-Ganz catheter, a triple lumen catheter, an oral gastric tube, a Foley catheter, and a matured colostomy. After the whirlpool treatment the patient was wrapped in sterile sheets and returned to her room where her dressings were reapplied under strict surgical aseptic technique.

Concurrent with the therapy were hyperbaric oxygen (HBO) treatments. Because of the patient's hemodynamic instability the initial HBO treatments occurred sporadically. Eventually these treatments became well tolerated, and they were increased to 90 minutes, two times a day, and continued until satisfactory wound coverage was achieved.

By the fifth day postinjury, mesh grafts were applied as the first stage of wound coverage. Porcine grafts were next applied on the 12th day postinjury, with the first split-thickness skin grafts (STSG) attempted 2 days later. The grafting process took several months to complete and included autografts, heterografts, homografts, cadaver grafts, and muscle flap procedures.

Additional wound-related complications included abdominal dehiscence on the 9th day postinjury, right knee disarticulation on the 14th day postinjury, cecal perforation on the 20th day postinjury, spontaneous rupture of the right iliac artery on the 32nd day postinjury, and cecal bypass on the 36th day postinjury. During the initial 4-month stay, this patient received more than 700 blood products and required more than 50 operative procedures.

Despite a 95% mortality estimation, this patient survived. She had received an unprecedented amount of blood products and suffered what should have been a fatal amount of tissue, muscle, and bone loss, and still she survived. After 11 months in a rehabilitation facility she returned to light work, was walking with a prosthetic leg and walker, enrolled in college, and lectured on safety measures for fire departments across the nation.

## 1. What is the pathophysiological basis for this patient's injury?

There are four mechanisms of traumatic injury: direct impact, deceleration, rotary force, and shearing force. A degloving injury is a shearing force injury that is usually the result of the tangential entrapment of a part of the body between two surfaces, one mobile and the other fixed. This entrapment can result in injuries ranging from partial-thickness skin avulsion, which involves the pulling away of the epidermal and parts of the dermal layers of the skin, to full-thickness circumferential loss of tissue down to and including the bone. These injuries can be viewed in terms of third-degree burns, and are often treated as such (1).

This case of degloving presented as a full-thickness injury manifested in a manner similar to a third-degree burn. In a third-degree burn, epidermis, dermis, nerve endings, hair follicles, and sweat glands are lost; subcutaneous tissue, muscle, and bone also can be lost. Regeneration will not occur, and grafting is necessary (2).

Historically, degloving injuries involved the upper extremities in the form of wringer injuries. Today most degloving injuries occur as lower extremity injuries and are accompanied by fractures and other associated injuries. The extent of injury, which depends on the amount of body surface area involved, can range from minor local skin disruption to loss of function, loss of limb, or loss of life if extensive tissue disruption occurs (1).

The pathophysiology of the injury is based on the traumatic tissue destruction and the acute phase of the inflammatory reaction. The acute phase of inflammation is not just a local reaction. It is a chemically mediated response resulting from a highly complex interaction of organs and systems involving the liver, spleen, kidneys, and brain along with the neurological, metabolic, vascular, lymphatic, and endocrine systems (3). Each patient's prognosis depends on the amount of tissue involved and the severity of associated injuries (1).

When the skin's integrity is severely disrupted, actual spillage of blood and serum occurs. This spillage triggers the initial phase of the inflammatory process in which the entire microcirculation experiences a sustained reaction in response to the injury (4, 5). The area of inflammatory response contains three distinct regions: central, mixed, and peripheral. The central region, which is a result of direct injury, is surrounded by a mixed region, where direct trauma and chemically mediated trauma overlap. These first two regions are then surrounded by an area of only chemically mediated injury, which forms the periphery of the lesion (4).

At the site of disruption, chemical mediators (histamine, bradykinin, and serotonin) are released, initially triggering vasoconstriction, which is shortly followed by vasodilatation and increased capillary permeability. This dilatation and increased permeability results in the localized pooling of serum and fibrinogen in adjacent tissues. The accumulation of edema fluids perpetuates the cycle of tissue damage by compromising capillary circulation and supporting the development of tissue hypoxia (5). A vicious cycle of tissue death can occur when hemoconcentration develops as a result of fluid loss and edema formation. Hemoconcentration leads to increased blood viscosity, which can impede flow through the capillaries, and even occlude them. When the capillaries become occluded, anaerobic metabolism and acidosis results, leading to tissue hypoxia and cell death (6).

Kudsk et al. report the management of degloving injuries with two surgical procedures. These two procedures involve the simple reattachment of the avulsed tissue or the removal of the damaged skin segment with subsequent skin graft coverage. When performing reattachment, it has been found that immediate defatting of the tissue, before covering the debrided muscle, produced the greatest graft survival rate. In cases where the avulsed tissue cannot be reattached, it is recommended that, when possible, the avulsed tissue be harvested for later grafting procedures (1).

When a degloving injury involves a large area with varying degrees of wound depth, as in the case of this patient, the healing process will proceed at different rates. It is essential to the healing process that optimal wound control, through removal of necrotic tissue and debris, be achieved (7). The presence of a healthy granulation bed is evidenced by a thin layer of light-colored tissue that bleeds readily and is easily controlled with light pressure. Once this bed has been achieved it is important to graft immediately, which will prevent the progression of the granulation process to a chronic stage that is unsuitable for grafting (7). Cocke et al. recommend that these heterogenous wounds be managed with the placement of small mesh grafts over those areas able to support the graft and that the established dressing routine be continued on the remainder of the wound. The mesh encourages the migration of the epithelial cells in the granulation bed and supports the healing process (7). Once an area is revascularized, STSG are applied. In areas where extensive loss of dermis has occurred, a full-thickness skin graft may be necessary. Where muscle destruction has occurred, full muscle grafts may be required (2).

In this specific case, the area of damage and limb loss was so extensive that donor sites were scarce. Therefore, donor mesh grafts and porcine grafts were used. The thicker grafts were then taken autologously from the few available sites and homologously from suitable cadaver donor supplies. The goal of the grafting process during the acute stage was wound coverage. The areas of the wound requiring full thickness or muscle donors were grafted at a later stage of the reconstructive process. During the acute stage of the grafting process with this patient, it was necessary to induce paralysis through the use of Pavulon, morphine, and Valium to prevent her from disrupting the young grafts.

## 2. What are the nursing diagnoses of highest priority?

A. Potential for infection and delayed wound healing
B. Impaired physical mobility

## 3. What are the goals of nursing care?

### A. Nursing Diagnosis

Potential for infection and delayed wound healing related to altered skin integrity

## Goal of Care

Wounds will be infection free and begin to heal.

## Nursing Interventions

- Change dressings using wet-to-dry or moist-to-moist dressings as ordered.
- Change dressings sequentially, from most clean area to most contaminated area.
- Maintain aseptic technique; gown, glove, and mask for all wound care.
- Sterilize all bed linens.
- Administer antibiotics as ordered.
- Coordinate whirlpool and hyperbaric treatments.
- Keep grafted areas moist.
- Expose graft donor sites to heat lamp every 4 hours for 20 minutes for each exposure.
- Maintain fluid and electrolyte status with necessary replacements as ordered.
- Monitor laboratory values as ordered, specifically the white blood cells, hematocrit and hemoglobin, prothrombin/partial thromboplastin time, and electrolytes.
- Monitor nutritional needs and provide supplemental nutritional support as ordered.
- Maintain patient comfort; sedate as needed.
- Protect the patient from excessive exposure.

## Rationale

Wound healing occurs in three phases: defense, reconstruction, and maturation (8). The goal of all wound care is to establish optimal wound control for the promotion and augmentation of the healing process (7). Open wounds require dressings that protect the wound from further trauma, absorb accumulated drainage that could inhibit the healing process, provide mechanical debridement of necrotic tissue, and supply gentle compression to control bleeding and edema formation without constricting circulation (5). The phases of the wound-healing process proceed at different rates, depending on the amount and extent of tissue injury. Dressing types must, therefore, be specific to the needs of the wound (7). Wounds with areas of necrosis will not begin to heal until effective wound control is achieved through debridement (5, 7). Major debridement requires surgical intervention. Minor debridement, however, can often be achieved mechanically through the use of wet-to-dry saline dressings of coarse-mesh gauze. Areas of the wound supporting young granulation tissue require moist-to-moist saline dressings of fine-mesh gauze. The fine mesh prevents disruption of the delicate new tissue beds. It is important that all wound types remain moist. If the wounds dehydrate, tissue necrosis will extend beyond the area of injury, prolonging the healing process (5). The use of dressings soaked in hemostatic and/or vasoactive agents should be highly individualized and only on the order of a physician.

Cross-contamination can be minimized by the following measures: dressing the wounds in the order of the cleanest first; using protective isolation techniques and monitoring traffic in the patient area; providing as sterile an environment as possible, even using positive air-flow rooms where available; and maintaining antimicrobial therapy as ordered (9).

Whirlpool and hyperbaric oxygen treatments may be part of the treatment strategy. Hydrobaths help cleanse the wound of dead tissue and debris and gently stimulate the circulation in the wound area. Hyperbaric oxygen treatments provide hyperoxygenation and vasoconstriction, promote wound healing, and retard the growth of some microorganisms (10).

Grafting should occur as soon as the wound is ready for coverage (7). Once a graft has been applied, the donor tissue must be protected from dehydration and movement. Occlusive dressings are kept moist and held in place with staples to encourage graft survival (2). Donor sites are also subject to infection and can be painful. Heat lamps are used to dry the donor sites and prevent the collection of fluid mediums that could support the growth of bacteria. Fine-mesh gauze that has been impregnated with an antiseptic material, such as xerofoam gauze, may be used to cover donor sites. Donor sites that heal properly can be used again for further harvesting if needed (2).

Skin is rugged, elastic, and waterproof. It functions as a protector, a regulator, and a barrier. When the skin is seriously disrupted, these functions are lost. The host is then at risk for infection, fluid volume and electrolyte imbalances, and thermal regulation dysfunctions (11).

Hematological, coagulation, and electrolyte studies must be frequently monitored. A rise or fall in the white blood cell count can indicate the presence of infection or the inability of the body to fight infection. Abnormal coagulation studies may indicate continued hemorrhage, disseminated intravascular coagulation (DIC), or development of thrombus formations. Electrolyte studies in conjunction with hemoglobin and hematocrit levels are used to analyze the effects of the redistribution of plasma, hemoconcentration, and volume losses that occur from extensive destruction of skin. The total picture presented by these ongoing data establishes the basis for fluid, electrolyte, and blood product replacement (8).

Maintenance of adequate nutrition is vital for survival, healing, and recovery from massive tissue loss injuries. Protein and vitamin C are essential for collagen formation. Trace minerals are needed for re-epithelialization and development of tensile strength. Vitamin A is essential for granulation tissue formation. Caloric needs proportionately increase with the amount of injury and stress that the body experiences. In a situation where the patient is unable to maintain adequate intake of nutritional requirements, it becomes necessary to use hyperalimentation, augmented by intralipid administration, to meet these needs (8).

It is important to maintain adequate levels of sedation. Dressing changes, invasive procedures, and grafting procedures will all contribute to the patient's discomfort. The fear of disfigurement, sense of powerlessness, and constant presence of unfamiliar stimuli cause the patient to experience high levels of anxiety. Fear, anxiety, and pain must all be adequately managed to ensure patient cooperation; otherwise the patient may demonstrate behaviors that are detrimental to the healing process (8).

Excessive exposure is also a problem for the patient suffering massive skin loss. This problem is twofold. First, and most obvious, is the emotional stress produced by constant examination of the wound by many people. Second, is the loss of the thermal barrier function of the skin. Interference with body temperature regulation occurs with large dermal defects, and the patient can quickly become hypothermic. Providing extra blankets and using overhead heat lamps during dressing changes can help minimize this problem (12).

## B. Nursing Diagnosis

Impaired physical mobility with potential for atelectasis, contractures, constipation, and venous stasis

### Goals of Care

- Chest x-ray will be clear.
- Maintain joint mobility and prevent contractures.

- Prevent constipation.
- Prevent venous stasis.

## Nursing Interventions

- Perform chest physiotherapy with postural drainage as ordered.
- Suction and lavage intubated patients every 2 hours.
- Administer incentive spirometry with coughing and deep breathing exercises every 2 hours.
- Perform full range of motion (ROM) to unaffected limbs as ordered every 4 hours.
- Perform modified ROM to affected limbs as ordered every 8 hours.
- Maintain all joints in functional position.
- Turn patient every 2 hours.
- Place footboard when patient is in supine position.
- Maintain good body alignment.
- Maintain accurate intake and output records.
- Digitally check every day for impacted stool.
- Maintain fluid intake as ordered.
- Establish bowel regimen as soon as possible.
- Administer embolism prophylaxis as ordered, such as pneumatic pumps or Ace wraps.
- Instruct patient to move toes and ankles often throughout the day.
- Observe daily for calf pain or ankle edema.
- Elevate arms and legs if possible.

## Rationale

Immobility leads to retained secretions that pool in the lower airways, predisposing the patient to atelectasis. Vigorous pulmonary toiletry, hydration, and exercise will facilitate the removal of these secretions (13).

The function of the musculoskeletal system involves a highly complex interaction of its parts: the muscles, joints, and bones. Extensive deterioration of this system can occur with prolonged immobility. Muscles, joints, and bones require motion and stress to maintain their integrity (14). A full range of lengthening and shortening exercises for muscles and joints, every 4 hours during the day, is necessary to prevent the development of contractures. The use of a firm mattress and a footboard, good body alignment, and frequent turning will also help prevent the formation of contractures (14, 15).

Constipation can occur for many reasons. The atrophy and loss of muscle tone seen in the immobilized patient can interfere with elimination. A plan for bowel hygiene management should be started as soon as possible. This plan should include exercise, adequate nutrition, adequate fluid intake, and the ongoing assessment of the elimination process of the patient (14, 15).

Loss of muscle tone may predispose the patient to venous stasis and thrombus formation. Daily monitoring for signs of thrombus formation includes assessing distal pulses, assessing for the presence of a positive Homans' sign (calf discomfort behind the knee with forced dorsiflexion of the foot), and monitoring for signs of circulatory restriction (14, 15).

## ASSOCIATED NURSING DIAGNOSES

A. Potential for fluid volume excess secondary to acute renal failure related to myoglobinuria

B. Disturbances in sleep patterns
C. Body image disturbance

## REFERENCES

1. Kudsk KA, Sheldon GF, Walton RL. Degloving injuries of the extremities and torso. J Trauma 1981;21:835–839.
2. Wooldridge M, Surveyer JA. Skin grafting for full-thickness burn injury. Am J Nurs 1980;11:2000–2004.
3. Gordon AH, Koj A. The acute-phase response to injury and infection. New York: Elsevier, 1985:xxi–xxix.
4. Movat HZ. The inflammatory reaction. New York: Elsevier, 1985:77–89.
5. Sieggreen MY. Healing of physical wounds. Nurs Clin North Am 1987;22(2):439–447.
6. Hurley JV. Acute inflammation. London: Churchill Livingstone, 1983:48–107.
7. Cocke WM, White RR, Lynch DJ, Verheyden CN. Wound care. New York: Churchill Livingstone, 1986:1–19.
8. Bruno P. The nature of wound healing. Nurs Clin North Am 1979;14(4):667–681.
9. Pfaff SJ. Wound management. In: Miller S, Sampson L, Soukeys S, eds. AACN procedure manual for critical care. Philadelphia: WB Saunders, 1985:431–449.
10. Strass MB, Hart GB. Crush injuries and the role of hyperbaric oxygen. Top Emerg Med 1984;4:9–23.
11. Stanley JW, Clarice A, Francone A, Lossow W. Structure and function in man. Philadelphia: WB Saunders, 1982:5–47.
12. Neff J. Standard of care for the adult patient with thermal injury. J Emerg Nurs 1987;13(1):59–63.
13. McHugh JM. Chest physiotherapy. In: Miller S, Sampson L, Soukeys S, eds. AACN procedure manual for critical care. Philadelphia: WB Saunders, 1985:269–274.
14. Johnson BJ, Thompson LF, McCarthy JA, Schroeder LM, Wade M. The hazards of immobility. AJN 1967:780–796.
15. Powell M, Little M. Making an assessment, In: Van Meter M, ed. Managing the critically ill effectively. New York: Medical Economics Books, 1982:2–11.

# CHAPTER 27

# Chemical Burn: Initial Resuscitation

Victoria Marselek, RN, MS, CCRN
Mary Elizabeth Clark, RN

## Clinical Presentation

A 33-year-old man arrived via helicopter from his job site to the regional burn center at
4 AM on Wednesday following an explosion involving molten sodium alum fluoride at
approximately 595°C (1100°F). He arrived awake and oriented, moving all extremities.

The patient had sustained a 51% total body surface area (TBSA) burn according to the
Lund and Browder chart (Figs. 27.1 and 27.2). Thirty percent of the burn was third degree
to his left forearm, left flank, and circumferential to both legs (Tables 27.1 and 27.2). The
remaining 21% of the burn was second degree to the back and left thumb. His initial vital
signs were blood pressure (BP) 120/60, pulse 108, unlabored respirations at 18/minute, and
temperature 36.5°C (98°F). Popliteal and pedal pulses were positive by use of a Doppler
with good capillary refill. The patient was able to move his toes.

On admission a triple-lumen intravenous (IV) catheter was inserted in the right subclavian
artery, and placement was verified by chest x-ray. Admission laboratory studies were obtained. An intravenous infusion of Ringer's lactate was started en route in the helicopter
according to the Parkland formula, providing 100 cc of Ringer's lactate (Table 27.3).

A 12-lead ECG was obtained and continuous cardiac monitoring initiated. The central
venous pressure (CVP) was 4 mm Hg. A nasogastric Salem sump tube was inserted for
antacid therapy; a Foley catheter was also placed to monitor hourly outputs, and a urinalysis
was sent for baseline monitoring.

Morphine sulfate 5 mg was administered IV for pain and debridement of loose burned
tissue in the Hubbard tank. Silver sulfadiazine (Silvadene) cream was applied to all wounds
and covered with one layer of sterile dressings. The patient's legs were elevated on pillows
because of swelling. He stated he was allergic to tetracycline; his tetanus inoculations were
up to date. He was listed in critical condition.

By 10:45 the same morning, the patient's initial fluid resuscitation had been reached. The
IV of Ringer's lactate was turned down to 550 cc/hr. Urine output was adequate at 45 to
50 cc/hr, BP 123/92, pulse 105, respirations 12 to 22/minute, and CVP 5 mm Hg. However,
from 1:30 to 2:30 PM his urine output was 12 cc after having slowly dropped each hour since
the IV rate was decreased. Significant changes in vital signs were CVP decreased to 2 mm
Hg, and pulse increased to 120 beats/minute. His BP remained essentially the same. A bolus
of 500 cc of Ringer's lactate was given at 3:00 PM. The nasogastric tube was taken out, and
clear liquids were started. By 3:30 PM, the CVP increased to 4.5, and the pulse decreased
to 105 with a urine output of 22 to 40 cc/hr. By 9:00 PM, capillary refill in both feet was
poor, and the patient complained of loss of sensation. Doppler pulses were still present.
However, his skin color was documented as "dusky" and felt cool to the touch. Escharotomies (surgical incisions through eschar, or layer of necrotic tissue) were performed to both
legs to lessen constriction. Epinephrine soaks were applied to the escharotomy sites to control
bleeding. Both legs remained elevated on pillows. At 11:00 PM, the first of two ampules of
calcium chloride was given for a serum calcium of 7.2 mg/dl. Kayexalate 30 mg was
administered with 100 cc of sorbitol by mouth for a serum potassium of 6.6 mmol/liter. By

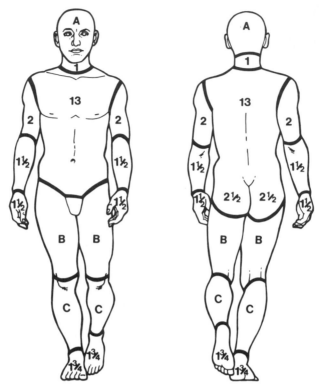

**Figure 27.1.** Determining percentage of body surface burn area using the Lund and Browder chart, which takes age and size differences into account.

Percentages of body surface areas affected by growth:

|  | Adult | 15 Years | 10 Years | 5 Years | 1 Year | Birth |
|---|---|---|---|---|---|---|
| A (half of head) | 3½% | 4½% | 5½% | 6½% | 8½% | 9½% |
| B (half of thigh) | 4¾% | 4½% | 4¼% | 4% | 3¼% | 2¾% |
| C (half of lower leg) | 3½% | 3¼% | 3% | 2¾% | 2½% | 2½% |

(Adapted from Strange JM. Shock trauma care plans. Springhouse, PA: Springhouse, 1987.)

midnight the second calcium chloride was given IV. A repeat Kayexalate dose was given at 2:00 AM Thursday.

Previous to IV fluid changes, there were significant variations in vital signs. CVP was 6, and urine output was 100 to 260 cc/hr. IV fluids were converted to D₅W at 100 cc/hr, Ringer's lactate at 275 cc/hr, and Plasmanate at 90 cc/hr. At 2:00 PM on Thursday, the Ringer's lactate was decreased to 100 cc/hr. Urine output at this time was 85 to 150 cc/hr, CVP was 9.5, and BP was 150/85.

The patient continued to have a urine output of 150 cc/hr throughout the night. On Friday at 6:30 AM, the patient was changed to maintenance fluids: normal saline was 20 mEq of potassium chloride/liter at 150 cc/hr. Later that morning, one dose of potassium chloride (10 mEq) was given IV piggyback for a serum potassium of 3.1 secondary to a high urine output. The IV fluids were also changed to half normal saline with 20 mEq of potassium chloride/liter at 150 cc/hr.

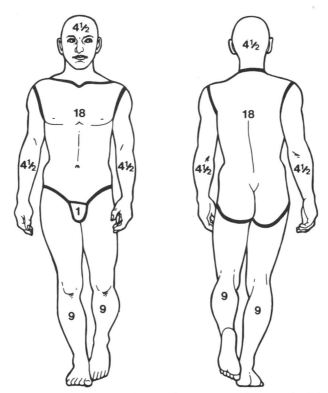

**Figure 27.2.** Estimating the percentage of body surface burn area using the "rule of nines." (Adapted from Strange JM. Shock trauma care plans. Springhouse, PA: Springhouse, 1987.)

## 1. What is the pathophysiological basis for this patient's problem?

The patient sustaining a chemical scald/burn injury may exhibit a combination of pathophysiological changes in fluid and electrolyte balance with potential multisystem organ involvement. Tissue damage from a thermal injury triggers an inflammatory response and vascular changes at both local and systemic levels. The larger the burn size, the more significant the systemic impact of these vascular changes (1, 2). Hyperdynamic fluid shifts are seen with a systemic response leading to hypovolemia, hyperkalemia, and massive interstitial edema known as burn shock (3).

Vascular changes at the site of burn injury are the result of direct capillary damage and the local release of chemicals mediating the inflammatory response (4). Damaged capillaries lose vessel wall integrity and leak plasma, which is rich in electrolytes and proteins, into the interstitial space. Damaged tissue cells release chemical mediators, such as serotonin, prostaglandins, histamine, and hyaluronidase as part of the inflammatory response. This release causes vasodilation and capillary bed leakage of fluids, electrolytes, and plasma proteins (1).

In patients with a burn size of approximately 20% TBSA or greater, these chemical mediators affect systemic vasodilation and increased capillary permeability. A significant fluid and electrolyte shift occurs from the intravascular to the interstitial space, while red blood cells remain within the vessel walls (3). Oxygen transport is then compromised

**Table 27.1.** Depth of injury[a]

| Characteristic | First Degree | Second Degree Superficial Partial Thickness | Second Degree Deep Partial Thickness | Third Degree Full Thickness |
|---|---|---|---|---|
| Morphology | Destruction of epidermis only | Destruction of epidermis and some dermis | Destruction of epidermis and dermis, leaving only skin appendages | Destruction of epidermis, dermis, and underlying subcutaneous tissue |
| Skin function | Intact | Absent | Absent | Absent |
| Tactile and pain sensors | Intact | Intact | Intact but diminished | Absent |
| Blisters | Present only after first 24 hours | Present within minutes, thin-walled, fluid-filled | May or may not appear as fluid-filled blisters; often is layer of flat, dehydrated "tissue paper" that lifts off in sheets | Blisters rare; usually is layer of flat, dehydrated "tissue paper" that lifts off easily |
| Appearance of wound after initial debridement | Skin peels at 24 to 48 hours, normal or slightly red underneath | Red to pale ivory, moist surface | Mottled with areas of waxy white, dry surface | White, cherry red, or black; may contain visible thrombosed veins; dry, hard leathery surface |
| Healing time | 3 to 5 days | 21 to 28 days | 30 days to many months | Will not heal; may close from edges as secondary healing if wound is small |
| Scarring | None | Present, influenced by genetic predisposition | Highest because slow healing rate increases scar tissue development, influenced by genetic predisposition | Skin graft scarring is minimized by early excision and grafting, influenced by genetic predisposition |

[a]*Source:* Reprinted with permission from Cardona VD, Hurn PD, Bastnagel-Mason PJ, et al. eds. Trauma nursing: from resuscitation through rehabilitation. Philadelphia: WB Saunders, 1988.

**Table 27.2.** American Burn Association: Definitions of injury extent[a]

| Minor Burn Injury | Moderate Uncomplicated Burn Injury | Major Burn Injury |
|---|---|---|
| Second-degree burn of less than 15 percent TBSA in adults or less than 10 percent TBSA in children | Second-degree burns of 15 to 25 percent TBSA in adults or 10 to 20 percent in children | Second-degree burns of greater than 25 percent TBSA in adults or 20 percent TBSA in children |
| Third-degree burn of less than 2 percent TBSA not involving special care areas (eyes, ears, face, hands, feet, perineum) | Third-degree burns of less than 10 percent TBSA not involving special care areas | All third-degree burns of 10 percent TBSA or greater |
| Excludes electrical injury, inhalation injury, complicated injury (fractures), all poor-risk patients (e.g., at extremes of age, with intercurrent disease) | Excludes electrical injury, complicated injury (fractures), inhalation injury, all poor-risk patients (e.g., at extremes of age, with intercurrent disease) | All burns involving hands, face, eyes, ears, feet, perineum |
| | | All inhalation injury, electrical injury, complicated burn injury involving fractures or other major trauma |
| | | All poor-risk patients |

[a]*Source:* Reprinted with permission from Cardona VD, Hurn PD, Bastnagel-Mason PJ, et al. eds. Trauma nursing: from resuscitation through rehabilitation. Philadelphia: WB Saunders, 1988.

**Table 27.3.** The Parkland formula[a]

| | |
|---|---|
| First 24 hr | Ringer's lactate: 4 cc/kg of body weight/TBSA (%)<br>One-half in the first 8 hr<br>One-half in the next 16 hr |
| Second 24 hr | Colloid: 0.5 cc/kg of body weight/TBSA (%)<br>$D_5W$ 2000 cc<br>One-half of the first day's Ringer's lactate |

Patient's weight on admission: 87.3 kg
TBSA: 51%
Time of Burn: 3:00 AM
Time of admission: 4:00 AM
Requirement for the first 24 hr:
  4 cc × 87.3 × 51 = 17,809.2 cc = 17,800 cc
    First 24 hr = 8900 cc
    minus 100 cc given in the helicopter
    Left to give in the first 24 hr = 8800 cc
Because the patient arrived 1 hour postburn, the fluid due in first 8 hours postburn must be given over a 7-hour period.
Rate of Ringer's lactate from 4:00 AM to 11:00 AM will be 1257 cc/hr. The rate of Ringer's lactate for the following 16 hours will be 550 cc/hr.
Requirement for the second 24 hr:
  Colloid:  0.5 cc × 87.3 × 51 = 2226 cc
       Rate of colloid = 90 cc/hr
  $D_5W$:    2000 cc
       Rate of $D_5W$ = 93 cc/hr
       (We increased the rate to 100 cc/hr to give the patient a little more free water).
Ringer's lactate: 8800 cc
       Rate of the Ringer's lactate = 366 cc/hr
       (We decreased the rate to 275 cc/hr because of the $K^+$.)

[a]*Source:* Adapted from Artz CP, Moncrief JA, Pruitt BA, eds. Burns: a team approach. Philadelphia: WB Saunders, 1979:182.

as red blood cells become clogged within the intravascular space with little liquid medium to facilitate blood flow.

The increased capillary permeability and fluid shifts continue for the first 18 to 24 hours postburn. Once the capillary integrity stabilizes, the fluid shifts follow the gradients created by oncotic and hydrostatic pressures as fluid returns to the vascular space (5). Within 2 to 3 days, a homeostatic fluid distribution between interstitial and intravascular spaces is re-established.

Electrolyte disturbances in potassium and sodium balance may occur in patients experiencing burn shock. Hyperkalemia can result during the first 24 to 48 hours postburn as the result of the release of intracellular potassium from damaged blood and tissue cells (6). Hypernatremia can be seen following crystalloid fluid replacement as the patient attempts to equilibrate intravascular and interstitial fluid distribution (6). Serum sodium concentration may remain high because of the large quantity of sodium administered during intravenous fluid repletion.

Exposure to sodium alum fluoride (an industrial fluoride compound) by chemical scald can produce two toxic effects. One effect is cell membrane disruption when the fluoride ion denatures proteins through salt formation (7). The second effect occurs when fluoride ion binds with accessible calcium ions, leading to cell death and decalcification of bone and hypocalcemia (8).

## 2. What are the nursing diagnoses of highest priority?

A. Fluid volume deficit
B. Potential for altered tissue perfusion
C. Potential for electrolyte disturbances

## 3. What are the goals of nursing care?

### A. Nursing Diagnosis

Fluid volume deficit related to 51% TBSA second- and third-degree burn shock and insensible water loss

### Goal of Care

Restore and maintain normal body fluid volume.

### Nursing Interventions

- Titrate administration of intravenous fluids to maintain adequate urine output and vital signs.
- Assess heart rate (HR), BP, CVP, and sensorium every 1 to 2 hours.
- Strictly monitor intake and output hourly throughout fluid resuscitation.
- Obtain admission weight and monitor daily.
- Auscultate breath sounds every 4 hours and report signs of pulmonary edema.
- Assess extent of interstitial edema at least every 8 hours.

### Rationale

The chemical scald/burn injury victim often requires a large volume of intravascular fluid replacement during the first 3 to 5 days after injury. Parkland Formula guidelines are used for estimating volumes of fluids needed for crystalloid repletion; however, the patient's clinical response should guide the actual volumes and administration rates. Urine output is the most helpful clinical tool for assessing the adequacy of the patient's resuscitation. The patient who excretes urine at a rate of 0.5 to 1.0 cc/kg/hr is receiving adequate resuscitation (6). Other useful information includes the patient's sensorium, heart rate, BP, central venous pressure, daily weight, and extent of interstitial edema. The patient receiving adequate fluid resuscitation will be alert, with a heart rate of less than 120, blood pressure within normal range, central venous pressure between 2 and 12 mm Hg, and a moderate amount of edema that does not compromise circulation (3). Monitoring of daily weight should demonstrate an increase of no more than 5 kg concurrent of large volumes of fluid during the initial 24 hours postburn and a gradual decrease to admission weight accompanied by progressive excretion of excess interstitial fluid and progressive decrease in dependent edema (1).

### B. Nursing Diagnosis

Potential for alteration in tissue perfusion related to circumferential third-degree burns

### Goal of Care

Maintain adequate tissue perfusion and limit tissue damage.

### Nursing Interventions

- Make neurovascular checks of circumferentially burned extremities every 1 to 2 hours in the first 24 hours postburn.
- Report findings of diminished peripheral circulation immediately.
- Teach patient and family about escharotomies.
- Assess escharotomy incisions every 4 to 8 hours for evidence of bleeding.

- Apply epinephrine-soaked gauze pads to escharotomy sites initially and at least every 12 hours.
- Elevate extremities.

### Rationale

Circumferential third-degree burns result in full-thickness destruction of skin, leaving an eschar with limited capacity to expand (2, 6). As the burn-injured patient develops interstitial edema, the circumferential eschar expands minimally, resulting in fluid compression of the underlying tissues and potentially compromising nerve function, blood flow, and movement. Neurovascular assessment of circumferentially burned extremities facilitates early detection of compromised circulation, sensation, and/or movement, thus allowing for timely escharotomies to optimize viable tissue perfusion (3).

Escharotomies facilitate expansion of underlying viable tissue as interstitial edema continues (6). The procedure can be completed at the patient's bedside using sterile technique. Anesthetic agents are unnecessary, as the eschar is insensate. The escharotomy incisions may be packed with epinephrine-soaked gauze to accomplish hemostasis of small bleeding capillaries. A recommended solution of 1:100,000 can be prepared by adding 10 ampules of 1:1000 epinephrine to 1000 ml of normal saline (9, 10). The vasoconstrictor action of epinephrine may control superficial bleeding if applied topically, but only against bleeding from arterioles and capillaries, not venous oozing or bleeding from larger vessels (9, 10). Other methods of hemostasis (such as electrocautery, suture material, silver nitrate sticks) may be necessary to stop bleeding when epinephrine soaks fail. The use of dressings impregnated with hemostatic and/or vasoactive agents should be highly individualized and only on the order of a physician.

Fasciotomies (surgical incision through the fascia) may be necessary when escharotomies fail to restore adequate circulation; however, they should be completed in a controlled, sterile environment such as an operating room (1). The patient and family will need repeated explanations of the reason for the procedure and reinforcement that the appearance of the wound with a deep surgical incision is temporary. Escharotomy and fasciotomy incisional defects are usually treated by secondary closure or covered with split-thickness skin grafts (11).

### C. Nursing Diagnosis

Potential for electrolyte disturbances related to burn shock, insensible fluid loss, and wound healing

### Goal of Care

Maintain homeostatic intravascular electrolyte concentration.

### Nursing Interventions

- Monitor electrolyte levels daily and as needed.
- Administer electrolyte supplements and related medications.
- Check neurovascular function every 8 hours.
- Administer nutritional therapy as prescribed.
- Monitor intake and output every 8 hours.

### Rationale

Hyperkalemia, hypernatremia, and hypocalcemia are the three significant electrolyte disturbances that the patient sustaining a sodium alum fluoride chemical scald/burn is most likely to exhibit. All three of these problems can be avoided or controlled through close monitoring, astute assessment, and timely intervention. The treatment for hyperkalemia will usually include the use of the exchange resin agent Kayexalate for removal of excess potassium by excretion through the gastrointestinal tract (6). Kayexalate is administered orally by suspension in sorbitol or administered as an enema suspended in warm normal saline. An alternative more rapidly effective treatment for hyperkalemia is the administration of insulin with 10% dextrose intravenously to facilitate movement of potassium into the cells. Bowel function should be monitored frequently along with intake and output to assess for potential hinderances to potassium excretion.

Hypernatremia is resolved by the administration of free water intravenously and/or orally. The patient should be given fluids intravenously that are free of all sodium chloride until the serum sodium concentration returns to normal (5). Close monitoring of daily serum sodium levels along with intake and output will provide information regarding the patient's sodium and water balance.

The patient's hypocalcemia is attributable to his contamination with the sodium alum fluoride compound. The treatment of choice is intravenous administration of calcium supplement. Either calcium chloride or calcium gluconate can be used to total 1 to 1.5 gm/day depending on the patient's replacement needs (5). Monitoring of the patient's serum calcium levels on a daily basis is crucial in determining the adequacy of treatment.

## ASSOCIATED NURSING DIAGNOSES

A. Impairment of skin integrity
B. Potential for infection
C. Potential for ineffective thermoregulation
D. Altered comfort: acute pain
E. Impaired physical mobility
F. Anxiety
G. Fear
H. Body image disturbance
I. Alteration in nutrition: less than body requirements

**REFERENCES**

1. Artz CP, Moncrief JA, Pruitt BA. Burns: a team approach. Philadelphia: WB Saunders, 1979.
2. Kravitz M. Thermal injuries. In: Cardona VD, Hurn PD, Bastnagel-Mason PJ, et al, eds. Trauma nursing: from resuscitation through rehabilitation. Philadelphia: WB Saunders, 1988:707–745.
3. Hills SW, Birmingham JJ. Burn care. Bethany, CT: Fleschner, 1981.
4. Strange JM. Shock trauma care plans. Springhouse, PA: Springhouse, 1987.
5. Stroot VR, Lee CAB, Barrett CA. Fluids and electrolytes: a practical approach. 3rd ed. Philadelphia: FA Davis, 1984.
6. Feller I, Archambeault C. Nursing the burned patient. Ann Arbor: Institute for Burn Medicine, 1974.
7. Fitzpatrick KT, Moylan JA. Emergency care of chemical burns. Postgrad Med 1985;78:192.
8. Stewart CE. Chemical skin burns. Am Fam Physician 1985;31:153.
9. Heimbach DM, Engrav LH. Surgical management of the burn wound. New York: Raven, 1984:14.
10. Gilman AC, Goodman LS, Gilman A. The pharmacological basis of therapeutics. 6th ed. New York: Macmillan, 1980:168.
11. Wagner MM. Care of the burn-injured patient: multidisciplinary involvement. Littleton, MA: PSG Publishing Co., 1981:190–191.

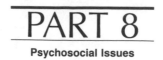

# PART 8
**Psychosocial Issues**

# CHAPTER 28

## Families in Sudden Crisis

Margaret M. Epperson-Sebour, MSW, ACSW, CSW

## Clinical Presentation

Mr. and Mrs. Smith (fictitious name), the middle-aged parents of two teenagers, were awakened by an early-morning phone call from the state police. John, their 19-year-old son, had been in a serious car accident and was being flown by helicopter from the accident scene to the hospital. One of the car's occupants had been killed. By police estimate, John appeared to be in critical condition.

The Smiths and their 17-year-old daughter, Lisa, drove from their home in western Maryland to the hospital in Baltimore, a 2-hour trip. They were met in the family waiting area by a social worker trained in family process. The way they spoke, their body language, and their agitated behavior indicated that these family members were under severe stress.

Mr. Smith began pacing the floor, shouting, "Where's my son?" and "Can't someone do something?" Mrs. Smith sat on the edge of a chair with her hands clasped between her thighs, repeating over and over "My God, what happened? I hope he's all right!" Lisa, with red eyes and nose, quietly wove a torn facial tissue around her fingers as she sat tensely in the corner of the couch.

Because many families are "fragmented" families (i.e., families with one or more members temporarily or permanently absent), and because of the currently differing views of the sociological composition of the so-called modern family grouping, the definition of *family* used in this paper is based on that of the philosopher–theologian Thomas Aquinas: Family is the community of one's household—the person or persons one is living with.

The phrase "sudden, severe stress due to life-threatening situations of family members" describes the state of acute crisis the family experiences when a family member is in critical physical condition due to multiple injuries as a result of a catastrophic event. Families must deal with the reality that one of their members is suddenly in danger of death because of a road accident, violent criminal assault, industrial mishap, recreational miscalculation, or some domestic tragedy.

Caplan defines *crisis* as "an upset in a steady state" (1). This definition rests on the systems-theory concept that an individual, a family, or any social system strives to maintain a state of equilibrium through a constant series of adaptive maneuvers and characteristic problem-solving activities that allow for basic need fulfillment to take place. Whether a situation or event becomes a "crisis" depends greatly on how the family defines or interprets the event in light of its own cultural and historical experiences. What may be a crisis for one family may not be so for another.

Throughout a system's life span, many situations or events occur that can lead to sudden

This article, "Families in Sudden Crisis," has been adapted by permission of the publisher, Haworth Press, from *Social Work in Health Care* (Spring) 1977;2(3):265–273.

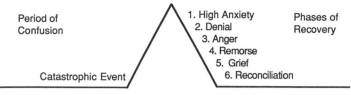

**Figure 28.1.** Families under sudden, severe stress in life-threatening situations undergo a six-phase recovery process.

breakdowns in the system's functioning. One event that can disrupt the usual homeostatic state of a family system is the sudden, catastrophic illness of one of its members. The Smith family is typical of a family thrown into a sudden crisis state.

It is postulated that in a state of crisis the system's usual problem-solving mechanisms are insufficient and do not rapidly lead the system back to a state of equilibrium. Often, a family must find new solutions to deal with situations that, up to the current crisis state, had been outside the realm of their family system's life experience (2). The Smiths needed external help in coping with their situation until they could mobilize their own adaptive capacities and activate their inner resources that would eventually help re-establish the family's precrisis "steady state."

# Description of Process

Families under sudden, severe stress appear to go through, or at least touch on, six distinct phases before the family system is able to reorganize, reintegrate, and regain its homeostatic state. It is to be understood that families differ in regard to both the sequence of phases and the rate by which family members pass through the various stages. Also, it is to be noted that some families skip over stages and eliminate them altogether in the adaptive process. Furthermore, all family members do not go through the phases at the same time, and each member is unique in his or her completion of the process. Each family member, like each family group, is individualistic in his or her pattern of the adapting process. However, despite this diversity, there remains a distinct, identifiable method of recovery to a "steady state" (see Fig. 28.1).

## High Anxiety

A period of high anxiety is most often the phase families go through first, and it is usually experienced by most family members at the same time. The high-anxiety phase is characterized by great physical agitation, a high-pitched voice, tight neck and shoulder muscles, and other body reactions, such as fainting, nausea, and diarrhea, found to be typical of persons under severe stress. On their arrival at the hospital, Mr. and Mrs. Smith overtly demonstrated many of these physical signs of stress. Lisa sat quietly to the side; only her body language revealed her stressful state. Sometimes anxiety is manifested by withdrawal and body tenseness as if the person is using all his or her energies in body containment. This acute anxiety can last anywhere from a few minutes to several hours.

Three things are done to help diminish the family's anxiety:

1. Brief, accurate information is given about the patient. The family is told where the patient is at the moment—the admitting area, the operating room, or the critical care area. They are also told the general condition of the patient, for example, "His condition at the moment appears to be serious." The family is assured that a physician and nurse will be in to give a complete medical report as soon as the physician team has done a thorough examination and x-rays have been read—usually within an hour.

2. Life-saving methods and advanced technology are explained. This seems to reassure the family that the patient has every advantage modern medicine can offer.

3. The family members are encouraged to ventilate about the initial impact of the news of this sudden catastrophe, such as where they were, what they were doing, and what they were told about the accident.

These three steps, coupled with definite information from the physician's report, are most often sufficient to relieve the anxiety to a level at which the family members can begin to consider other issues, such as, what this means, what they should do now, and other pragmatic considerations that lead to another phase, usually that of denial.

## Denial

John was severely injured in the car accident. He had multiple fractures and several lacerations that could heal over time, but a spinal-cord injury would leave him permanently paralyzed from the waist down. After a lengthy discussion with the family, the doctor left and Mrs. Smith began to cry. Her husband tried to comfort her, saying, "Everything will be all right. You know John; he's a tough kid. He'll be walking again, you'll see." He repeated this statement to Lisa and to the therapist. Later he told the nurse about spinal-cord-injured army buddies who had learned to walk again and that there was no reason why John couldn't do the same. Mr. Smith's denial of the situation was real.

The denial phase is important because it seems to act as a psychological preparation for any further bad news the family may receive about the patient. It also seems to have in it the essential element of hope needed to carry on. Further, denial is a regression to a comfortable childhood stage of "magical thinking" that says "in spite of what happened everything will be all right."

It is important for the therapist to maintain a balance in this situation by recognizing the need for denial as well as the need for the family to deal with the reality of what has happened and what the situation now is. Statements such as "Mr. Smith, John was such a healthy boy, it must be difficult for you to believe that he is now paralyzed" are often helpful. Appropriate reiterating of like statements to the family conveys to them that the therapist understands and accepts their struggle with reality. These statements also act as a reminder of what is, without removing the denial defense.

Often, the denial phase lasts until the family is able to speak to the patient, usually after a 48-hour stabilization period. Some family members hold on to their denial for long periods of time, and special efforts must be made through follow-up sessions to help these persons deal with the reality of the situation.

## Anger

Anger expressed by families under sudden, severe stress seems to be amoeboid, taking many different shapes and directions. During this phase, anger can be directed toward oneself or another family member in an apparent attempt to place the blame, or part of the blame, for what has happened. It can be directed toward the physician and nursing staff, the state police, the emergency medical technicians, the therapist, and others. Often, it is a diffuse kind of anger that lashes out at society or at life in general for allowing to exist circumstances such as high speeds, lack of gun controls, or lenient drunk-driving laws that may have contributed to the tragedy.

Often families unite in their expressions of anger. In the Smith's case, Lisa was the first to articulate her angry feelings. In response to her father's statements of denial, she began to accuse him of always having to be in control, of telling everyone what they could or could not do: "You're always telling everyone what they're going to do. Just because you say he is going to walk again doesn't mean he is going to." She began to blame him for the accident: "You're the one who told him to 'get out.' This wouldn't have happened if he was at home." (John was living outside the parental home.) Mrs. Smith lashed out at Lisa for being disrespectful to her father. After siding with her husband, Mrs. Smith began to express angry feelings about the inefficiency of the state police. He husband joined her in her accusations. Lisa began to criticize society in general.

During this phase, the therapist encourages ventilation of angry feelings. It is the therapist's task to help the family focus on the real cause of their anger. When families have a chance to really listen to their accusations, they often see the illegitimacy of their charges. Eventually, the family comes to realize that they are angry at the patient himself or herself for disrupting the family routine and causing great stress and disorganization within the family system. It must be noted, however, that there are times when outside agents are legitimately responsible, at least in part, for the accident.

In families that appeared to have good, open patterns of communication, the expressed anger was often immediately directed toward the patient for being so "careless," "dumb," or "stupid" in putting himself or herself in the dangerous situation that was now causing the family such stress. But these same families often expressed feelings of guilt for blaming the sick person for what had happened.

All families who express anger toward the injured member, whether immediately or through a circuitous route, need reassurance that they are not "bad" persons for feeling angry. Often, individual members need repeated "permission" from the therapist to say their angry words. Our society says that it is not nice to be mad at sick, helpless individuals. Consequently, some members experience a sense of uneasiness for blaming the injured member. It is the experience of this writer that, unless the anger family members feel toward the patient is expressed and dealt with, it can cause further destruction to the family system by being later expressed in passive–aggressive behavior toward the patient during his or her rehabilitation.

## Remorse

The sense of guilt families feel for blaming the patient for the current crisis is different from what is considered to be a period or phase of remorse. Guilt feelings say "Somehow I have done wrong; I am culpable." Remorse, on the other hand, includes the elements of both guilt and sorrow. Remorse seems to describe best what family members feel about the part they may have played in contributing to the accident. They regret not only that the incident occurred, but that they did not, or could not, do more to prevent it. It is the "if only . . ." stage.

With great sorrow, the Smith family expressed their remorse with such statements as "If only I had not bought him that car, this would never have happened"; "If only he had still been living at home, he would not have been out so late"; and "If only I had given him the money to get that car fixed, this might not have happened."

It is important to listen to these expressions of remorse and to try to inject some reality as to how much blame the family members can take for the accident. What is it that the family members actually could have done to prevent this tragedy from happening? Usually, there is little, if anything, they could have done to prevent it, but the family can come to this reality only by open discussion.

What family members seem to need and want most during this phase is a reassurance that they are good people in spite of what has happened. Often, the news media compound this problem by giving inaccurate reports that appear to show negligence on the part of the family. Families find it very difficult to cope with this public censure as well as that of other systems with which they must interact, such as in their job situations, school, clubs, and church groups. It is the task of the therapist to help the family relieve themselves of the burden of taking responsibility for the accident, as, in the judgment of the investigator, it was a rare case that a family member could or should have taken legitimate blame for what had happened.

## Grief

During the second interview with the Smith family, Mrs. Smith began to express the meaning of her loss. As is characteristic of family members beginning to deal with their grief, Mrs. Smith began by talking about how others would miss her son. "He's such a good boy. The other kids really depend on him to help them out. If anything happens to him, I don't know what they'll do." Eventually, after much discussion about how others would feel about John's temporary absence from his social groups and how they would be affected by his paralysis, both Mrs. Smith and Lisa were able to internalize their feelings of loss. Through her tears Mrs. Smith was able to say "I love him so much—he's my oldest baby; he's always been such a comfort to me. Why did this have to happen?" Lisa's statement showed a recognition of at least temporary loss of old, familiar family patterns and the need for role reversal: "He has always taken care of me. I guess now I'll have to take care of him."

The grief phase usually follows the period of remorse, but not always. It is to be remembered that each family system and each family member differs when going through the phases. The family, at one time or another, experiences an intense period of sadness, a grieving time when their sense of loss, even temporary loss, becomes almost overwhelming. At this time, tears and deep sobbing are frequent. Some family members withdraw into privacy. Tears shed during this phase are different from those that offer a cathartic release of tension in the anxiety phase. This stage is the beginning of a grieving process, the duration and intensity of which depend on such factors as the medical condition of the patient, the length of hospitalization, the family solidarity, and the degree of remorse experienced by the family.

During the grief phase, the therapist remains with the family. Grief cannot be taken away, nor should there be any attempt to do so. Grief is a natural, human response to the loss, or threatened loss, of a loved object or person. Most often, the therapist just sits quietly with the family members, offering silent support. Many times physical closeness, holding a trembling hand or embracing limp shoulders, conveys an empathy for and an understanding of what the family members are experiencing. These empathic gestures are often all that are needed to begin the flow of copious tears that give some release to the deep emotional feelings of loss.

## Reconciliation

Reconciliation usually occurs last, and it seems to be a culmination point in the therapist's intervention during the acute family crisis. At this time the high state of anxiety is diminished, the reality of the situation is clear or is becoming clearer to the family, anger and remorse have usually been expressed, and the grieving process has begun.

Choosing an accurate word to describe what transpires during this phase is a problem of semantics. The word *reconciliation* is used because it differs from *acceptance* or *acquiescence* in that it connotes a "bringing together" or "bringing into harmony" all that has taken place. Reconciliation is not acceptance of what has happened; most families cannot accept the tragedy, especially if it appeared to be a senseless occurrence. This is a phase of putting things in place, of being reconciled to the fact that something terrible has happened that deeply affects, and will continue to affect, the total family unit. Included in this period of reconciliation is a realistic sense of hope that, whatever hardship this tragedy may impose, the family can and will survive.

This period is the time when mobilization of the family system's resources begins, if it hasn't already, to enable the family to adapt to the current situation and cope with whatever is to come. During this phase, a family solidarity seems to emerge and concretize through a concerted effort on the part of the family to plan for the future.

The Smiths gave evidence that they were becoming reconciled to the tragic reality of John's injuries by such statements as "We've been through hard times before and we've made it"; "There's no reason we can't ride this storm out"; "Tragedy is nothing new to us"; and "We'll have to pull together to take each day as it comes."

During this phase, the social worker helps the family to start thinking about and begin to develop a feasible plan of action: What needs to be done now? Who will be able to do these things? What are the available resources that can be used? Who and what helped the family pull through previous crises? For a variety of reasons, either current or long standing, some families appear unable to activate adequate coping mechanisms and must rely heavily on outside resources. Other families are better able to cope but require minimal outside support. In both cases, appropriate referrals to community agencies must be made.

## REFERENCES

1. Caplan G. Formulated in seminars at the Harvard School of Public Health, 1959–1960.

2. Spiegel JP. The resolution of role conflict within the family. Psychiatry 1957;20(1):15.

## SUGGESTED READINGS

Brodland GA, Andreasen NJ. Adjustment problems of the family of the burn patient. Social Casework 1974;55(1):13.

Fahy TJ, Irving MH, Millac P. Severe dead injuries— a six-year follow up. Lancet 1967;2(7509): 475.

Mueller AD. Psychologic factors in rehabilitation of paraplegic patients. Arch Physical Med 1962;43(4):151.

Parad HJ, Caplan G. A framework for studying families in crisis. Social Work 1960;5(3):34.

West ND. Stresses associated with ICUs affect patients, families, staff. J Am Hospital Assoc 1975;49(49):63.

# CHAPTER 29

# Family Considerations in the Rehabilitation of the Closed Head Injury Patient

Adrianne E. Avillion, RN, MS, CCRN, CNA

## Clinical Presentation

A 20-year-old man was admitted to a rehabilitation facility following a 5-week acute care hospitalization for the treatment of a closed head injury. The police report at the time of his trauma concluded that the patient was driving at a high rate of speed when he lost control of the car, hit a tree, and struck his head on the windshield on impact. The patient was alone in the car and was not wearing a seat belt.

During acute care hospitalization, the patient progressed from Rancho Los Amigos classification Level I to Level IV (Table 29.1) (1). On admission to the rehabilitation hospital, the patient remained at Level IV for 10 days. He had no other injuries except for some minor facial lacerations; he never required a tracheostomy. He was able to ambulate and to eat with supervision. The patient was in a confused and agitated state and had a markedly decreased ability to process information; his attention span was almost nonexistent. He was unable to perform self-care activities without maximum assistance. The patient also displayed aggressive behavior and often attempted to strike staff members. Throughout this period only his mother's presence had a calming influence over his behavior.

The patient progressed through Level V to Level VI during the next 4 weeks. He plateaued at Level VI and remained at that level for 1 month, at which time final discharge plans were made.

As a Level VI head-injured patient, he was able to follow simple directions and had an attention span of 20 to 30 minutes. He was continent of bowel and bladder and could perform self-care activities with minimal supervision. He was able to recognize his family and a few close friends but was oriented inconsistently to time and place. His short-term memory remained moderately impaired, and his safety awareness was quite poor. His speech was slow and halting, and he exhibited emotional lability, crying and laughing inappropriately. He spoke of returning to college "next week" and displayed little insight regarding his injury and its consequences.

The patient is the eldest of three children, with a 16-year-old sister and a 10-year-old brother. His parents both work full-time; his father is a college professor, and his mother is a buyer for a major department store. The patient was a college sophomore, an A and B student, majoring in psychology. He was described by family and friends as an outgoing, popular young man who studied hard, maintained a part-time job in a fast-food restaurant, and had close relationships with his parents and siblings. He lived at his parents' home and commuted to a local college. There was no known history of substance abuse.

The accident placed great strain on the family unit. The patient's mother took an unpaid leave of absence from her job and spent most of her time at the hospital with her son. She considered quitting her job because the patient's lack of safety awareness made it risky to leave him alone. The decrease in the family income began to cause some financial problems.

The patient's father maintained his job and began to tutor students as an income supplement. Both parents were therefore away from home a great deal, and the patient's 16-year-old sister had to assume more and more responsibility for running the household and supervising

**Table 29.1.** Rancho Los Amigos classification[a]

| | |
|---|---|
| *Level I*<br>No Response | Patient is completely unresponsive to any stimuli presented to him. |
| *Level II*<br>Generalized Responses | Patient responds inconsistently and non-purposefully to stimuli. The earliest response is often to deep pain. |
| *Level III*<br>Localized Responses | Patient reacts specifically but inconsistently to stimuli. He may follow simple commands in a delayed, inconsistent manner. |
| *Level IV*<br>Confused-Agitated | Patient is in an increased state of activity and responds primarily to his own internal confusion. Behavior is frequently bizarre and may be aggressive. Verbalization is frequently incoherent and/or inappropriate to the environment. Attention span is very short. Maximum assistance may be needed for self-care activities. |
| *Level V*<br>Confused-Inappropriate | Patient appears alert and is able to follow simple commands but is unable to follow more complex commands. He has gross attention to the environment but is highly distractible and needs frequent redirection. Verbalization is often inappropriate and memory is severely impaired. He may be able to perform previously learned tasks when structured for him, but is unable to learn new information. If the patient is physically mobile he may wander off either randomly or with the idea of "going home." |
| *Level VI*<br>Confused-Appropriate | Patient shows goal-directed behavior, follows simple directions consistently, and shows carry-over for tasks he has relearned. He no longer wanders and is inconsistently oriented to time and place. He has an increased awareness of self, family, and basic needs in an appropriate manner as contrasted with Level V. |
| *Level VII*<br>Automatic-Appropriate | Patient appears appropriate and oriented within hospital and home settings, goes through daily routine automatically, but frequently robot-like, with minimal-to-absent confusion. He shows increased awareness of self, body, family, foods, people, and interaction in the environment. He has superficial awareness of, but lacks insight into his condition, has decreased judgment and problem solving abilities and lacks realistic planning for his future. He requires at least minimal supervision for learning and for safety purposes. He is independent in self-care activities but requires supervised in home and community skills for safety. |
| *Level VIII*<br>Purposeful and Appropriate | Patient is alert and oriented, is able to recall and integrate past and recent events, and is aware of and responsive to his culture. He shows carry-over for new learning if acceptable to him and his life role, and needs no supervision once activities are learned. Within his physical capabilities, he is independent in home and community skills. His social, emotional, and intellectual capacities may continue to be at a decreased level for him, but functional in society. |

[a]*Source:* Rancho Los Amigos Hospital. Rehabilitation of the head injured adult—comprehensive management. Palm Springs, CA: Professional Staff Association of the Rancho Los Amigos Hospital, Inc., 1980:8–11.

her younger brother. She resented these additional tasks and described her brother as "embarrassing, not the same person as before." She also commented that it would have been better if her brother had died in the accident.

The patient's 10-year-old brother was also angry and bewildered by the changes in the family unit. He attempted to run away from home on several occasions, and his schoolteacher reported that his grades dropped and his behavior became increasingly argumentative and belligerent.

The patient's parents quarrelled frequently over finances and their children's various problems. The father began to question the family's ability to supervise the patient continuously postdischarge. The mother insisted that her son would be "back to normal as soon as we can get him home where he belongs." She talked of looking for a tutor so the patient wouldn't be too far behind "when he goes back to college next semester." The family unit was close to breaking down completely, and the rehabilitation team attempted to support the family during this especially difficult time.

## 1. What is the psychological basis for this patient's problems?

The process of recovery from head injury is lengthy, uneven, and unpredictable. Families, anxiously looking for reasons to maintain hope, sometimes find them in small signs of improvement and in uncertain prognoses from professionals (2 [pp. 102–109]). Rosenthal and Muir use the phrase *mobile mourning* to describe the extended grieving process that families of head-injured patients must face (3).

The family's emotional readjustment to the impact of the head injury often requires an extensive time period; they may just begin to face the implications at the time of his discharge from the rehabilitation center. Furthermore, many families are still struggling to adjust to these factors 2 or more years later (2 [pp. 102–109]).

Health care professionals involved in the treatment of head-injured patients should provide a regularly repeated educational lecture series, as well as written educational materials, to supplement individualized contacts with patient and family. Topics that may be offered in a lecture series include pathophysiology of head injury, safety needs, sexuality, a plan of care based on the Rancho Los Amigos classification, and vocational retraining. A family-centered support group may also provide much-needed emotional support and a means of helping families of head-injured patients to network and solve problems.

## 2. What are the nursing diagnoses of highest priority?

A. Grieving—family
B. Alterations in family process
C. Ineffective family coping

## 3. What are the goals of nursing care?

### A. Nursing Diagnosis

Grieving—family: related to an unpredictable, lengthy recovery process compounded by cognitive deficits

### Goal of Care

Regain and/or maintain psychosocial functioning throughout the grieving process.

### Nursing Interventions

- Provide consistent, accurate information regarding the patient's progress and participation in the rehabilitation program. Such information should be shared at regularly scheduled family conferences. All nurses must be aware of the patient's care plan so that there is consistency in the reporting process.

- Encourage attendance at educational classes, and support group meetings.
- Encourage ventilation of feelings.
- Respect the family's concerns, hopes, and fears. Be objective.

### Rationale

Lezak (4) found that families of head-injured patients go through a series of reactions similar to the response to terminal illness identified by Kübler-Ross (5): denial and isolation, anger, bargaining, depression, and acceptance. Lezak noted that early in the rehabilitation process families were hopeful and often anticipated a complete recovery. This hope deteriorated to anxiety, confusion, and even guilt and anger, as recovery did not meet their expectations.

Early in the rehabilitation process families should be told that some feelings of anxiety, guilt, and anger are normal responses to tragedy. The professional staff can help families deal with, and put into perspective, such feelings by providing information about these emotional reactions and about the patient's conditions so families can make well-informed decisions. In the instance of anger, it is especially important for the staff to understand the grieving dynamics and to respond with respect and support rather than with defensiveness (2 [p. 106]).

### B. Nursing Diagnosis

Alterations in family process related to changes in responsibilities

### Goal of Care

Assist family members to attend to their personal needs while adjusting to alterations in the family process.

### Nursing Interventions

- Explain to family members that they need not devote all of their time to the patient.
- Urge family members to attend to their own needs and provide information regarding support services that may assist them in meeting needs.
- Provide a format for family therapy as needed.
- Encourage support-group attendance.
- Provide a means of postdischarge follow-up for at least 1 year.

### Rationale

Family members, especially parents, have difficulty detaching themselves from the overwhelming needs of the head-injured patient. Other family concerns and activities are often sacrificed to meet the patient's needs. Marital stress, in both healthy and troubled marriages, can be a problem throughout the rehabilitation period and beyond. The importance of ongoing dialogue, open communication, and mutual support should be stressed by the health care team.

Siblings are often the most neglected family members (2 [p. 109]). They may feel neglected, embarrassed by the patient's behavior, resentful toward the patient for being the center of attention, and angry for being burdened with additional responsibilities. Group discussions for siblings of head-injured patients provide understanding of head injuries and help in dealing with changing roles and responsibilities.

A discharge follow-up that ensures contact with patients and families helps provide support, guidance, and information as the family unit continues the adjustment process. Complete realization of the patient's deficits may take place after discharge. Families should be taught to anticipate this realization and encouraged to maintain follow-up contact.

## C. Nursing Diagnoses

Ineffective family coping related to ongoing stress

### Goal of Care

Regain coping mechanisms to promote effective family functioning.

### Nursing Interventions

- Give information simply, directly, and consistently.
- Anticipate the need for repetitive education sessions.
- Encourage attendance at family therapy and support groups.
- Provide objective, empathetic support and clarification of family responses.
- Monitor for signs of breakdowns in health status.

### Rationale

Family members can cope with their extremely difficult feelings better if they recognize them as normal responses to catastrophic injury. The best professional interventions include empathetic concern, good listening, and objective support. It is critical to give the family honest, consistent information while respecting their need to maintain hope. The care plan serves as the basis for communication between patient, staff, and family. By keeping the plan current, staff will be able to share consistent, up-to-date information regarding the patient's progress.

A particularly difficult family reaction is that of denial of the patient's deficits. Denial may be used as a defense mechanism that allows families time to absorb the implications of catastrophic injury. However, it becomes pathological when treatment is disrupted, when patient welfare is threatened, or when denial continues to the point of disrupting the family unit. In this case, confrontation, combined with support from the staff, may be necessary for the welfare of the patient and family (2 [p. 105]). Confrontation may be carried out with primary caregivers from each discipline meeting with the family. The setting should be private, with minimal distraction. A staff member who has established good rapport with the family should sit next to them, thus avoiding the adversarial feeling of all family members on one side of a conference table and all staff members opposite them. Facts about the patient's progress and the family's reaction (i.e., disruption of therapy) should be openly discussed. Time must be allowed for the family to ventilate concerns and for the entire team, including the family, to discuss the care plan and propose alternative options that fit within that therapeutic care plan.

## ASSOCIATED NURSING DIAGNOSES

1. Anxiety
2. Fear
3. Knowledge deficit
4. Social isolation

**REFERENCES**

1. Rancho Los Amigos Hospital. Rehabilitation of the head injured adult: comprehensive management. Palm Springs, CA: Professional Staff Association of the Rancho Los Amigos Hospital, Inc., 1980:8–11.
2. Polinko PR, Barin JJ, Backman KM. Working with the family. In: Ylvisaker M, ed. Head injury rehabilitation—children and adolescents. San Diego: College-Hill Press, 1985.
3. Rosenthal M, Muir CA. Methods of family education. In: Rosenthal M, Griffith ER, Bond MR, Miller JD, eds. Rehabilitation of the head injured adult. Philadelphia: FA Davis, 1983:407–419.
4. Lezak MD. Unpublished data, 1984.
5. Kübler-Ross E. On death and dying. New York: Macmillan, 1969.

# CHAPTER 30

# Psychosocial and Sexual Aspects of the Spinal Cord Injury Patient

Mary Murphy-Rutter, RN, MSN
Valerie May Summerlin, RN, MSN, CNAA

## Clinical Presentation

Bill is a 32-year-old man who sustained a complete spinal cord injury after falling from a second-story roof. His 2½-year-old daughter witnessed the accident. Bill was admitted to the emergency department with complete motor paralysis and complete sensory disruption at and below the level of thoracic vertebra number 4. He had immediate placement of Harrington rods to stabilize the fracture and was transferred to a rehabilitation facility 4 weeks later.

Bill and his wife have been married 8 years and have a 6-year-old son in addition to their daughter. Bill is the eldest of three children; his parents and his in-laws live nearby. Bill is self-employed in the construction industry and is away from home for long periods during the day; his wife teaches school part-time at the local community college. Bill is described by family and friends as an outgoing, hard working, and athletic individual. His marriage has been what friends consider the "ideal" relationship. Bill has been the major financial support for his family.

Since Bill's accident his wife has attempted to manage the construction business, which has placed a strain not only on the family but on her own job as well. Homeowners and contractors are being delayed because of the wife's inability to respond to their inquiries because of her job, family, and hospital commitments. Both sets of parents assist somewhat; however, the main burden of responsibility is the wife's, and she is experiencing coping difficulties.

Bill's son is exhibiting some problems in school. He is not completing his classwork, and his homework is not always correct or neat. He is very angry because his father has been away from the home for such a long time, and he wonders why Dad is not home, since he is not "sick." Bill and his son have a close relationship; the mother's support is new, and their relationship is not as close.

The little girl is very independent. She enjoys going to day school where she receives support and love. She misses her Dad and has, on occasion, found her way into her parents' room to sleep at night. Since Bill's accident the daughter is terrified when she hears the sound of a siren, as she recalls the accident.

## 1. What are the pathophysiological and psychological bases for this patient's problems?

A complete injury at the T4 level results in loss of sensation below the nipple line and in paraplegia. Patients with such an injury are able to transfer to and from a wheelchair, bed, or automobile using a transfer/sliding board; to drive an automobile equipped with special hand controls; and to roll over and independently sit up in bed using an overhead trapeze (1) (see Table 30.1). They can also achieve independence in hygiene, grooming, and bowel/bladder care through re-education via an individualized program specifically designed to meet the patient's needs. We can compare the physical deficits associated with a spinal cord injury (SCI), but we cannot compare individual responses to the injury

**203**

**Table 30.1.** Spinal cord levels of function[a]

| Level | Peripheral Nerves | Muscle Innervation | Action | ADL and Mobility: Level of Independence | Adaptive Devices |
|---|---|---|---|---|---|
| C1, 2, 3 | Phrenic | Partial of—sternocleidomastoid, upper trapezius, spinal accessory C3—partial diaphragm | Shrug shoulders (weak) | Dependent in all activities of daily living (ADL) Head and trunk support needed when sitting | Electric wheelchair (w/c) with high back Mouth stick for writing |
| C4 | | Partial of—middle trapezius, slight deltoids, weak diaphragm, absent intercostals | Rotate head Shrug shoulders (stronger) | As for 1–3 May have more head control | Electric w/c with high back Ballbearing feeder |
| C5 | Spinal Accessory | Full of—trapezius, sternocleidomastoid, deltoids, diaphragm Partial of—biceps, brachioradialis, rhomboids, internal and external rotators | Gross arm Shrug shoulders Abduct arms Rotate head (full) Diaphragm excursions Strong shoulder shrug Slight flexion of arm Slight rotation of arm Slight rotation of forearm | Moderate to maximum assistance with ADL One-man transfers May self-feed with adaptive devices Manual locomotion over level surface for short distances | Electric w/c with support to shoulder level Regular w/c with quad pegs Sling device on w/c |
| C6 | Axillary Musculocutaneous Radial | Full of—rotator cuff, biceps Partial of—serratus anterior, intissimus dorsi, pectoralis major, pronator, supinator, extensor carpi radialis and ulnaris | Full flexion and rotation of arm Weak shoulder depression flexion, adduction and medial rotation of arm Some wrist extension and rotation | Weak "pincer" grasp—gross hand control Minimal assistance with ADL Can drive in adapted car or van Roll side to side—raise self to supine position on elbows Transfers may be independent with sliding board Manual locomotion on level surface for short distances | Manual w/c with quad pegs Sliding board Adaptive utensils for eating |

| Level | Nerve | Muscles | Function | Functional outcome | Equipment |
|---|---|---|---|---|---|
| C7 | Radial | Full of—shoulder depressors; Partial of—triceps, common finger extensors, long finger flexors, flexor carpi, radialis and ulnars | Full shoulder depression; Weak hand grasp and release; Wrist flexion; Forearm extension | Independent in ADL; Weight shift and full sitting push-ups makes transferring independent; Level surfaces for long distances, good endurance; rough surfaces may require assistance; May be able to stand with assistance and with knee-locking full-leg braces | Manual w/c with quad pegs or mits |
| T1–4 | Mediun ulnar | Intrinsic and extrinsic hand muscles, segmental trunk muscles, diaphragmatic breathing, partial intercostals | Good hand grasp and release; Upper trunk stability | Independent transfers; May be able to go from floor to wheelchair (T2–4); Independent in all ADL | Elevated toilet seat |
| T4–10 | Thoracic and lumbar | Full—more segmental muscles; Some abdominal muscles intercostals; Abdominal reflexes T12; T6–12 spastic paralysis | Can lift body; Improved respiratory exchange; More trunk stability | Independent in w/c and ADL; Improved endurance | |
| T11–L2 | Sacral Femoral | Oblique abdominals; Rectus abdominus; Transverse abdominals; Thoracic muscles; Quadiatus lumborum; Iliopsoas; Sartorius; L2—bladder, bowel; Sexual loss—depends on nerve roots | Abdominal support; Trunk flexion; Flexion of thigh; Lateral and medial rotation of thigh | Continued independence; Ambulation possible but unrealistic because of need for heavy leg braces; hands needed for support; high energy spent for short distances; slow movement; most people prefer to remain in w/c | Long leg braces; Crutches/walker |

**Table 30.1.** Spinal cord levels of function[a] (continued)

| Level | Peripheral Nerves | Muscle Innervation | Action | ADL and Mobility: Level of Independence | Adaptive Devices |
|---|---|---|---|---|---|
| L4 | Deep peroneal sciatic | Erector spinae<br>Primary hip flexors<br>Quadiceps femoris<br>Hamstrings<br>Biceps femoris | Hip and trunk flexion and rotation<br>Leg extension; thigh flexion | Continued independence<br>Ambulation functional for short distances (i.e., household)<br>Stairs possible<br>W/C for long distances (i.e., community) | Short leg braces<br>Crutches |
| L5 | Tibial | Gluteus maximus<br>Ankle, foot, and hip muscles | Improved function in legs | Good potential for independent ambulation | Braces |
| S1–5 | Pudendal | Sphincters | Plantar flexion<br>Some sphincter control | Lower leg weakness | Braces<br>Bowel regimen<br>Bladder regimen |

[a]*Sources:* Adapted from Clark U. University of Maryland Hospital. Department of Nursing Teaching Tool; and Ricci MM. Spinal trauma. In: Core curriculum for neuroscience nursing. Park Ridge, IL: American Association of Neuroscience Nurses, 1984:57.

**Table 30.2.** Problems encountered by 25 SCI clients classified according to Maslow's hierarchy of needs[a]

| Need | Problems |
|---|---|
| Physiological | Paralysis |
| | Loss of sensation |
| | Renal dysfunction |
| | Soft tissue damage |
| | Respiratory problems |
| | Bowel incontinence |
| | Muscle spasticity and contractures |
| | Inadequate body temperature control |
| | Osteoporosis |
| | Autonomic dysreflexia |
| | Weight control |
| Security | Loss of mobility |
| | Inability to escape from danger |
| | Fear of intruders |
| | Increased susceptibility to hazards |
| | Financial insecurity |
| | Transportation problems |
| | Insecurity over long-term care |
| Love and belonging | Role reversal |
| | Sexual love adjustments |
| | Limitations in social effectiveness |
| | Limitations in touching |
| | Family conflict |
| | Limitations in social and religious activities |
| Self-esteem | Discomfort in asking for help |
| | Frustrations with architectural barriers |
| | Alteration in body image |
| | Dissatisfaction with education or occupation |
| Self-actualization | Barriers to career fulfillment |
| | Boredom and apathy |
| | Lack of spontaneity |
| | Dissatisfaction with amount of responsibilities |
| | Dissatisfaction with meaning and purpose in life |
| | Unresolved anger and hostility |

[a]*Source:* Reprinted from ARN Journal 5(5):18, with permission of the Association of Rehabilitation Nurses, © September/October 1980.

and rehabilitation process (see Table 30.2). Psychologically, patients with SCI must adapt to forced changes in virtually every aspect of their lives (see Table 30.3) (1). For Bill, who has been unexpectedly injured, rehabilitation involves far more than teaching techniques for physical care; it also involves developing a new identity as a person with

**Table 30.3.** Factors that influence reaction to a crisis[a]

1. Having little or no time to prepare
2. Having little or no time experience with this type of stressor
3. The perceived danger to and emotional impact of the injury on the family
4. The amount of time spent in the crisis situation
5. Loss of control and feelings of helplessness
6. The description of family roles, responsibilities, and routine functioning
7. Having little guidance regarding what is expected of them

[a]*Source:* Adapted from Figley CR. Catastrophes: an overview of family reactions. In: Figley CR, McCubbin AL, eds. Stress and the family, Vol. II: Coping with catastrophe. New York: Brunner/Mazel, 1983.

a disability. Bill is going to experience conflict between caring for his increased physical needs and the strained personal relationships with his family.

The rehabilitation program must address Bill's adjustment to his injury, as well as the adjustment of those who are significant to him. Bill's preinjury personality is an important determinant in predicting his adjustment. Also important are support systems available, previous coping mechanisms, and knowledge of his injury.

## 2. What are the nursing diagnoses of highest priority?

A. Ineffective family/individual coping
B. Potential for anxiety and grief

## 3. What are the goals of nursing care?

### A. Nursing Diagnosis

Ineffective family/patient coping related to ongoing stress and alterations in family process

### Goal of Care

Patient/family will participate in goal setting with the health care team.

### Nursing Interventions

- Encourage family and patient participation in care by involving them in goal setting prior to and during team conferences.
- Assist the patient and family to develop or improve decision-making skills.
- Invite or schedule family members to attend various therapy sessions and to meet team members.
- Encourage/enroll the family/patient in educational programs that provide information on SCI. Validate the patient and family understanding of information taught.

### Rationale

The patient's perceived outcomes postdischarge will influence his rehabilitation program. The key to psychological adjustment to a disability is to encourage the patient and family to participate in the rehabilitation goal setting and decision making. This process enables the patient and family to have more control over the environment, and establishes a less stressful atmosphere for adaptation to the rehabilitation process at their own pace.

The role of the nurse is to assist the patient in minimizing physical dependency as much as possible. The higher the degree of physical dependency the more difficult the psychological adjustments (see Table 30.2).

### Goal of Care

Develop and restore appropriate coping mechanisms to promote effective family and patient functioning.

### Nursing Interventions

- Refer concerns to appropriate team members (i.e., primary nurse, psychiatrist, and so on).
- Encourage patient and family to make changes related to care.
- Negotiate care with patient and family and set limits as indicated.
- Assist the patient and family in identifying healthy coping mechanisms to minimize stress and to allow for participation in the rehabilitation program.
- Explore with the patient and family the consequences of the patient's behavior.
- Identify barriers to learning.

- Explain to the family that a functional trial visit (FTV) is part of the goal-setting process and a mechanism to evaluate the goals set by the patient, family, and team.
- Encourage the attendance of the patient/family not only within the therapies but with internal/external support groups as well.
- Monitor the family for crisis situations.
- Assess available support systems.

### Rationale

The patient's and family's repertoire of coping skills and support systems may aid their adjustment to this high degree of stress (2). Figley outlined seven factors that influence reaction to a crisis (see Table 30.3) (3).

Successful coping keeps stress manageable within acceptable limitations established by the patient, the family, and the health care team. It also helps the patient maintain self-esteem and feelings of personal worth; redevelops personal relationships with significant others; assists the patient through the rehabilitation recovery phase, maximizes functional recovery following physical disability; and establishes an acceptable social life postdischarge (2, 4). The patient and family will be able to deal with the rehabilitation process if they are better prepared to deal with the stress involved. Coping enables one to remove or re-establish those stressors so needs are met and goals can be achieved (5).

Family members may have difficulty adjusting to a loved one's disability, relative to their own dependency on that individual and his or her role in the family. Referrals and support are provided so the family can develop a new role for the patient and themselves. At times, depending on their current roles, family members are unable to assume added responsibility; therefore, external assistance may be needed, or a restructuring of their family system may be necessary. Other issues, such as child dependency, will also need to be explored.

### Goal of Care

Regain and/or maintain psychosocial functioning throughout the grieving process.

### Nursing Interventions

- Maintain communication with family/patient by keeping all informed of progress and encourage participation in the rehabilitation program.
- Encourage attendance at support group meetings.
- Encourage the family to vocalize their own feelings regarding the accident.

### Rationale

It is well documented that the spinal cord injured patient and the family go through a period of depression or "mourning" in their effort to work through grief over their loss (6). Responses to grief are dependent on the significance of the loss (7). Each family member, as well as the patient, will progress at his or her own rate; the varying levels of acceptance of the disability may create conflict within the family.

The family and the patient should be reassured that their feelings of shock, mourning, dependency, depression, and anger are all normal responses to an unexpected, tragic accident. The nurse must allow expression of these feelings to enable them to progress to acceptance of the disability.

### B. Nursing Diagnosis

Potential for profound anxiety and grief related to major alterations in sexual functioning.

## Goal of Care

Lessen the extent of anxiety and grief that stem from disrupted sexual functioning.

## Nursing Interventions

- Introduce the topic of sexuality in a low-key fashion by letting the patient know that it is a legitimate topic for discussion whenever he is ready to talk about it.
- Take the time to listen to the patient's sexual concerns, creating a soothing, accepting atmosphere wherein the patient feels free to talk about his disability and the meaning it has for him.
- Respond to the patient's concerns with a balance of gentle reassurance and realism about the difficult adjustments that lie ahead.
- Offer the patient as much or as little information about sexuality as he requests.
- Encourage the patient to adopt a broad definition of sexuality and intimacy, a definition that is not limited to the genital sex act (8). Assist the patient to explore other options for sexual pleasure, such as foreplay involving stimulation of secondary erogenous zones, massage, oral sex, use of sexual aids such as vibrators or dildos, and creative use of fantasy and erotic imagery.
- Encourage experimentation in lovemaking (9). Tell the patient to try new positions, new caresses.
- If a patient is experiencing reflex erections, make him aware that this is happening.
- A patient may experience a decrease in libido during his recovery. Offer him reassurance that this is not unusual and that the libido frequently returns with the passage of time and the return to familiar surroundings (10).
- Be aware that masturbation is an important sexual option for the disabled individual. Share this information with the patient if it is appropriate.
- Arrange for a newly disabled person to talk with someone who has made a successful adjustment to a similar disability. Such an individual can be a valuable source of information and inspiration.
- Offer positive comments about the disabled person's body, such as "Your skin looks beautifully clear. There are no signs of any pressure areas." Such comments are comforting because they counteract the "body as enemy" stigma that many disabled individuals experience (11).
- Use the technique of "behavioral rehearsal" if it is appropriate (11). This technique entails helping the patient to consider ahead of time how to handle certain situations that may occur when he resumes sexual activity. For example, the nurse might say, "Pretend that I am a new partner and we are on our way to your bedroom. How would you explain your urinary catheter to me? What would you do if you had a bowel accident?" The goal of behavior rehearsal is to lower some of the tremendous anxiety associated with such situations by considering various coping strategies and explanations in advance.
- Allow the patient to spend quiet, private time with his spouse or significant other.
- Refer the patient to a more highly trained professional for sexual counseling if necessary. A patient may have questions about fertility, sexual response, birth control, and so on, that may best be answered by someone with advanced background in this area.
- Recognize that *all* of the above interventions, with the exception of the one concerning reflex erections, are equally important for the woman with a spinal cord injury and for the spouse or significant other of the patient with cord trauma.

The sexual concerns of these two groups are often mistakenly downplayed or forgotten.

## Rationale

Patients with an upper motor neuron lesion cannot achieve psychogenic erections or vaginal lubrication, but may experience nipple erection, tachycardia, and an increase in blood pressure (12). Approximately 90% of males with upper motor neuron injuries do, however, experience reflex erections that occur either spontaneously or in response to external stimuli to the penis or pelvic area, such as pinching or stroking the inside of the upper thighs, pulling pubic hair, or anal stimulation (13). In females, direct genital stimulation produces vaginal lubrication and pelvic engorgement. Autonomic dysreflexia may occur with genital stimulation or with priapism. Orgasm can occur on a sensory subjective level in genital and nongenital erogenous zones. Ejaculation is rare (12).

Most patients with lower motor neuron lesions can achieve psychogenic erection due to intact thoracolumbar sympathetics; 25% with complete lesions have reflexogenic erections as well. Ejaculation may also occur (10, 12).

Fertility is low because of difficulties with erections, ejaculation, low sperm counts, and decreased sperm motility. In females, menses may cease for a few months after injury, but after this period, female fertility is unaffected. Onset of labor may go unrecognized because of a lack of subjective sensations unless it precipitates autonomic dysreflexia; however, contractions can be seen on a fetal monitor.

Autonomic dysreflexia is a life-threatening complication for SCI patients that is caused by a variety of stimuli that would be painful or noxious if the patient did not have sensory loss. Examples would be a full rectum, bladder distension, decubiti, injury below level of sensation, and priapism. An exaggerated reaction of the sympathetic nervous system occurs, as there is no control from higher centers. Symptoms include severe headache due to the sudden onset of hypertension, which if not controlled may lead to cerebral hemorrhage or myocardial infarction. Other symptoms include sweating and flushing above the level of sensation, pallor and coolness below, nasal congestion, severe apprehension, and bradycardia or tachycardia. Autonomic dysreflexia may occur any time after the resolution of spinal shock, usually within the first year after injury, but it may be a lifelong problem. Nursing care is aimed at prevention, but should autonomic dysreflexia occur, the patient should be placed in high Fowlers, his blood pressure controlled with antihypertensives, and the offending source of the syndrome identified and removed (12).

It has long been recognized that patients who sustain a spinal cord injury experience profound turmoil with respect to their sexuality. The source of this turmoil is not difficult to discern in a "body beautiful" society, in which physical attractiveness is a major component of one's sexiness. A society with such values makes it difficult for a disabled person to initiate and sustain intimate relationships. Newly disabled individuals may consider themselves asexual, unaware of the possibilities that are still available to them as sexual, intimate persons. They may experience intense fear of rejection and wonder, "How will I ever meet someone who will love and accept me?" Such feelings pose a threat to one's self-esteem and can indeed overwhelm an individual with anxiety and grief. Yet, disabled patients can be assisted to attain rich and satisfying intimate relationships with partners who learn to accept and appreciate their bodies. The warm support of a concerned, informed nurse can positively influence the lives of such individuals.

The nurse begins the helping process by realizing that patients will rarely communicate their sexual concerns in a direct, forthright manner. Instead, such concerns are often conveyed in a veiled fashion, through subtle or symbolic language or through general behaviors. For example, one patient remarked, "My pilot light is out." Another asked, "What kind of future is there for half a man?" Such statements provide important clues about how patients view their postinjury sexual impairment (10). Other clues to the existence of sexual concerns might include behaviors such as patting or pinching the nurse, telling dirty jokes, exposing oneself, and reading books or magazines or watching videos with sexual content.

Some patients may provide none of the above clues and yet may harbor tremendous anxieties about their furture sexual potential. For many, the perceived inability to function sexually is such a profound loss that the patient cannot begin to talk about it without help. Thus, the nurse has a responsibility to initiate the discussion, to let the patient know that sexual concerns are a legitimate topic for him or her to talk and ask about. An excellent way to initiate such a discussion is to say, "After an injury such as yours, many people have questions about their future capabilities. These questions often include concerns about sexual function. I would be happy to talk with you any time about any questions you might have." Introducing the topic of sexuality in this gentle manner does not overwhelm or threaten the patient who may still be employing a significant amount of denial about the permanency of his or her injury (14). Also, discussing sexuality in the context of the variety of problems the patient faces does not make the subject uncomfortably conspicuous by singling it out for separate handling (13). This approach can be used even during the early, acute postinjury phase, when patients may already be experiencing tremendous turmoil about their future sexual role. Unless acknowledged quickly, this turmoil can build and may limit progress in all areas of rehabilitation (15). Often just the simple explanation that it is natural and understandable to feel anxious about sex is, in itself, reassuring (16).

Once the nurse has succeeded in initiating a discussion of sexual concerns, what next? At this point, the importance of listening cannot be underestimated. By listening to a person describe his or her sexual concerns, the nurse affirms that the person is, indeed, still seen as a sexual person. Also, once a patient shares his feelings, he no longer has to bear them alone. It is important to remember that the ties to a lost part or to a function that has been drastically altered are represented by hundreds of separate memories that must be worked through. This is part of the "work of mourning" (17). It helps to talk about these memories and the feelings they invoke to a receptive listener.

Providing the spinal cord injured patient with consistent caregivers is another vital intervention. Such consistency facilitates the growth of trust between nurse and patient. Discussions of an intimate, sexual nature occur more readily within the security of a trusting relationship. Also, consistent assignment helps the nurse to become familiar with the patient's family background, moral and religious attitudes, sexual orientation, and so on. Such information is critical to any discussion of sexuality, since the nurse must work within the patient's framework when offering sexual counseling and support.

When providing factual information about sex and spinal cord injury, offer the patient as much or as little detail as he or she desires. Often, in the acute phase after injury, many patients simply need reassurance that they are not "finished" sexually. Actual details may not be important at a time when the patient must deal with many other concerns. But some patients may want more specific information and may ask, "What can I actually do?'' Although genital intercourse may still be possible, it is important to remember that sexuality is more than genitality. By helping the patient to explore other options for sexual pleasure, the nurse encourages a broader, richer concept of sexuality and intimacy. Tell the patient, ''Try anything you can think of,'' so that many possibilities are explored to achieve maximum enjoyment.

A discussion of sexual options following spinal cord injury would not be complete without noting the concept of masturbation, which may be possible depending on the extent of the injury. Masturbation is important to a disabled individual for several reasons (18). It can be an alternative outlet if one is without a partner for a while. Also, masturbation helps one to relearn his or her body's potential for sexual response. This can enable a person to communicate to a partner what feels best. Finally, masturbation can be a positive, pleasuring experience that may make a person feel better about his or her body in general. This is important, since the disabled body is so often a source of negatives, such as impaired mobility, bowel and bladder hassles, and pain.

A final consideration that the nurse should address when working with spinal cord injured individuals is his or her own comfort level regarding both sexuality and disability. Carrying one's personal taboos, prohibitions, and negative attitudes to the bedside can be a tremendous disservice to the patient. Such feelings can pose barriers to the formation of a rapport and openness that is so vital in the caring relationship. It is crucial for the nurse to take time for self-analysis in this regard. This analysis can be facilitated by taking courses on sexuality, reading the growing body of literature on sexuality and disability, or talking with a disabled friend or family member. Such efforts will enable the nurse to address a patient's sexual concerns in a respectful, honest, and compassionate manner.

## ASSOCIATED NURSING DIAGNOSES

A. Impaired adjustment
B. Anxiety
C. Fear
D. Hopelessness
E. Noncompliance
F. Powerlessness
G. Social isolation
H. Disturbance in self-concept: body image, personal identity, self-esteem
I. Potential for self-directed violence
J. Diversional activity deficit
K. Impaired home maintenance management
L. Altered health maintenance
M. Knowledge deficit
N. Potential for altered parenting
O. Posttrauma response
P. Altered role performance
Q. Self-care deficit: bathing/hygiene, dressing/grooming, feeding, toileting
R. Impaired social interaction

**REFERENCES**

1. Pallet P, O'Brien M. Textbook of the neurological nurse. Boston: Little, Brown, 1985:428–429.

2. Hamburg DA, Adams JE. A perspective on coping behavior. Arch Gen Psychiatry 1967;17:277–284.

3. Figley CR. Catastrophes: an overview of family reactions. In: Figley CR, McCubbin AL, eds. Stress and the family, Vol II: Coping with catastrophe. New York: Brunner/Mazel, 1983.
4. Stevens K. Alterations in psychosocial functioning coping with spinal cord injury. In: Matthews R, Carlson C, eds. Spinal cord injury: a guide to rehabilitation nursing. Rockville, MD: Aspen, 1987:49.
5. Gunther MS. The threatened practitioner: work under stress. In: Martin N, Holt NB, Hicks D, eds. Comprehensive rehabilitation nursing. New York: McGraw-Hill, 1981:113.
6. Bartol G. Psychological needs of the spinal cord injured person. Neurosurg Nurs 1978;10:171.
7. Fontaine PK. Physical, personal, and cognitive responses to trauma. Crit Care Nurs Clin North Am 1989;1(1):11–20.
8. Cole TM, Colass DP. Sexuality and physical disabilities. Arch Phys Med Rehabil 1977; 58:585.
9. Thornton CE. Sexuality counseling of women with spinal cord injuries. In: Bullard P, Knight S, eds. Sexuality and physical disability: personal perspectives. St Louis: CV Mosby, 1981:160.
10. Stewart TD. Sex, spinal cord injury, and staff rapport. Rehabil Lit 1981;42:347.
11. Bogle J, Shaw S. Body image and the woman with a disability. In: Bullard P, Knight S, eds. Sexuality and physical disability: personal perspectives. St Louis: CV Mosby, 1981:94.
12. Walleck CA. Central nervous system II: spinal cord injury. In: Cardona VD, Hurn PD, Basthagel-Mason PJ, et al, eds. Trauma nursing: from resuscitation through rehabilitation. Philadelphia: WB Saunders, 1988:444–446.
13. Cole TM. Sexuality and the spinal cord injured. In: Coreen R, ed. Human sexuality: a health practitioner's text. Baltimore: Williams & Wilkins, 1979:160.
14. Crigler L. Sexual concerns of the spinal cord injured. Nurs Clin North Am 1974;9:713.
15. Hanlon K. Maintaining sexuality after spinal cord injury. Nursing 1975;5:50.
16. Rudocker M, Bullard D. Basic issues in the sexual counseling of persons with physical disability: personal perspectives. St Louis: CV Mosby, 1981:244.
17. Siller J. Psychological situations of the disabled with spinal cord injuries. Rehabil Lit 1969;30:292.
18. Becker E. Sexuality and the spinal cord injured woman. In: Bullard P, Knight S, eds. Sexuality and physical disability: personal perspectives. St Louis: CV Mosby, 1981:18.

# PART 9

**Special Topics**

# CHAPTER 31

# Septic Shock in the Trauma Patient

Christy L. Crowther, RN, MS, ANP-C, CCRN
Nancy J. Hoyt, MA, CIC

## Clinical Presentation

A 36-year-old male construction worker was admitted to the hospital following a building collapse in which he fell 15 feet. He was noted to be quadriplegic at the scene. On arrival at the trauma center, he was alert and oriented to time, person, and place. His past medical history was nonsignificant.

Physical examination revealed a bruise at the bridge of the nose; tympanic membranes were without blood. There was no Battle sign. Pupils were equal and reactive to light. Cranial nerve examination was within normal limits. Motor and sensory examination and cervical spine x-rays were consistent with C4 and C5 sublaxation with deficit.

Vital signs were blood pressure (BP) 90/60; heart rate 118; respiration 28; and temperature 37°C (98.6°F). Breath sounds were diminished on the right. Chest x-ray revealed a right pneumothorax with right-sided rib fractures 9 through 12. The patient was intubated, and a chest tube was placed on the right. Diagnostic peritoneal lavage was positive.

The patient was taken to the operating room, where an exploratory laprotomy was performed, a small stellate liver laceration was repaired, and a retroperitoneal hematoma was noted. The patient's cervical spine injury was treated with 15 lbs of halo traction, which produced easy alignment. The plan at the time was stabilization and traction for 10 to 14 days and then a multilevel cervical laminectomy of C3 to C7 with a fusion of C4, C5, and C6.

During the first week, the patient progressed well except for persistent hypothermia of 35.5°C (96°F) and intermittent bouts of atelectasis. On the 11th day, it was observed that the patient was not absorbing enteral tube feedings. Bowel sounds had significantly diminished, and the abdomen appeared slightly distended. Vital signs were within the patient's previous baseline parameters at the 0800 hour nursing assessment. At this time his white blood cell (WBC) count was 16,300/mm$^3$. However, at 1000 hours the patient appeared confused and agitated, and both vital signs and arterial blood gases began to deteriorate. Tables 31.1 and 31.2 indicate the vital signs and arterial blood gases at 1000 hours and during the subsequent 3 hours. The patient was started on dopamine at 15 μg/kg/minute, on dobutamine at 20 μg/kg/minute, and on Isuprel at 10 μg/minute. At 1100 hours epinephrine was added at 10 μg/minute and was increased to 15 μg/minute, then to 20 μg/minute at 1200 hours.

Physical examination at 1000 hours remained consistent with the 0800 assessment. Chest x-ray was clear, and sputum gram stain was not significant. All intravascular lines were changed, and sites were noted to be free of inflammation or purulence. Microscopic examination of the urine was not significant. Blood cultures were drawn by percutaneous

**215**

**Table 31.1.** Vital signs[a]

| Hour | BP | MAP | T | HR | PAWP | CO | SVR | UO |
|------|-------|-----|------|----|------|------|------|----|
| 1000 | 92/60 | 84 | 35.8 | 88 | 27 | 14.3 | 504 | 20 |
| 1100 | 88/42 | 66 | 36 | 92 | 20 | — | — | 15 |
| 1200 | 82/40 | 59 | 36.9 | 90 | 28 | 5.6 | 1487 | 15 |
| 1300 | 92/50 | 65 | 37 | 80 | 23 | — | — | 30 |

[a]Key: BP = blood pressure; MAP = mean arterial blood pressure; T = temperature (degrees centigrade); HR = heart rate; PAWP = pulmonary arterial wedge pressure; CO = cardiac output; SVR = systemic vascular resistance (normal 800–1200 dynes/sec/cm$^{-5}$; UO = urinary output (cc/hr).

puncture. The patient was empirically placed on amikacin sulfate 500 mg every 6 hours and Ceftazidime 2 gm every 8 hours.

Clinical manifestations were thought to be consistent with an intra-abdominal septic focus. Emergent laparotomy was performed with subsequent removal of the gallbladder. The next day, blood cultures became positive for gram-negative rods. *Klebsiella pneumoniae* was identified as the causative organism from both blood and gallbladder cultures.

On the 16th day, the patient underwent a cervical spine laminectomy and fusion. He was discharged to a rehabilitation facility on the 32nd day after his admission.

## 1. What is the pathophysiological basis for this patient's problem?

Septic shock is a severe, often life-threatening manifestation of invasive infection and/ or the toxic effects of tissue necrosis. Although septic shock has been most commonly associated with endotoxins from gram-negative bacillary organisms, it may result from infection from a variety of other microorganisms, such as gram-positive bacteria, anaerobic bacteria, viruses, rickettsia, and fungi. Exotoxins produced by anaerobic clostridia, and gram-positive organisms, such as coagulase-positive staphylococci and pneumococci can cause the same detrimental consequences (1). Exotoxins such as lecithinase (alpha-toxin), hemolysins, enterotoxins, coagulases, and hyalonidases destroy cellular membranes, alter vascular permeability, and induce tissue necrosis. The release of exotoxins is directly responsible for the progression of disease (2). In cases where septic shock is associated with tissue necrosis, the progression of disease is rapid. Septicemia results when either bacteria or toxins invade the bloodstream. Therefore, septicemia may be blood culture negative.

Septicemia produces a constellation of symptoms, including fever, shaking chills, and confusion as well as signs and symptoms of shock—hypotension, tachycardia, tachypnea, and oliguria. Hypovolemia is caused by the release of the bacterial toxins. These toxins

**Table 31.2.** Arterial blood gases

| Hour | PaO$_2$ | pH | PaCO$_2$ | Ventilator Settings |
|------|------|------|-------|---------------------|
| 1000 | 67 | 7.20 | 35 | 70% (18 PEEP[a]) changed to 100% (18 PEEP) |
| 1030 | 85 | 7.15 | 45 | 100%—18 PEEP changed to 20 PEEP with rate 20/minute |
| 1100 | 111 | 7.20 | 39 | No change in settings |
| 1200 | 76 | 7.25 | 32 | 100%—20 PEEP changed to 18 PEEP |
| 1300 | 86 | 7.25 | 45 | 100%—20 PEEP |

[a]PEEP = positive end-expiratory pressure.

induce increased vascular permeability, resulting in significant losses of plasma fluid into the interstitial spaces, specifically third-spacing (3–5). The net result is inadequate circulatory volume, circulatory collapse, and shock.

The clinical presentation of septic shock is directly dependent on the patient's underlying volume status (6). Septic shock in the normovolemic patient creates a hyperdynamic state with elevation of cardiac output, low systemic vascular resistance, wide pulse pressure, tachycardia, and warm, flushed extremities ("warm shock"). On the other hand, the hypovolemic patient presents hypodynamic parameters—the blood pressure decreases, the pulse rate increases, and the skin becomes cold and clammy ("cool shock"). In the hypovolemic patient, the determination of the etiology of the shock state can be difficult (6–8).

Decreased perfusion of nonvital tissues produces deranged cellular metabolism (1). Tissue anoxia results in the anaerobic metabolism of glucose with increased production of lactic acid. The production of lactic acid is the primary cause of metabolic acidosis in the patient with hypovolemic septic shock. This alteration of cellular metabolism, coupled with the destructive effects of the bacterial toxins inducing the lungs to compensate for these, results in hypoxia and acidosis. The patient's respirations will become more rapid and shallow as the disease progresses. Respiratory insufficiency can develop and ultimately lead to acute respiratory failure.

Treatment of septic shock is directed toward the correction of hypovolemia and the removal of the septic focus. Fluid replacement, inotropic drugs, ventilatory support, and immediate initiation of antimicrobial therapy are the first steps of therapy. Antibiotics should begin after blood cultures are obtained by percutaneous puncture. It is important to remember that septic shock can develop from a myriad of infections, clinical conditions, or organisms. Therefore, the removal or control of the septic focus is a key determinant of the patient's outcome. The patient must be carefully examined, wounds and intravascular sites inspected, chest x-rays and appropriate diagnostic scans obtained, and purulent exudates and drainage sent for culture and gram stain (9). Mortality rate from septic shock is more closely related to the underlying disease than to the severity of infection (10). Factors most associated with mortality include persistent acidosis, low or normal temperature, azotemia, leukopenia, or persistent bacteremia.

Infection in the trauma patient is influenced by a variety of factors, including the nature of the underlying injuries, the magnitude of the trauma, the use of multiple invasive devices and therapeutic procedures, the loss of the anatomical defense mechanisms, the microorganisms of the body's resident flora, the hospital environment, the use of antibiotics, the clinical scenarios of resuscitation, and the amount of attention paid to infection control principles (9). Therefore, prevention of septic shock in the trauma patient is a challenge, since the diagnosis of infection in this population can be difficult and complex (9, 11, 12). Patients frequently cannot communicate or sense their symptoms because of a decreased level of consciousness, disorientation, sedation, endotracheal intubation, or central nervous system injury. Physical examination can be hindered by multiple indwelling devices, casts, traction, fixation devices, bandages, and the necessity for immobilization. Diagnostic tests may be less valuable because it may be risky or difficult to transport the patient to the appropriate department for a particular evaluation, or it may be impossible to place the patient in the optimal position for the study.

Classic indicators of infection, such as leukocytosis and fever, may not be useful in the critically ill trauma patient (9). Inflammatory responses can be triggered from a variety of mechanical and chemical sources as well as from the development of an infectious process. Similarly, fever patterns can be abnormal as the result of atelectasis, drug reactions, transfusion reactions, hematoma formation, presence of necrotic tissue, central nervous system injury, or inflammation alone. In addition, these patients can be hemodynamically unstable and in shock due to hemorrhage, cardiac and pulmonary dysfunction, or neurological dysfunction, and not necessarily from sepsis. It is this undercurrent of multiple underlying clinical conditions that must be differentiated from infection.

The above case presentation illustrates some of these problems. Development of septic acalculus cholecystitis has been reported to be a latent complication of blunt abdominal injury, especially when the liver is involved (13). Adynamic ileus can be induced by the shock state, sepsis, or the presence of a retroperitoneal hematoma (14). This patient was quadriplegic and could not sense abdominal pain, which would have been a common complaint in a person who had not sustained this injury. Suspicion of an intra-abdominal focus was based on physical examination, confusion and agitation, loss of gastric motility, and appropriate risk factors that could be associated with the underlying injury. In addition, he was hypothermic secondary to his central nervous system dysfunction. His highest recorded temperature was 37°C (98.6°F), which is considered normal temperature. This temperature, however, was a sudden spike of 2°C within a 3-hour interval. It is this sudden change in the patient's baseline fever pattern that often signals the onset of septic shock.

## 2. What are the nursing diagnoses of highest priority?
A. Alteration in tissue perfusion
B. Potential/actual impaired gas exchange
C. Potential/acutal fluid volume deficit

## 3. What are the goals of nursing care?
### A. Nursing Diagnosis
Alteration in tissue perfusion related to effects of endotoxins and decreased cardiac output

### Goal of Care
Maintain adequate tissue perfusion

### Nursing Interventions
- Monitor hemodynamic parameters:
  – BP
  – Pulmonary artery wedge pressure (PAWP)
  – Heart rate
  – Cardiac output
  – Urine output
  – Systemic vascular resistance (SVR)
- Administer medications, fluids

### Rationale
The release of endotoxins by bacteria (frequently gram-negative organisms) has several effects, including selective vasoconstriction, peripheral vasodilation, and an increase in capillary permeability. As circulating blood volume leaks out of the capillaries into the interstitial spaces, there is less circulating volume; this process, combined with peripheral vasodilation, results in a relative hypovolemia (3). The body attempts to compensate by increasing cardiac output, blood pressure, and heart rate. Initially, cardiac output and blood pressure may be at or above normal, with a widened pulse pressure, rapid heart rate, bounding periperhal pulses and low SVR. As shock progresses, these compensatory measures begin to fail, with the

net effect at the cellular level being uneven perfusion and interference with gas and nutrient exchange (3).

For these reasons, close monitoring of trends in hemodynamic parameters provides vital information regarding the progression of shock. As the shock state continues, blood pressure falls, the pulse pressure narrows, peripheral pulses become weak and thready, and the SVR increases.

Antibiotics must be started as soon as cultures have been obtained. Fluids, both colloid and crystalloid, are given to combat the relative hypovolemia incurred in septic shock. Inotropic agents are used to improve cardiac contractility and cardiac output. Other vasoactive agents may be used to reduce preload and afterload and to improve perfusion to the kidneys and other vital organs.

## B. Nursing Diagnosis

Impaired gas exchange related to poor tissue perfusion and the direct effect of endotoxin on the lung

### Goals of Care

- Maintain adequate ventilation, $PaO_2$.
- Prevent/correct acidosis.

### Nursing Interventions

- Assess rate, quality, and character of respirations.
- Note increasing dyspnea, tachypnea.
- Monitor arterial blood gases, particularly pH.

### Rationale

Respirations are initially rapid, both as a direct effect of the endotoxin on lung tissue and as an effort to compensate for hypoxia; they become more shallow and rapid as acidosis progresses (3, 15). Respiratory insufficiency develops and may progress to acute respiratory failure.

Frequent assessment of respiratory rate, character of respirations, and arterial blood gases provides information on the adequacy of ventilation. Hypoxemia is a common early finding in septic shock (3). Supplemental oxygen, whether by mask or mechanical ventilation, is necessary to prevent or correct hypoxemia. Hypoxia associated with septic shock can cause cardiac output to fail.

## C. Nursing Diagnosis

Potential/actual fluid volume deficit related to a relative hypovolemia from vasodilation and capillary leaking

### Goal of Care

Maintain normal vital signs, urine output >0.5 ml/kg/hr.

### Nursing Interventions

- Monitor hemodynamic parameters (BP, cardiac output, PAWP, SVR).
- Accurately record intake/output amounts.
- Monitor laboratory values.
- Administer IV fluids.

### Rationale

In the early stages of septic shock, a systemic inflammatory response occurs in response to the effects of endotoxin on the immune system. Numerous vasoactive chemical mediators, including histamine, prostaglandins, and kinins are released, causing peripheral vasodilation and an increase in cardiac output. Initially, SVR may be normal and the skin may even be dry and appear flushed ("warm shock").

Bradykinin (the most abundantly released kinin) contributes to increased capillary permeability, in addition to its vasodilatory properties. As the capillaries leak fluid and protein into the interstitial spaces, there is less circulating volume and a relative hypovolemia ensues. The body attempts to compensate for this hypovolemia by stimulation of the sympathetic nervous system.

Blood pressure, pulmonary artery pressures, and cardiac output provide information about circulating blood volume. As circulating volume decreases, these parameters begin to fall. Sympathetic nervous stimulation allows the cardiac output to be maintained or even elevated for a time. As septic shock progresses, continued low cardiac output may be a sign of myocardial depression. Peripheral vasoconstriction causes the skin to feel cool and clammy, and tachycardia continues with the presence of a weak, thready pulse ("cool shock").

This combination of falling cardiac output, vasodilation, and capillary leaking, as well as the endotoxin's direct effects on cell tissue, hampers the delivery of nutrients and oxygen to the cells. Large volumes of crystalloids (such as 5% dextrose in water and normal saline) and colloids (blood and blood products) are generally required to compensate for the circulating volume deficit.

Intake/output records provide a way of assessing both volume replacement and adequacy of renal function. Positive fluid balances and weight gain may indicate continued third-spacing. Colloids may be useful in mobilizing fluids back into the intravascular space. Renal function is sensitive to changes in volume; decreased output with an increased specific gravity may indicate worsening shock as the body attempts to compensate by retaining fluid. Decreased urine output with a normal specific gravity may be a sign of renal failure as the kidneys lose their ability to concentrate urine.

White blood cell counts are usually grossly elevated but may also fall to subnormal levels. Platelet counts may decrease as pooling and sludging of blood occurs in the capillary circulation. Hematocrit/hemoglobin changes reflect alterations in hydration, blood viscosity, or hemolysis. Electrolyte imbalances, especially potassium, are associated with fluid shifts and may interfere with myocardial functioning (15). Other blood chemistries, such as sudden glucose intolerance, may provide early warning signs of sepsis.

Vasoactive drugs are given to improve cardiac output, systemic vascular resistance, blood flow to vital organs, and blood pressure. Positive inotropic agents increase myocardial contractility; vasodilators reduce SVR; and in combination, they are used to reduce preload and afterload. Table 31.3 illustrates the major effects of some of these agents. Sodium bicarbonate may be used to counteract metabolic acidosis. Opiate antagonists, such as Narcan, have been used to block endorphin-mediated vasodilation. The use of steroids in septic shock is controversial (16–18).

## ASSOCIATED NURSING DIAGNOSES

A. Decrease in cardiac output
B. Alteration in body temperature
C. Impaired gas exchange

**Table 31.3.** Selected cardiovascular drugs and their effects

| Drug | Usual Dose (IV infusion) | Receptor Site | | | Hemodynamic Effect | | | |
|---|---|---|---|---|---|---|---|---|
| | | α | β₁ | β₂ | MAP | CO | PCWP | SVR |
| Dobutamine | 2.5–5.0 μg/kg/minute | + | +++ | + | ↓→ | ↑ | ↓ | ↓ |
| Dopamine | 1–3 μg/kg/minute (renal) | | | | | | | |
| | 5–15 μg/kg/minute (heart) | ++ | ++ | + | ↕ | ↕ | ↓ | → |
| | 15–20 μg/kg/minute (heart) | +++ | ++ | | ↑ | ↑ | ↑ | ↑ |
| Epinephrine | 0.01–0.1 μg/kg/minute (low dose) | | +++ | ++ | ↑ | ↑ | ↓ | ↓ |
| | Dose dependent (high dose) | +++ | ++ | | | | ↑ | ↑→ |
| Isoproterenol | 0.02–0.1 μg/kg/minute | | ++++ | ++ | ↓ | ↑ | ↓ | ↓ |
| Metaraminol | 1.5–10 μg/kg/minute (variable with dose) | ++ | + | | ↑ | ↕→ | ↑ | ↑ |
| Norepinephrine | 2–10 μg/minute (dose dependent) | ++++ | + | | ↑ | ↕→ | ↑ | ↑ |
| Phenylephrine | Variable with dose | +++ | | | ↑↕ | → | ↑ | ↑ |

aKey: MAP = mean arterial pressure; CO = cardiac output; PCWP = pulmonary capillary wedge pressure; SVR = systemic vascular resistance.

## REFERENCES

1. Schumer W. General treatment of septic shock. In: Cowley RA, Trump BF, eds. Pathophysiology of shock, anoxia, and ischemia. Baltimore: Williams & Wilkins 1982:479–482.
2. Caplan ES, Kluge RM. Gas gangrene—a review of 34 cases. Arch Intern Med 1976;136:788–791.
3. Emanuelson SD. Shock. In: Emanuelson KL, Rosenlicht JM, eds. Handbook of critical care nursing. New York: John Wiley & Sons, 1986:417–431.
4. Muller-Eberhand HJ. The serum complement system. In: Miescher PA, Muller-Eberhand HJ, eds. Textbook of immunopathology. New York: Grune & Stratton, 1976:45–73.
5. Shumer W. Septic shock. JAMA 1979;242:1906.
6. McQuillan KA, Wiles CE. Initial management of traumatic shock. In: Cardona VD, Hurn PD, Bastnagel-Mason PJ, et al, eds. Trauma nursing: from resuscitation through rehabilitation. Philadelphia: WB Saunders, 1988:161.
7. Committee on Trauma, American College of Surgeons advanced traumatic life support course (student manual). Chicago: American College of Surgeons, 1985.
8. Shires GT. Principles and management of hemorrhagic shock. In: Shires GT, ed. Principles of trauma care. New York: McGraw-Hill, 1985:3–42.
9. Hoyt NJ. Infection and infection control. In: Cardona VD, Hurn PD, Bastnagel-Mason PJ, et al, eds. Trauma nursing: from resuscitation through rehabilitation. Philadelphia: WB Saunders, 1988:224–262.
10. Hruska JF, Hornick RB. Treatment of infection in septic shock. In: Cowley RA, Trump BF, eds. Pathophysiology of shock, anoxia, and ischemia. Baltimore: Williams & Wilkins, 1982:482–497.
11. Caplan ES, Hoyt NJ. Infection surveillance and control in the severely traumatized patient. Am J Med 1981;70:638–640.
12. Hoyt NJ, Caplan ES. Identification and treatment of infection in the critically ill trauma population. CCQ 1983;6:17–24.
13. DuPriest RW, Khaneja SC, Cowley RA. Acute cholecystitis complicating trauma. Ann Surg 1979;189:84–89.
14. Bastnagel-Mason PJ. Abdominal trauma. In: Cardona VD, Hurn PD, Bastnagel-Mason PJ, et al, eds. Trauma nursing: from resuscitation through rehabilitation. Philadelphia: WB Saunders, 1988:491–524.
15. Moorehouse MF, Geissler AC, Doenges ME, eds. Critical care plans: guidelines for patient care. Philadelphia: FA Davis, 1987:329–342.
16. Balis JV, Paterson JF, Shelley SA, et al. Glucocorticoid and antibiotic effects on hepatic microcirculation and associated host responses in lethal gram-negative bacteremia. Lab Invest 1979;40:55–65.
17. Dale DC, Petersdorf RG. Corticosteroids and infectious diseases. Med Clin North Am 1973;57:1277–1288.
18. Greisman SE, DuBuy JB, Woodward CL. Experimental gram-negative bacterial sepsis: prevention of mortality not preventable by antibiotics alone. Infect Immun 1979;25:538–557.

# CHAPTER 32

# Disseminated Intravascular Coagulation

Anne G. Hopkins, RN, BSN, CCRN

## Clinical Presentation

A 41-year-old man was transported to the emergency department by helicopter following a serious motor vehicle accident. Paramedics at the scene stated that the patient was the unbelted driver of a vehicle that struck a telephone pole; a 20-minute extrication was required. Initial vital signs in the field were blood pressure (BP), 80/40 mm Hg; heart rate, 120/minute; and respiratory rate, 28/minute. The patient was moaning and able to move all extremities on command, the left leg being weaker. Abdominal distension was noted, and the pelvic area was very painful to palpation. Medical antishock trousers (MAST) were inflated, and an intravenous (IV) line of lactated Ringer's was started; a slight improvement of blood pressure to 100/50 was noted.

On arrival at the emergency department, the patient's blood pressure was 90/50 and heart rate was 115. Rapid fluid resuscitation was continued via central lines. A diagnostic peritoneal lavage was grossly positive. Pelvic x-ray films demonstrated an unstable pelvic fracture with dislocation of the sacroiliac (SI) joint. The patient was transported to surgery, where an exploratory laparotomy revealed a deep liver laceration, which was packed; a small bowel avulsion, which was repaired; and a large retroperitoneal hematoma. Orthopedic surgeons applied a pelvic Hoffman fixation device, and a Steinman pin was inserted in the left tibia for traction. Throughout surgery the patient was hypotensive and required multiple blood products of packed red cells, fresh frozen plasma, and platelets in addition to crystalloids.

On admission to the intensive care unit (ICU), the patient was mechanically ventilated via an endotracheal tube. Vital signs were blood pressure, 110/60; heart rate, 110; respiratory rate, 12; and temperature, 98°F (36.1°C) rectally. A subclavian pulmonary artery line; radial arterial line; and saphenous, jugular, and antecubital lines were in place. A Foley catheter and oral gastric tube had also been inserted. The abdominal incision was oozing bloody drainage, as were the pelvic Hoffman pin sites.

Over the next several days, the patient remained unstable with episodes of hypotension and required multiple transfusions of blood products and crystalloids. A dopamine drip at 5 μg/kg/minute was started for inotropic support, and cardiac outputs were measured twice a day. On the fourth postoperative day, the primary nurse noted increased ecchymosis in the pelvic area and petechiae scattered on the abdomen and back. There were mottling in the toes of both feet. All line and wound sites were oozing bloody drainage. During the first 3 days of hospitalization, this patient had received 45 units of packed cells, 26 units of fresh frozen plasma, and 15 units of platelets. Clotting studies produced the following results: prothrombin time (PT): control, 11 seconds, and patient, 16 seconds; partial thromboplastin time (PTT): control, 27 seconds, and patient, 33 seconds; platelets: 35,000; fibrinogen: 50 mg/dl; and fibrin degradation products: >40 μg/ml.

The health care team determined that the patient's hospital course was now complicated by disseminated intravascular coagulation (DIC).

## 1. What is the pathophysiological basis for this patient's problem?

DIC does not occur as a primary problem; it is a complication of a variety of disease processes. It is most frequently associated with infection, surgery, trauma, burns, malignancy, and obstetrical complications (1).

DIC is a consequence of tissue-damage-induced activation of the coagulation cascade. Excessive amounts of thrombin are generated, which overwhelm the body's normal antithrombin activities and result in the consumption of certain clotting elements. Mechanisms within the fibrinolytic system acting concurrently with the consumption of clotting factors lead to varying degrees of thrombosis and hemorrhage (2 [pp. 311–313]).

Reviewing the coagulation process is helpful in understanding the pathology that triggers DIC. Coagulation can be divided into the intrinsic and extrinsic pathways. Clot formation begins with the interaction of platelets and exposed subintimal collagen of disrupted vessels (3 [p. 329]). The coagulation proteins are referred to as factors I (figrinogen), II (prothrombin), V, VII, VIII, IX, X, XI, and XII (Hageman factor). These coagulation proteins circulate in the bloodstream until they are activated (4 [p. 369]).

A phospholipid released by active platelets in conjunction with factor XII, kallikrein, and kininogen activates the intrinsic system cascade: factor XI → IX → VIII. These sequential reactions then trigger the common pathway of coagulation: factor X → V → prothrombin → thrombin → fibrinogen → fibrin (3 [p. 329]). The common pathway may also be activated by the extrinsic pathway. When plasma proteins come in contact with tissue thromboplastin released from injured cells, factor VII is activated. Factor VII in turn activates factor X of the common pathway (4 [p. 370]). The extrinsic and intrinsic pathways are complementary in the formation of thrombin and fibrin (Fig. 32.1).

The formation of the fibrin clot then activates the fibrinolytic system. Plasmin is produced to dissolve and lyse the clot. Plasmin is a proteolytic enzyme that digests fibrin, fibrinogen, factor V, factor VIII, prothrombin, and factor XII. The resulting fibrin degradation products (FDP) (or fibrin split products) exert an anticoagulant effect.

DIC involves an interplay between fibrin formation and fibrinolysis. Signs and symptoms caused by clotting result from ischemic damage secondary to occlusion of the microvasculature, whereas those caused by fibrinolysis result from hemorrhage (2 [p. 313]) (Fig. 32.2). The continual activation of the coagulation cascade leads to depletion of the coagulation factors at a rate greater than they can be generated, resulting in bleeding (Fig. 32.3). This depletion or consumption of clotting factors has been also referred to as a consumptive coagulopathy.

DIC manifests as prolongation of prothrombin time and partial thromboplastin time, hypofibrinogenemia, thrombocytopenia, and elevation of fibrin split products (5). No single test confirms DIC. Normal laboratory values will vary institutionally. Treatment of DIC should be directed toward alleviation of the underlying cause. Without this approach, the stimulus for continued clotting and bleeding persists.

DIC within the first 10 days of the traumatic insult is more likely associated with liver injuries, pelvic fractures, and intracranial injuries. Later development of DIC is more commonly associated with infection (6). The most common nonmechanical cause of trauma-induced coagulopathy is dilution of the clotting factors due to massive blood and crystalloid infusion (3 [ p.334]).

Primary treatment is replacement of clotting factors with fresh frozen plasma and

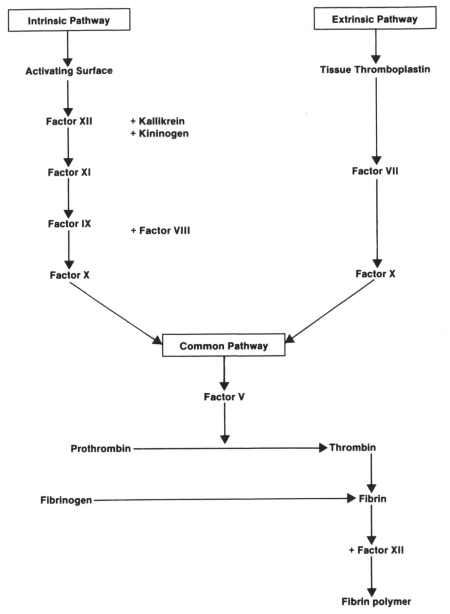

**Figure 32.1.** Activation of blood coagulation.

fibrinogen with cryoprecipitate. Platelet transfusions are used for thrombocytopenia associated with bleeding conditions when the platelet count is less than 50,000 and in nonbleeding conditions when the count is less than 30,000 (5 [pp. 37–38]). Vitamin K is administered for hypoprothrombinemia. The use of heparin in DIC remains contro-

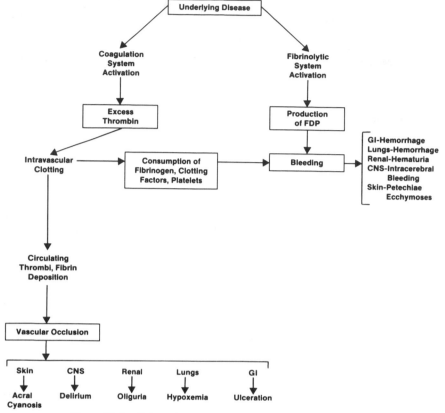

**Figure 32.2.** Balance between coagulation and fibrinolysis in DIC.

versial. Heparin is advocated on the principle that prevention of further intravascular generation of thrombin will result in decreased deposition of fibrin in the microvasculature (2 [pp. 318–320]).

## 2. What are the nursing diagnoses of highest priority in this situation?

A. Potential for alteration of tissue perfusion
B. Potential for fluid volume deficit
C. Potential for impairment of skin integrity

## 3. What goals of care and nursing interventions are appropriate for the above diagnoses?

### A. Nursing Diagnosis

Potential for alteration in tissue perfusion related to hemorrhage and accelerated capillary clotting

### Goal of Care

Maintain optimal tissue perfusion.

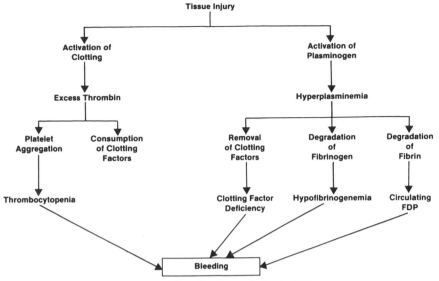

**Figure 32.3.** Bleeding evolution in DIC.

## Nursing Interventions

- Monitor cardiovascular status by documentation of blood pressure and heart rate.
- Assess skin color, temperature, and capillary refill time.
- Monitor hemodynamic status if indicated. Record central venous pressure (CVP), pulmonary artery pressure (PAP), pulmonary capillary wedge pressure (PCWP), and cardiac outputs.
- Obtain serial blood samples for arterial blood gases, hemoglobin, and hematocrit.
- Identify bleeding sources and volume loss.
- Check urine, stool, and gastric drainage for occult blood. Record intake and output.
- Assess and document petechiae, ecchymosis, mottling, and peripheral cyanosis.
- Administer blood and blood components as ordered. Ensure availability of cross-matched blood.

## Rationale

Ongoing cardiovascular assessment and hemodynamic monitoring reflect the degree of shock and impaired tissue perfusion. Serial laboratory testing is necessary for trend analysis. Arterial blood gases are indicator of hypoxemia and determine whether oxygen therapy is adequate. Blood loss decreases the amount of oxygen-carrying red blood cells, which in turn decreases tissue perfusion. Intake and output trends reflect the adequacy of volume replacement.

The presence of petechiae, ecchymosis, and occult blood is evidence of undetectable bleeding (2 [pp. 313–316]). Mottling and cyanosis may reveal clotting in the microvasculature in addition to ischemia due to poor tissue perfusion.

## B. Nursing Diagnosis

Potential for fluid volume deficit related to hemorrhage and coagulopathy

## Goal of Care

Restore adequate circulatory blood volume and correct coagulopathy.

## Nursing Interventions

- Infuse blood, blood products, and crystalloids through large-bore intravenous line.
- Type O (RH +) red blood cells are infused in cases of profound hemorrhage until typed and cross-matched blood is available.
- Use autotransfusion to replace blood if indicated.
- In massive transfusion, 1 to 2 units of fresh frozen plasma may be administered for every 5 units of packed cells, or a fresh frozen plasma continuous infusion may be started.
- Infuse fresh frozen plasma as soon as possible after thawing.
- Infuse platelets as indicated by the platelet count and as ordered by physician.
- Warm blood and fluids prior to administration in massive transfusion.
- Monitor serum calcium and pH.
- Obtain serial PT, PTT, fibrogen, platelet counts, and FDP, preferably from a nonheparinized line.
- Use plain normal saline flush rather than heparinized normal saline if platelet count is low.

## Rationale

In resuscitative transfusion, the goal is to restore the intravascular volume as rapidly as possible. In the multiple trauma patient in whom the main cause of hypovolemia is blood loss, blood component therapy is the procedure of choice. Blood component therapy restores intravascular volume, maintains adequate oxygen-carrying capacity of blood, and maintains coagulability of the blood.

Dilutional coagulopathy is associated with massive transfusion (7). Serial coagulation testing will determine the degree of coagulopathy. Coagulation studies may be distorted by heparin used to flush the arterial cannula. If possible, do not draw blood for these studies from a heparinized line. (Policies for obtaining coagulation studies vary among institutions.)

The PT tests the extrinsic clotting system. A prolonged PT in the presence of a normal PTT implies a factor VII deficiency. An elevated PTT but normal PT signifies a problem in the intrinsic system involving factors XII, XI, IX, and VIII. FDP confirm the consumptive process (3 [pp. 332–333]). Infusion of fresh frozen plasma restores clotting factors. Two units of group-specific fresh frozen plasma are usually administered with every 5 to 6 units of red blood cells, but administration should be based on coagulation parameters and clinical evaluation of bleeding. If the fibrogen level is less than 100 mg/dl and there is no response to fresh frozen plasma, cryoprecipitate is given (5 [p. 38]). Infusion of platelets is dictated by the platelet count in combination with the clinical presentation.

Heparin can cause acute thrombocytopenia. It therefore should be avoided in flush solutions of patients with low platelet counts (8).

Hypothermia is commonly associated with massive infusion. The degree of hypothermia is proportional to the rapidity and volume of stored blood infused. Hypothermia induces platelet sequestration and inhibits the coagulation process by decreasing enzyme activity (3 [p. 330]). Blood should be warmed through coiled tubing prior to transfusion. Citrate used to maintain anticoagulation of the blood during blood bank storage is calcium binding. During massive transfusion there is a potential for the development of hypocalcemia. Monitoring serum calcium levels will identify this problem. Whole blood is acidic and can contribute to the metabolic acidosis of hypoperfusion in the shock patient, but acidosis is not generally associated with red blood cell transfusion alone (9). Some blood additives may also bind calcium, resulting in a decreased serum calcium level; normal calcium levels are necessary for clot formation.

## C. Nursing Diagnosis
Potential for impairment of skin integrity secondary to coagulation disorder

### Goal of Care
Protect patient from further blood loss and unnecessary trauma.

### Nursing Interventions
- Administer medications by IV or oral route. Minimize intramuscular injections and use the smallest gauge needle possible.
- Suction gently.
- Provide gentle oral hygiene.
- Use electric razor to shave patient.
- Avoid vigorous activity and chest physiotherapy.
- Use tape sparingly. Paper tape is preferred. Use Stomadhesive or a similar product to protect skin from tape burns.
- Withdraw laboratory specimens through arterial or existing IV line.
- Do not remove clot formations.
- Initiate nutritional support.

### Rationale
The patient with DIC is particularly vulnerable to friction, irritation, and local trauma. Even slight trauma may cause hemorrhage because of impaired clot formation. Inadvertent removal of existing clots can also precipitate bleeding. Nutritional support through tube feedings or hyperalimentation is imperative because an adequate supply of protein, vitamin K, and calcium is required for generating clotting factors (10).

## ASSOCIATED NURSING DIAGNOSES
A. Fear
B. Potential for infection
C. Altered comfort
D. Alteration in nutrition
E. Potential for hypothermia

### REFERENCES

1. Rutledge R, Sheldon GF. Bleeding and coagulation problems. In: Mattox KL, Moore EE, Feliciana DV, eds. Trauma. Norwalk, CT: Appleton & Lange, 1988:809–819.
2. Carr ME. Disseminated intravascular coagulation: pathogenesis, diagnosis, and therapy. J Emerg Med 1987;5:311–320.
3. Silva R, Moore EE, Galloway WB. Reducing coagulopathy after trauma. Infect Surg (May) 1985:329–334.
4. Hubner CA. Altered clotting. In: Carrieri VK, Lindsey AM, West CM, eds. Pathophysiological phenomena in nursing human responses to illness. Philadelphia: WB Saunders, 1986:369–370.
5. Cowley RA, Dunham CM, eds. Shock trauma/critical care manual: initial assessment and management. Baltimore: University Park Press, 1982:35–38.
6. Dawson RB. Acute coagulation disorders after trauma. In: Siegel JH, ed. Trauma emergency surgery and critical care. New York: Churchill Livingstone, 1987:748–749.
7. McQuillan KA, Wiles CE. Initial management of traumatic shock. In: Cardona VD, Hurn PD, Bastnagel-Mason PJ, et al, eds. Trauma nursing: from resuscitation through rehabilitation. Philadelphia: WB Saunders, 1988:167–173.
8. Dunham CM, Cowley RA. Shock trauma/critical care handbook. Rockville, MD: Aspen, 1986:63–64.
9. Hollar DL. Hemorrhagic shock. In: Strange JM, ed. Shock trauma care plans. Springhouse, PA: Springhouse, 1987:14–18.
10. Hollar DL. Disseminated intravascular coagulation (DIC). In: Strange JM, ed. Shock trauma care plans. Springhouse, PA: 1987:278–281.

## SUGGESTED READINGS

Bart JB, Dear CB. Hematopoietic disorders. In: Kinney MR, Dear CB, Packa DR, Voorman DM, eds. AACN's clinical reference for critical-care nursing. New York: McGraw-Hill, 1981:591–597.

Guyton AC. Textbook of medical physiology. 7th ed. Philadelphia: WB Saunders, 1986:76–86.

# CHAPTER 33

## Ocular Trauma

### Barbara J. Keyes, RN, BSN

## Clinical Presentation

Following an automobile accident, a 42-year-old man was admitted to the emergency department of a large university hospital. Physical examination, supported by routine laboratory work, x-ray films, and a computerized tomography scan, revealed that he had sustained isolated ocular injuries. Specifically, these included an orbital floor blow-out fracture on the left, a left ruptured ocular globe, a right corneal abrasion, and multiple small eyelid lacerations. The remaining physical and medical history assessment determined that the patient had no other injuries, no significant health problems or history, and no allergies and that he was currently taking no medication. He presented in the emergency department with stable vital signs and was neurologically intact. His chief complaints were acute visual loss in the left eye, photophobia in the right eye, and ocular pain bilaterally.

Both an opthalmologist and plastic surgeon were consulted for treatment. The first priority was to save the integrity of the left ocular globe and therefore its vision. Surgery was then performed in an attempt to repair the ruptured globe and the blow-out fracture. The fracture was easily repaired; however, the prognosis for retaining vision in the left eye was still questionable. Plastic surgeons debrided and sutured the eyelid lacerations. Following stabilization in the recovery room, the patient was admitted to the hospital's ophthalmology floor.

His immediate postoperative nursing care on the floor was routine and uncomplicated. This care included monitoring vital signs, administering intravenous (IV) therapy, taking intake and output measurements, conducting physical assessments, initiating prophylactic antibiotics (topical and/or IV), administering pain medications as needed, coordinating routine postoperative lab work, administering respiratory care, and providing psychological assessment and support. The patient was awake and alert and able to participate with his postoperative care. Both eyes were bandaged; a protective shield covered the left eye. The eyelids were swollen and ecchymotic, especially the left.

Within 24 hours, the corneal abrasion on the right eye had healed and the patch had been removed; it was determined that no vision had been lost in the right eye. The left eye was monitored closely for infection and visual activity. The patient's stable condition allowed him to assume almost total self-care with some assistance. On the sixth postoperative day, his left eye appeared to be healing well without signs of infection. No further surgical intervention, specifically enucleation, was deemed necessary.

The patient was discharged from the hospital 8 days after the accident. Both he and his wife were taught eye care as well as how to observe for signs of complications. The patient was then followed by his family ophthalmologist and office nurse.

### 1. What is the pathophysiological basis for this patient's problem?

Each year an estimated 1.3 million people in the United States suffer ocular injuries. More than 40,000 of these injuries result in some degree of visual loss (1).

The priorities of care in ocular injury are (a) protection of the intact portions of the visual system and prevention of further damage to undamaged structures; (b) assessment of the extent of injury with referral of the patient for immediate repair of injured tissue to prevent further damage; and (c) initiation of therapeutic measures that achieve first, optimal function and second, optimal cosmetic results (2).

Perforating ocular injuries are the major cause of traumatic visual loss. When such an injury is suspected, the ocular globe requires extensive exploration and surgical repair while the patient is under general anesthesia. Every attempt should be made to save the ocular structures. If unsuccessful, an enucleation can be performed at a later date. A major indication for an enucleation is to prevent sympathetic ophthalmia, a complication characterized by a severe, bilateral, granulomatous uveitis, or inflammation of the entire uveal tract, iris, ciliary body, and choroid (2). Symptoms appear as early as 9 days following the injury or can be delayed for years. The exact cause of sympathetic ophthalmia is unknown; however, it is believed that the inflammation in the noninjured eye is an autoimmune response to the retinal S antigen from the injured eye. Left untreated, the inflammatory response will result in bilateral loss of vision. Sympathetic ophthalmia is not reversible, and enucleation will not improve this condition after the immune response has occurred. Aggressive oral steroid therapy is used prophylactically. In situations where enucleation is considered, such as a blind eye or one with severe irreparable damage, the enucleation generally should be performed within 9 days following the initial injury to prevent an autoimmune response.

Clinical observations of orbital fractures include periorbital swelling, ecchymosis, proptosis, chemosis, crepitus, subconjunctival hemorrhage, ophthalmoplegia (caused by swelling and muscle entrapment), infraorbital and buccal anesthesia, and palpable deficits in the bony orbital rims. The extent of orbital fractures is determined by radiological studies. The importance of repairing orbital fractures is twofold: functional correction and cosmetic appearance. Medical indications for surgery include (a) diplopia in primary gaze and downward gaze that shows no sign of spontaneous improvement and (b) enophthalmos or recession of the eyeball within the orbit. Surgical repair is generally accomplished by an open reduction with wiring. Complications, including permanent loss of vision, persistent enophthalmos and diplopia, scarring, and eyelid retraction, can occur following the surgical repair. Orbital fractures can be corrected surgically even weeks after trauma.

Corneal abrasions are usually the result of the introduction of a foreign body into the eye. Clinical findings include photophobia, pain, excessive tearing, the feeling of something in the eye, redness, and irritation. Fluorescein staining, which outlines the abrasion with fluorescein dye, facilitates examination and diagnosis. Management includes administering topical anesthetic and antibiotic drops and pressure patching the eye for 24 to 48 hours. Length of treatment is determined by the rapidity of the healing process and the severity of the abrasion. Minor corneal abrasions heal within 24 to 72 hours; more severe injuries will usually heal within 10 days. Scarring and infections are complications that can occur with this injury.

## 2. What are the nursing diagnoses of highest priority?

A. Potential for infection
B. Potential for loss of visual activity
C. Potential for feelings of powerlessness

## 3. What goals of care and nursing interventions are appropriate for the above diagnoses?

*A. Nursing Diagnosis*

Potential for infection related to the loss of skin, structural integrity

*Goal of Care*

Wound healing without infection

### Nursing Interventions
● Monitor for signs of infection.
● Perform wound/dressing care every 4 hours (or as otherwise ordered).
● Administer antibiotics as ordered.

### Rationale
The importance of keeping wounds clean and free of blood and drainage cannot be overstated. Both provide an excellent medium for bacterial growth and infection, which could result in loss of vision. Unless otherwise specified, routine care is to cleanse periorbital sutures, incisions, lacerations, and abrasions thoroughly with a half-strength mixture of normal saline and hydrogen peroxide. A thin layer of an ophthalmic antibiotic ointment should then be applied to the wounds. No dressing is necessary if drainage is absent. The use of iodine-based ointments should be avoided for three reasons: the products can damage cells responsible for tissue repair, thus impeding granulation and antimicrobial defenses; cause preventable scarring; and be inflammatory to the sclera (2).

### B. Nursing Diagnosis
Potential for further loss of visual activity related to possible extension of injury

### Goal of Care
Maintain maximum functional potential.

### Nursing Interventions
● Restrict activities to minimize ocular pressure.
● Institute safety precautions (prevent accidental injury).
● Monitor visual acuity for changes.

### Rationale
Every effort should be made to prevent the extension of an ocular injury, since complications can result in more permanent visual loss than the original injury. Increased ocular pressure (resulting from hemorrhage or edema following surgical repair) can damage ocular structures as well as the optic nerve, with residual loss of sight. Activities that increase intraocular pressure (bending, lifting, coughing, chest physiotherapy) should be curtailed; bed rest for 24 hours is preferable. It is also important to protect the eye from accidental injury. A metal shield can be taped over a gauze eyepatch for additional protection. With impaired vision from trauma, patients require additional safety measures to prevent falls, tripping, and blows to the head. Careful monitoring of visual acuity (using hand-held eye cards and wall eye charts; discernment of objects, lights, colors) is essential to determine visual progress or deterioration, regardless of etiology.

### C. Nursing Diagnosis
Potential for feelings of powerlessness related to visual impairment

### Goal of Care
Increase feelings of independence.

### Nursing Interventions
● Introduce persons in patient's presence.
● Explain all procedures and noises.
● Allow for choices when appropriate.
● Encourage patient assistance with activities of daily living and treatments.
● Orient as needed.
● Consult occupational/physical therapy as needed.

## Rationale

Sudden loss of vision is a frightening and incapacitating experience. It affects every aspect of an individual's being. Patients are rendered dependent on others for all activities. Psychologically, this can be devastating to an individual, and efforts to promote independence and to increase self-esteem must be initiated. The existence and magnitude of this concern needs to be acknowledged, especially if the visual impairment is permanent.

## ASSOCIATED NURSING DIAGNOSES

A. Alterations in sensory perception related to visual impairment
B. Disturbances in self-concept and body image
C. Potential for sleep pattern disturbances
D. Alterations in comfort

### REFERENCES

1. America Academy of Ophthalmology, San Francisco, CA, 1985.
2. Karesh JW, Keyes BJ. Ocular trauma. In: Cardona VD, Hurn PD, Bastnagel-Mason PJ, et al, eds. Trauma nursing: from resuscitation through rehabilitation. Philadelphia: WB Saunders, 1988: 616.
3. Holler DL. Maxillofacial injuries. In: Strange JM, ed. Shock trauma care plans. Springhouse, PA: Springhouse, 1987:202.

### SUGGESTED READINGS

Cowley RA, Dunham CM, eds. Shock trauma/critical care manual: initial assessment and management. Baltimore: University Park Press, 1982:76–77, 90–91.

Deutsch TA, Feller DB. Paton and Goldberg's management of ocular injuries. 2nd ed. Philadelphia: WB Saunders, 1985.

Dunham CM, Cowley RA. Shock trauma/critical care handbook. Rockville, MD: Aspen, 1986:103–108.

Karesh JW, Keyes BJ. Ocular trauma. In: Cardona VD, Hurn PD, Bastnagel-Mason PJ, et al, eds. Trauma nursing: from resuscitation through rehabilitation. Philadelphia: WB Saunders, 1988:598–619.

Newell SW. Management of corneal foreign bodies. Am Fam Phys 1985;31:149–156.

Welch J, Tyler J. Emergency! Dealing with eye injuries. RN 1984;47:53–54.

Wright BR. Eye injuries. In: Strange JM, ed. Shock trauma care plans. Springhouse, PA: Springhouse, 1987:211–220.

# CHAPTER 34

## Trauma in the Elderly

### Judith K. Bobb, RN, MSN

## Clinical Presentation

Patrick, age 82, was injured when his automobile slipped out of gear and rolled over him. He arrived at the hospital awake and alert, with moderate respiratory distress. A full-thickness burn was noted on the left posterior shoulder as well as ecchymosis over the left anterior chest. Also noted were a deformity of the right wrist and previous partial amputations of both feet.

Blood pressure at admission was 60/40 with a heart rate of 104. He had cool skin, diaphoresis, and weak major pulses. A grade I systolic murmur was present, and an electrocardiogram showed left anterior hemiblock and occasional atrial and ventricular ectopic beats. His blood pressure rose to 120/60 in response to infusion of 300 ml of lactated Ringer's solution.

Shortly after admission, increased respiratory distress was treated with endotracheal intubation and mechanical ventilation. Upright chest x-ray films revealed clear lung fields and fractures of right ribs 4 through 8 and left ribs 6 and 7. A second episode of hypotension also responded to fluid administration. Diagnostic peritoneal lavage was negative.

Patrick reported a medical history of insulin-dependent diabetes, hypertension, and peripheral vascular disease. His medications included NPH insulin 40 units daily, cardiazem, and digoxin.

He was stabilized and admitted to the intensive care unit (ICU) with diagnoses of fractures of ribs 4 through 8 on the right and of 6 and 7 on the left, a 1% body surface area full-thickness burn, and a comminuted fracture of the left radius and ulna, which was reduced and casted. Pulmonary contusion and myocardial contusions were ruled out.

Over the next several hours, Patrick continued to have ectopy and hypotensive episodes in response to morphine sulfate (1 to 2 mg IV) administered for pain. Blood pressure was restored easily with fluid administration. A Swan-Ganz catheter was introduced for hemodynamic monitoring. Initial cardiac output was 3.4 liters/minute with a pulmonary capillary wedge pressure (PCWP) of 4 mm Hg and a systemic vascular resistance of 1257 dynes/sec. He was also started on dopamine (2 μg/kg/minute) and dobutamine (3 μg/kg/minute) for urinary output of 20 to 40 ml/hr.

### 1. What is the pathophysiological basis for this patient's problem?

The most common cause of hypotension in a multiple system trauma patient is hypovolemia secondary to hemorrhage. However, this patient showed little evidence of significant occult bleeding. Both the chest x-ray film and the peritoneal lavage were negative, and the fractured left wrist was unlikely to hide a volume of blood large enough to produce hemorrhagic shock.

The second most likely reason for hypotension in this patient is nonhemorrhagic hypovolemia. Hypovolemia could be due to diminished intake of fluids antedating the injury, a common finding in elderly patients. Evidence of hypovolemia includes Patrick's rapid response to administration of lactated Ringer's solution and his low urinary output. He also experienced hypotension following administration of low doses of morphine for pain. The vasodilating effects of morphine may have induced a relative hypovolemia, which also responded to administration of fluid volume.

Another possible cause of this patient's hypotension, given his age and history, is pre-existing impaired myocardial function or myocardial contusion sustained at the time of injury. There is evidence that this patient has previously experienced a myocardial infarction. He shows a left anterior hemiblock and abnormal Q waves on the electrocardiogram, as well as a low-grade systolic murmur. The indications of myocardial contusion include ecchymosis on the left chest, ectopy, atrioventricular (AV) block, and hemodynamic instability.

Even if a primary cardiac cause of hypotension is ruled out, Patrick should be monitored closely to assess the impact of his injuries on his cardiac function. The elderly may be slower to respond to injury than the young, may be unable to respond adequately because of age-related decreases in cardiovascular function (1), and have a significantly higher mortality associated with low to moderate degrees of injury (2). It is necesary to initiate intensive monitoring early in the hospital course to avoid undertreatment or inappropriate treatment of the elderly trauma patient (3).

A Swan-Ganz catheter was introduced to provide better assessment of left ventricular function. Initial measurements were within normal limits. Subsequent episodes of hypotension were corrected with fluid boluses while PCWP was monitored closely. Blood pressure stabilized at approximately 170/90. PCWP was also stable in the range of 8 to 13 mm Hg, urinary output increased to 40 to 50 ml/hr, and ectopy diminished in frequency. The final diagnosis was hypovolemia of undetermined cause. Later studies revealed that Patrick had a myocardial infarction sometime in the past, leaving him with slight dyskinesis of the left ventricle.

## 2. What are the nursing diagnoses of highest priority?

A. Potential fluid volume deficit
B. Altered patterns of urinary elimination
C. Ineffective airway clearance
D. Potential for infection.

## 3. What are the goals of nursing care?

### A. Nursing Diagnosis

Potential fluid volume deficit secondary to inadequate replacement and related to aging

### Goal of Care

Maintain adequate intravascular volume.

### Nursing Interventions

- Monitor vital signs and urinary output.
- Monitor pulmonary artery pressures and cardiac output.
- Monitor peripheral pulses.

### Rationale

Because no single parameter measures intravascular volume directly, the nurse must assess its status from a collection of parameters. Blood pressure alone may give misleading information. Normal blood pressure may be present even when the patient is hypovolemic if compensatory vasconstrictive responses are intact. In addition, it is difficult to estimate the volume losses that typically accompany trauma, even when the injury appears to be mild. The combination of blood pressure, heart rate, and volume of peripheral pulses is more accurate. Patients who have tachycardia persisting after resuscitation, peripheral pulses weaker than expected, and cool skin are giving evidence of inadequate perfusion.

Urinary output provides a "window" into volume status, since the same compensatory responses that maintain blood pressure will reduce renal water losses if hypovolemia is present. However, changes in renal function are to be expected following trauma even in the absence of renal injury. For approximately 24 hours after resuscitation, the kidney has diminished concentrating ability. In order to excrete the usual load of waste products, a greater than normal volume of urine is required. Nurses should expect an output volume in the range of 50 to 100 ml/hr (4). This volume of urine output indicates adequate intravascular volume and perfusion.

When difficulty is anticipated in either assessment or perfusion therapy, hemodynamic parameters from a pulmonary artery catheter permit more discrete measurement of the status of cardiovascular function. In Patrick's case, measuring PAWP helped determine that his left ventricle was capable of tolerating fluid loads.

The PCWP is a measure of left ventricular filling pressure and, indirectly, of the volume of blood entering the left ventricle. The normal range is 10 to 14 mm Hg. It results from the ventricle contracting around a normal volume of blood. When the PAWP is low (Patrick's was 4 mm Hg), it indicates that the volume of blood entering the ventricle is less than normal and that the contractile state of the ventricle is adequate. Because a low volume reduces cardiac output, and therefore perfusion, a goal of therapy is infusion of additional volume until the filling pressure is normalized.

Additional values of the Swan-Ganz catheter are determination of cardiac output and measurement of venous oxygen tension. Once the cardiac output has been measured, additional calculations can be performed to assess the cardiovascular system. Both pulmonary and systemic vascular resistance can be calculated to determine the vasomotor tone against which the ventricles must contract. Although some vasoconstriction is expected as part of the compensatory response to injury, excessive amounts can precipitate heart failure if contractility is impaired. Measurement of the venous oxygen tension after the blood is mixed in the right ventricle reflects the amount of oxygen consumed by the tissues. Oxygen consumption can then be calculated using the Fick principle. A simpler assessment of oxygen consumption is derived from determining the difference between arterial and venous oxygen contents, the $C(a-v)O_2$. Use of the Swan-Ganz catheter in this manner provides the clinician with increased assessment accuracy when volume and/or contractility is in question.

## B. Nursing Diagnosis

Altered patterns of urinary elimination

### Goal of Care

Maintain adequate urinary output.

### Nursing Interventions

- Monitor urinary output.
- Monitor renal laboratory indices.
- Monitor perfusion status.

### Rationale

The literature documents decreased renal function as a consequence of aging (5). These changes include reduced renal blood flow, glomerular filtration rate, urine flow, and concentrating ability. Renal adjustment to acid or alkaline loads are also slowed with age. Generally, the unstressed kidney shows little laboratory evidence of aging, with the exception of a slightly elevated blood urea nitrogen (mean, 21.2 mg/dl) (5). Following trauma, it is probable that defects in concentrating ability and waste clearance will become manifest.

Anecdotally it is not uncommon for the aged patient to show reduced creatinine clearance and slight elevation in serum creatinine (1.2 to 1.5 mg/dl) and blood urea nitrogen. Most appear to be capable of maintaining adequate urine volume. Attention to volume output alone can lead to a false sense of security, since diminished concentrating ability is a potential cause of excess water losses. The most helpful assessment of renal function in the elderly seems to be urinary sodium. That is, the aged kidney can conserve sodium appropriately even in situations in which it is unable to elaborate a concentrated urine, such as hypovolemia.

The elderly are also at increased risk for acute renal failure as a result of trauma, because renal blood flow is reduced as a function of aging. As a consequence, particular attention must be paid to the adequacy of renal perfusion, and decreases in urine volume should be investigated promptly. Some patients in the author's experience have developed nonoliguric renal failure, which responded well to conservative management.

## C. Nursing Diagnosis
Ineffective airway clearance

## Goal of Care
Prevention of retained secretions

## Nursing Interventions
- Maintain patent airway.
- Monitor breath sounds.
- Monitor oxygen tension.
- Institute chest physical therapy as indicated.
- Mobilize the patient as early as possible.

## Rationale
Advancing age produces changes in respiratory function, which predispose the elderly to pulmonary complications even in the absence of chronic lung disease (6). Beginning in middle age, there is progressive loss of patent alveoli and a reduction in lung volume and elasticity. Gag and cough reflexes are less sensitive and muscular force is reduced. There is also less force available for respiration, but the work of breathing increases by approximately 10%. The small airways are less stable, leading to early airway closure, especially at low tidal volumes. Oxygen tension falls at approximately 4 mm Hg per decade, from a normal of 97 mm HG at age 20 to approximately 70 mm Hg at age 80. Because the changes occur gradually over the years, little impairment in function is noted under normal conditions. Under conditions of stress, however, the loss of pulmonary reserve predisposes the aged patient to retention of secretions.

When instrumentation of the airway is necessary following trauma, the older patient's risk of pulmonary compromise increases proportionately. Use of artificial airways bypasses the natural barriers to bacterial invasion and limits the patient's ability to clear secretions. Mechanical ventilation further impedes removal of secretions and appears to have an adverse effect on respiratory muscle strength, although this phenomenon has not been documented.

Allen and Schwab (7) have shown that elderly patients with single system injuries can be managed successfully without ventilatory support if pain is well managed.

Unfortunately, they also demonstrated that those with multiple system involvement invariably failed nonventilatory trials. From these data, we can conclude that ventilatory support is essential in the elderly multisystem trauma victim, that it should be instituted early when required, and that it carries an increased risk of additional pulmonary complications.

Once ventilatory support is instituted, the nurse must anticipate that it will be of longer duration in the elderly than in the young. Intensive tracheobronchial toilet for extended periods is the norm rather than the exception. The patient must be monitored closely for worsening hypoxemia and diminished breath sounds.

The nursing care plan should emphasize mobility as the first line of defense against atelectasis. Routine changes of position (i.e., every 2 hours) are probably inadequate for the elderly patient, but this must be evaluated individually in the absence of research supporting another strategy. Mobilizing the patient out of bed should be done at the first opportunity, even while ventilatory support is in place. This will help to reduce the potential for airway closure when the patient is supine.

Coughing and deep breathing should be done on a frequent basis; however, the need for suctioning should be evaluated each time. Test the patient for cough strength using the suction catheter initially only as a stimulus. If the patient can clear the airways adequately, avoid application of negative pressure. When suctioning is required (i.e., when secretions are mobilized within reach of the catheter and the patient cannot expel them), particular care must be exercised to minimize damage to the tracheal muscosa. Suction flow rates less than the standard 140 to 150 mm Hg, application of intermittent negative pressure, and "twirling" the catheter should reduce trachael trauma (8,9).

## D. Nursing Diagnosis
Potential for infection

## Goal of Care
Reduce pneumonia potential.

## Nursing Interventions
- Maintain patent airway.
- Monitor sputum for purulence.
- Institute chest physical therapy as indicated.
- Mobilize the patient as early as possible.

## Rationale
Since the advent of antibiotics, pneumonia has become almost exclusively a disease of the aged and a major cause of and/or contributing factor to elderly mortality (8). Aging changes associated with increased susceptibility to pulmonary infection include diminished immune competence; decreased volume, force, and flow rate during coughing; slowing of the mucociliary escalator for removal of foreign particles; and decreases in levels of immunoglobulin A (8). The risk of pneumonia appears to increase with advancing age as well as in the presence of additional health stresses such as trauma.

Recent studies of geriatric trauma patients have confirmed the risk of pneumonia in the elderly. Horst et al. (10) documented sepsis secondary to pneumonia in 67% of elderly trauma patients who died. DeMaria et al. (11) found pneumonia in 19% of elderly trauma survivors and a 35% incidence in nonsurvivors.

The elderly patient may not always show typical signs of pulmonary infection, such as fever and leukocytosis. Often the initial onset is marked by an altered mental status, tachypnea, fatigue, and purulent sputum. In the intensive care setting, clinical findings may be masked by other treatment modalities, such as intubation and mechanical ventilation. Chest x-ray findings can range from infiltrates and consolidation to abscess and cavitation. Pneumonia in the elderly may progress rapidly depending on the organism involved and the overall condition of the patient.

Nursing care is directed toward limiting the patient's risk through the measures to reduce secretion retention as outlined above. Additional attention should be placed on the appearance of purulent sputum, which is characteristic of pulmonary infection. If pneumonia is confirmed by sputum culture, narrow-spectrum organism-specific antibiotics are recommended.

## ASSOCIATED NURSING DIAGNOSES

A. Pain
B. Potential for aspiration
C. Impaired verbal communication
D. Potential impaired skin integrity
E. Potential activity intolerance
F. Potential for disuse syndrome
G. Impaired physical mobility

**REFERENCES**

1. Beard OW. Age-related physiological changes in the cardiovascular system. In: Cape RDT, Coe RM, Rossman I, eds. Fundamentals of geriatric medicine. New York: Raven Press, 1983:63–69.
2. Baker SP, O'Neil B, Haddon W, Long WB. The injury severity score: a method for describing patients with multiple injuries and evaluating emergency care. J Trauma 1974;14:187–196.
3. DelGuercio LRM, Cohn JD. Monitoring operative risk in the elderly. JAMA 1980;243:1350–1355.
4. Wilson RF, ed. Principles and techniques of critical care, Vol 1. Kalamazoo, MI: Upjohn.
5. Papper S. The effects of age in reducing renal function. Geriatrics 1973;28:83–87.
6. Harrell CV. Age-related changes in the respiratory system. In: Matteson MA, McConnell ES, eds. Gerontological nursing. Philadelphia: WB Saunders, 1988.
7. Allen JA, Schwab CW. Blunt chest trauma in the elderly. Am Surg 1985;51:697–700.
8. Kleiber C, Krutzfield N, Rose EF. Acute histologic changes in the tracheobronchial tree associated with different suction catheter insertion techniques. Heart Lung 1988;17:10–14.
9. Chulay M, Graeger GM. Efficacy of a hyperinflation and hyperoxygenation suctioning intervention. Heart Lung 1988;17:15–22.
10. Horst HM, Obeid FN, Sorensen VJ. Factors influencing survival of elderly trauma patients. Crit Care Med 1986;14:681–684.
11. DeMaria EJ, Kenney PR, Merriam MA, Casanova LA, Gann DS. Survival after trauma in geriatric patients. Ann Surg 1987;206:738–743.

# CHAPTER 35

## Organ Donation

Margaret K. Aberg-Cocchia, RN, BSN

## Clinical Presentation

As the rain beat against the windshield, J.M. swerved suddenly to avoid hitting a deer. His car crashed at 50 miles/hr into a large tree along the road. An unknown time lapsed before an ambulance arrived at the scene and found J.M., a 33-year-old man, to be unresponsive and cold to the touch. He had a heart rate of 50 beats/minute (bpm), a shallow respiratory rate of 32/minute, and systolic blood pressure (SBP) of 90 mm Hg by palpation. Before extricating J.M. from the car, a cervical collar was placed around his neck, and J.M. was moved to a backboard. A long linear laceration was noted on the right frontal area of his skull, which had exuded approximately 150 ml of blood. The left pupil was fixed and dilated, whereas the right pupil constricted to pinpoint. Blood was draining from his ears bilaterally. Following intubation with an esophageal obturator airway (EOA), 100% oxygen was applied via an Ambu bag. Decreased breath sounds were auscultated in the right lower lobe. Chest wall movement was symmetrical, and the trachea was in a midline position. Subcutaneous air was palpated over the right distal anterior portion of the chest. Two 16-gauge catheters were inserted into the antecubital fossa veins bilaterally to maintain intravenous infusions of Ringer's lactate at a rapid rate. Having no other obvious sources of physical trauma, J.M. was rushed to the local emergency department.

On presentation in the emergency department his vital signs were stable with a heart rate of 75 bpm, a blood pressure of 90/60 mm Hg, and a temperature of 95°F (35°C) rectally. Routine laboratory work was drawn and sent, including a urine toxicology screen for the presence of alcohol and drugs. An orogastric tube was inserted through the mouth to drain the stomach contents, and a Foley catheter was introduced into the bladder to monitor urine output. The neurological assessment demonstrated a Glasgow Coma Scale score of 3. However, both pupils were now fixed and dilated. Mannitol (50 gm) was given by intravenous push, and a 20% mannitol drip was begun at 25 ml/hr (5 gm/hr). Hyperventilation was initiated by placing the patient on a ventilator for mechanical ventilation. The ventilator settings were $FiO_2$, 1.00; tidal volume, 800; synchronous intermittent mandatory ventilation (SIMV), 20; and positive end-expiratory pressure (PEEP), 5. The respiratory assessment revealed decreased breath sounds in the right lower lobe. An imprint of the seat belt and steering wheel was noted across his chest and abdomen. A chest tube was inserted for a pneumothorax in the right lower lobe visualized on chest x-ray film. A diagnostic peritoneal lavage was negative for blood return. Further assessment revealed a fractured left clavicle and right tibial/fibular fracture. Cervical spine x-ray series were negative for fractures and dislocations. Scattered cuts and bruises were also present throughout the torso and extremities. The computerized tomography (CT) scan results indicated an epidural hematoma over the right frontal-temporal lobes and an intraventricular bleed. Massive cerebral edema existed with a right-to-left shift. The neurosurgeons created emergency burr holes in an attempt to relieve intracranial pressure. The family was updated and informed of the seriousness of the situation. J.M. was transferred to the intensive care unit (ICU). In the ICU, an arterial line was placed in the right radial artery. A pulmonary artery line was inserted into the left subclavian vein. Initial pulmonary artery (PA) pressure was 20/07 with a pulmonary capillary wedge pressure (PCWP) of 6 mm Hg. After approximately 7 hours in the ICU, the patient

**241**

had an episode of tachycardia and hypotension immediately followed by bradycardia and hypertension. With the unconfirmed diagnosis of brain-stem herniation, a neurosurgeon and an intensivist performed clinical testing for brain death at the bedside. J.M. failed to respond to any of these tests. A negative brain-flow study confirmed the occurrence of the herniation and therefore brain death. The attending physician and nurse explained the concept of brain death to the family. After this discussion, the subject of organ donation was presented to them. In compliance with federal law, the coordinator from the local organ procurement agency was contacted and arrived at the hospital to assess the possibility of donation. Following additional discussion with the organ procurement coordinator, the family agreed to donate the heart, liver, kidneys, corneas, skin, and bone for transplantation purposes.

## 1. What is the pathophysiological basis for this patient's problem?

Head trauma often produces cerebral edema, resulting in increased intracranial pressure (ICP). The increasing amount of edema as well as elevated ICP may lead to brain-stem herniation, which, in turn, causes a reduction of cerebral blood flow. When blood flow is impaired, cells die, and brain death occurs (1).

*Brain death* is defined as the irreversible cessation of all cortical and brain-stem function in accordance with reasonable medical standards (2). The possibility of metabolic central nervous system (CNS) depression must be excluded before brain death can be declared. Potentially reversible conditions that may impair brain function are drug and alcohol overdose/intoxication, hypothermia, hypoxia/shock, hypoglycemia, and fluid electrolyte imbalance (3 [p. 317]). After the mechanism of injury is established, the process of brain death declaration can begin.

Clinical criteria have been identified to pronounce a person legally and medically brain dead. The tests for these criteria must be performed by a physician. These criteria are absence of spontaneous movement, absence of reaction to internal and tactile/noxious external stimuli, total absence of respirations confirmed by an apnea test, and absence of cranial nerve reflexes. When performing the apnea test, 100% oxygen is applied for approximately 5 minutes and then the ventilator is turned to the continuous positive airway pressure (CPAP) mode. The arterial $CO_2$ level is allowed to rise to approximately 65, which should take 3 to 4 minutes. If the patient does not breathe during this time, then the apnea test is confirmed. This test should not be performed on any patient who is hemodynamically unstable and should be the last fulfilled clinical criterion. The cranial nerve reflex tests include the pupillary light response, corneals (blink), oculocephalic (doll's eyes), oculovestibular (cold water calorics), and otopharyngeal (cough and gag). Since spinal reflexes may remain intact because of the reflex arc in the spinal column (4 [p. 1391]), they are not a criterion for brain death. A reflex is a basic stimulus–response pattern that operates without voluntary or conscious control (5). After the clinical examination is completed, confirmatory studies, such as angiography or blood flow, may be performed if further documentation is needed to substantiate the results (4 [p. 1392]).

The brain stem controls all life-sustaining activities. Removing physiological ''life support'' from the patient after declaration of brain death would negate the possibility of organ donation. The heart would stop and the vascular organs would no longer be perfused. The state of brain death also promotes potential hemodynamic instability due to the loss of the autonomic nervous system controlled by the brain stem. Therefore, clinical management of a potential donor must be aggressive. After brain death is documented, the medical and nursing focus shifts from saving the life of the injured individual to procurement of the vascular organs and nonvascularized tissues.

Organs that may be donated are classified as vital and nonvital. Vital organs of donation include the heart, liver, lungs, kidneys, and pancreas. They must be harvested from brain-dead donors whose hearts are still beating. Nonvital organs or tissues include corneas, skin, bone, bone marrow, and inner ear structures. These may be harvested within established time constraints from cadaver donors whose hearts have stopped beating. Criteria for specific organ donation are listed in Table 35.1. Donor recipients are matched according to ABO blood group, human leukocyte antigen matching, antibody screening, and height and weight. Organ donation helps save, as well as improve, the lives of many other people in need.

Many health care professionals feel uncomfortable broaching the subject of organ donation with families. However, some studies have shown that grieving families may be comforted when they know that other people have improved lives because of the donation. Some families view donation as the highest form of charity, knowing that their loved one did not die in vain (6).

## 2. What are the nursing diagnoses of highest priority?

A. Fluid volume deficit
B. Impaired gas exchange
C. Hypothermia

## 3. What goals and nursing interventions are appropriate for the above diagnoses?

### A. Nursing Diagnosis

Fluid volume deficit related to dehydration and diabetes insipidus

### Goal of Care

Maintain normovolemic homeostasis as evidenced by stable vital signs, electrolytes within normal limits, and urine output >100 ml/hr.

### Nursing Interventions

- Assess intake and output (I & O) every hour.
- Monitor vital signs and hemodynamic parameters every hour and per physician's order.
- Use aggressive intravenous (IV) infusion of colloids and crystalloids (such as normal saline solution and lactated Ringer's) as ordered.
- Monitor serum electrolytes, hematocrit (Hct), hemoglobin (Hgb), and urine and serum osmolarity every 2 to 4 hours.
- If the SBP is <100 mm Hg and CVP is <10 mm Hg and/or PCWP is <8 mm Hg, administer aggressive fluid replacement first, then use low-dose dopamine (<5 to 10 μg/kg/minute) or dobutamine (<10 μg/kg/minute).
- Maintain urine output at 100 to 150 ml/hr.
- If Hct <30%, use packed red blood cells (PRBCs) for replacement.
- Give aqueous vasopressin (Pitressin) (IV drip, approximately 2.5 to 6 units/hr) as ordered if urine output >300 ml/hr (3 [p. 509]).
- If possible, avoid use of alpha stimulators, such as metaraminol, levarterenol, or Neo-Synephrine.

### Rationale

The goal of care for head-injured patients is to maintain a state of dehydration in an effort to decrease ICP. The goal of organ donor care shifts from dehydration to rehydration of potential organs, thereby minimizing ischemia and potential irreversible injury to the vascular organs (7). Diabetes insipidus is a deficiency in the release of antidiuretic hormone (ADH), resulting in an inability to conserve water. It is caused by neurological insults to the hypothalamus (8). Urine output can average

**Table 35.1.** Organ donation criteria[a]

| | Criteria for Donors | Unique Evaluation Requirements |
|---|---|---|
| All potential donors | Irreversible brain damage from trauma, hypoxia, or hemorrhage with brain death imminent or already pronounced<br>Negative medical history for specific organ to be donated<br>No signs of infection<br>No prolonged cardiac arrest<br>Stable vital signs without high doses of inotropic support<br>Cause of death established<br>No malignancy with exception of primary brain tumors<br>No history of intravenous drug abuse and not in a high-risk group for exposure to HIV<br>No signs of communicable disease | Electrolytes, serum glucose, creatinine, and urea nitrogen<br>Microscopic urinalysis<br>Urine cultures<br>Blood cultures<br>Toxicology screen<br>Hepatitis B surface antigen<br>ABO blood type<br>VDRL/RPR<br>HIV<br>Patient's height and weight |
| Liver | No history of drug abuse or alcoholism<br>No history of hepatitis<br>Under age of 50<br>No abdominal trauma | Liver function tests<br>Abdominal girth<br>Arterial blood gases<br>Coagulation studies<br>Hematocrit and hemoglobin |
| Pancreas | No history of hepatitis<br>No abdominal trauma<br>No burns >15% of body surface area<br>No history of diabetes mellitus in donor or first-degree relatives<br>No history of alcoholism<br>Between ages of 5 and 60 | Amylase level |
| Kidney | No overdose of nephrotoxic drugs<br>No history of hypertension<br>Between ages of 2 months and 65 years<br>Normal renal function:<br>  BUN, 11–23 mg/100ml<br>  Creatinine, 0.6–1.2 mg/100 ml<br>No violation of gastrointestinal tract | Two-hour urine creatinine clearance<br>Urine electrolytes<br>Serum level of nephrotoxic drugs |
| Heart | Under 50 years of age<br>No severe chest trauma<br>No intracardiac injections | 12-lead ECG<br>Chest x-ray film<br>Cardiology consult to evaluate cardiac condition<br>Arterial blood gases |
| Heart–lung | $PaO_2$ >400 torr on 100% $FiO_2$<br>Normal tidal volume<br>Approximate lung volume match by chest x-ray film<br>Normal chest x-ray film<br>No tracheostomy<br>Normal lung compliance | Same as heart donor<br>Sputum culture |
| Bone, skin, eye | Between the ages of 14 and 70<br>Time of death and recovery of tissue within 12 to 48 hours | |

[a]*Source:* Adapted from Murawski S. Making a miracle happen: organ donation and transplantation (self-instructional module). Baltimore: Maryland Institute of Emergency Medical Services Systems, 1988.

300 ml/hr to 1 liter/hr. Aqueous Pitressin is a short-acting ADH that can be titrated to decrease urine output. It is used in conjunction with fluid replacement to maintain a normal electrolyte balance. Frequent assessment of intake and output, vital signs, and serum electrolytes is recommended to facilitate trend analysis. Appropriate fluid and electrolyte management may necessitate replacement or removal of certain electrolytes such as potassium, sodium, and calcium as well as glucose. If hypotension occurs, the treatment of choice is replacement of fluids using colloids and crystalloids. If adequate intravascular volume is not successful in maintaining homeostasis, inotropic agents (such as dopamine and dobutamine) and/or vasopressors may be used at low doses not exceeding 20 μg/kg/minute. At higher doses these drugs, as well as other vasopressors such as epinephrine and isoproterenol (Isuprel), cause vasoconstriction, which reduces renal and hepatic perfusion, thereby causing organ ischemia. Fluid volume expansion often decreases serum Hct and Hgb levels. Infusion of PRBCs is needed to maintain adequate oxygenation of the vascularized organs and increase perfusion by replacing the lost blood volume. Arterial blood gases (ABGs) should be monitored and maintained within normal limits (9)

## B. Nursing Diagnosis

Impaired gas exchange related to pneumothorax, loss of respiratory mechanics (apnea), immobility, and neurogenic pulmonary edema

### Goal of Care

Maintain adequate gas exchange as evidenced by normal ABGs, normal breath sounds bilaterally, a normal chest x-ray film, and normal skin coloration.

### Nursing Interventions

- Maintain appropriate bedside emergency equipment (e.g., airway, Ambu bag).
- Monitor mechanical ventilation.
- Auscultate breath sounds every 1 to 2 hours.
- Maintain patent airway with tracheal suctioning every 2 hours as ordered.
- Observe sputum for amount, color, consistency, and odor; send cultures if ordered.
- Turn donor side to side every 2 hours.
- Monitor ABGs every 2 to 4 hours for effectiveness of ventilator changes.
- Obtain chest x-ray film as ordered.
- Use and increase PEEP as ordered.
- Increase $FiO_2$ as ordered.
- Administer furosemide (Lasix) if ordered.
- Maintain chest tube to 20 cm $H_2O$ suction as ordered.

### Rationale

The patient who has been declared brain dead does not have spontaneous respirations and requires mechanical ventilation. This may produce decreased alveolar ventilation, lung compliance, and oxygenation. Ventilation/perfusion mismatching and right-to-left shunting in the alveolar gas exchange decreases arterial oxygenation (9). Neurogenic pulmonary edema is caused by an increased ICP, which produces leakage of serous fluids from the pulmonary capillary beds into the interstitial tissue of the lungs. This edema may progress to a phenomenon similar to adult respiratory distress syndrome (ARDS). Increasing the $FiO_2$ and/or PEEP may be needed to improve alveolar gas exchange, thereby improving the $PaO_2$. Intravenous Lasix may be used to diurese excess fluid from the lungs (10).

## C. Nursing Diagnosis

Hypothermia related to CNS dysfunction

### Goal of Care

Maintain a normothermic state >97°F (36°C) rectally.

### Nursing Interventions

- Monitor rectal temperature every 2 to 4 hours.
- Place warming lights over donor as ordered.
- Apply warming blankets above and below the donor.
- Wrap head in blankets, if necessary.
- Increase temperature on the ventilator humidifier.
- Warm IV fluids and blood products.

### Rationale

The hypothalamus is nonfunctional when brain death occurs; therefore, internal body temperature regulation is not possible. Hypothermia may cause cardiac arrhythmias, including ventricular fibrillation and cardiac arrest. Hypothermia also produces vasoconstriction, which may decrease tissue and organ perfusion, resulting in ischemia (11). The head is wrapped because 80 to 85% of body heat can be lost through the scalp, particularly if the patient's head has been shaved for suturing head lacerations or craniotomy.

## ASSOCIATED NURSING DIAGNOSES

A. Potential for infection
B. Alteration in family process
C. Impaired tissue integrity

### REFERENCES

1. Goldsmith J, Montefusco CM. Nursing care of the potential organ donor. Crit Care Nurse 1986;6(6):24.
2. President's Commission for the Study of Ethical Problems in Medicine and Biomedical Behavior Research. Defining death: medical, legal, and ethical issues in the determination of death. Washington, DC: US Government Printing Office, 1981:61.
3. Dunham CM, Cowley RA. Shock trauma/critical care handbook. Rockville, MD: Aspen, 1986.
4. Polacek DJ, Grenvik A. Medical aspects of brain death. In: Shoemaker W, Ayres S, Grenvik A, et al, eds. Textbook of critical care. 2nd ed. Philadelphia: WB Saunders, 1989.
5. Nikas DI.. The neurologic system. In: Alspach JG, Williams SM, eds. Core curriculum for critical care nursing. 3rd ed. Philadelphia: WB Saunders, 1985:243.
6. Bartucci MR. Organ donation: a study of the donor family perspective. J Neurosci Nurs 1987;19(6):506.
7. Broznik B, Grenvik A. The logistics of organ transplantation. In: Shoemaker W, Ayres S, Grenvik A, et al, eds. Textbook of critical care. 2nd ed. Philadelphia: WB Saunders, 1989: 1353.
8. Gotch PM. The endocrine system. In: Alspach JG, Williams SM, eds. Core curriculum for critical care nursing. 3rd ed. Philadelphia: WB Saunders, 1985:468.
9. Gaul PP. The organ donor. In: Cardona VD, Hurn PD, Bastnagel-Mason PJB, et al, eds. Trauma nursing: from resuscitation through rehabilitation. Philadelphia: WB Saunders, 1988:790.
10. Baehrendtz S. Differential ventilation and selective positive end-expiratory pressure: effects on patients during anesthesia and intensive care. (Master's thesis.) Stockholm, 1983:3.
11. Boysen PG, Modell JH. Pulmonary edema. In: Shoemaker W, Ayres S, Grenvik A, et al, eds. Textbook of critical care. 2nd ed. Philadelphia: WB Saunders, 1989:516–518.

# CHAPTER 36

## Trauma and Pregnancy

Kathy A. Shane, RN, BSN, CCRN, CNRN

## Clinical Presentation

A 22-year-old pregnant woman, 24-weeks gestation, was a pedestrian struck by a motor vehicle traveling under 35 mph. She was transported by air to the regional trauma center where initial assessment of injuries revealed a stable pelvic fracture, blunt abdominal trauma, fractured right femur, and probable aspiration. Initial vital signs were pulse 110 beats/minute; blood pressure 98/60; labored, shallow respirations 32 breaths/minute; and fetal heart tones (FHTs) 160 beats/minute. The patient was intubated on admission and placed on $FiO_2$ of 0.50, tidal volume ($V_T$) 600, and synchronized intermittent mechanical ventilation (SMIV) 15. Open peritoneal lavage was carefully performed, and results were grossly positive. A Foley catheter was inserted with gross hematuric returns. Vital signs deteriorated rapidly, and the patient was fluid resuscitated with Ringer's lactate and Type O negative blood. FHT decreasd to 110 per continuous fetal monitoring for 2 minutes duration until return of adequate maternal blood pressure. The patient was taken to the operating room, where exploratory laparotomy revealed a ruptured spleen; a splenectomy was performed. FHTs remained 140 throughout the case. Initial arterial blood gases (ABGs) postintubation were 7.35, $PaO_2$ 110, $PaCO_2$ 32, $HCO_3$ 23, and $O_2$ saturation 97%. Her pelvic fracture was stable enough not to require treatment other than bed rest and logrolling. Surgical repair of her femur fracture was deferred, but was stabilized with 15 pounds of skeletal traction. Intravenous pyelogram (IVP) and cystogram were both negative for disruption of bladder integrity. Admission labs revealed the following: blood urea nitrogen (BUN) 9, creatinine 0.7, white blood cells (WBC) 17,000, prothrombin time (PT) 11.0/12.5, partial thromboplastin (PTT) 38, fibrinogen 450, platelets 250,000, hematocrit 28%, and hemoglobin 10.5. There was no sign of vaginal bleeding, and vaginal pH was 4.5.

Once stabilized, she was logrolled slightly to the left side and transferred to the intensive care unit (ICU) with continuous fetal monitoring for 24 hours. A pulmonary artery catheter was inserted for improved hemodynamic monitoring; initial readings were central venous pressure (CVP) 8, pulmonary artery pressure (PAP) 32/12 with mean of 22, pulmonary capillary wedge pressure (PCWP) 11. Chest x-ray 12 hours postinjury showed a patchy infiltrate in the right upper and middle lobes; ABGs at this time were 7.48, $PaO_2$ was 108, $PaCO_2$ was 28. A bronchoscopy on 100% oxygen was performed and was productive for large amounts of thick tan sputum. ABGs 3 hours postprocedure were improved at 7.47; $PaO_2$ was 150, $PaCO_2$ was 28; and the $FiO_2$ was decreased to 0.40. Chest physiotherapy treatments were initiated and performed every 4 hours.

The mother and fetus remained stable over the next 24 hours, and FHTs were changed to every hour by Doppler. Pneumatic compression devices were placed on the patient's legs for deep vein thrombosis prevention.

On day 3, maternal oxygenation deteriorated to 7.34; $PaO_2$ was 88; $PaCO_2$ was 36; and $O_2$ saturation was 96%. The chest x-ray was clear, and there were minimal endotracheal secretions. $FiO_2$ was increased from 0.40 to 0.50 with no improvement in oxygenation. A ventilation-perfusion (VQ) scan showed a moderate-to-high probability for pulmonary embolism. She was placed on a heparin drip at 900 units/hour.

On day 5, the patient spiked a temperature to 38.8°C (102.4°F), and ampicillin 500 mg,

IV every 6 hours was begun. On day 6, her temperature was 38.3°C (101°F), and FHTs remained stable.

The patient recovered from complications, and open reduction and internal fixation of her femur fracture was performed on day 11. The patient remained in the hospital 4 more weeks and was discharged home. She delivered a healthy 7-lb baby boy at 38 weeks gestation by cesarean (C-section).

## 1. What is the pathophysiological basis for this patient's problem?

Persons attending a pregnant trauma victim must remember that they are taking care of two patients; however, treatment priorities remain the same (1, 2). Fear of medicolegal issues should not result in diagnostic and therapeutic paralysis (2, 3).

Pregnancy causes major physiological changes and altered anatomical relationships that involve nearly every organ system. These changes may influence evaluation of the patient by altering signs and symptoms of injury, and may influence results of diagnostic or laboratory tests (2). Pregnancy may also affect the patterns and/or severity of injury (Tables 36.1 and 36.2) (2, 4).

Hemodynamic changes are the most numerous, and patient positioning has great impact on them. The supine position may result in profound hypotension, "supine hypotensive syndrome of pregnancy," or vena caval syndrome. The patient should be turned to the left side as soon as possible to prevent compression of the inferior vena cava. If diagnostic or treatment variables hinder this, the patient's uterus may be manually pushed to the left, or the backboard or table on which the patient is lying may be tipped to the left (5). All of the hemodynamic changes tend to make it difficult to assess blood loss and the diagnosis of shock (see Tables 36.1 and 36.2) (6). Increased pulse and decreased blood pressure, cardinal signs of shock, may be normal pregnant deviations. Hematocrit <30%, systolic blood pressure ≤80, and systemic vasoconstriction may each produce fetal hypoxia; therefore, the treatment of shock must be initiated immediately (7). Ringer's lactate and type-specific blood are preferred replacement solutions because they provide needed electrolytes and prevent sensitization of the mother. Type, cross-match, and direct Coombs' should be determined immediately to prevent Rh sensitization (2). Vasopressors should be avoided if at all possible because they may cause decreased uterine perfusion with resultant fetal hypoxia (8). However, if adequate volume replacement is not effective and a vasopressor is required, ephedrine is the drug of choice. It has many of the alpha and beta effects of epinephrine but with a duration of action 10 times as long. Ephedrine affects smooth muscle in the same manner as epinephrine, with the exception of the uterus, where activity is reduced (Table 36.3) (8, 9).

Alterations in blood cell composition occur as pregnancy advances. There is a greater tendency for coagulation during pregnancy because of increased clotting factors. The normal increase in clotting is a protective mechanism against blood loss during delivery, but it places the gravid individual at greater risk for developing thromboembolism from traumatic injuries, such as fractures, ecchymosis, and vascular damage. Disseminated intravascular coagulation (DIC) is associated with critical obstetric problems such as abruptio placenta, fetal demise, amniotic fluid embolism, shock, and ruptured uterus. Clotting factors are rapidly depleted in the body's attempt for hemostasis with resultant abnormal bleeding. Abruptio is frequently accompanied by decreased fibrinogen. It must be remembered that normal nonpregnant fibrinogen levels of 250 to 400 are abnormal in pregnant individuals (10).

Respiratory changes increase as pregnancy progresses because of the enlarging uterus. Maternal hypoxia ≤60 torr can produce fetal hypoxia. Fortunately the fetus is more resistant to an acute asphyxial event than is the mother. This is probably due to the

**Table 36.1.** Physiological changes in pregnancy[a]

| Changes | Implication |
|---|---|
| *Neurological* | |
| Increased risk of fainting | More susceptible to falls and injury |
| Increased fatigue | |
| *Cardiovascular* | |
| Vena caval syndrome; Hypotension and diminished right ventricular return that results from gravid uterus compressing the vena cava when the patient is supine; can decrease the cardiac output by 30 to 40% | Affects perfusion during evaluation; keep patient on left side. If not possible to keep patient on left side, manually displace uterus to the left and recheck blood pressure |
| Increased pulse by 15 to 20 beats/minute | Presents difficulty in assessing blood loss and treatment of shock; may be normal deviation of pregnancy, particularly if patient is supine |
| Decreased central venous pressure | |
| Cardiac output increased to 6 to 7 liters/minute by term; after 10 weeks gestation, increases by 1 to 1.5 liters/minute | Not to be confused with hyperdynamic state. Supine position will decrease |
| By 34 weeks gestation, circulating blood volume has increased by 50% | |
| 5 to 15 mm Hg decrease in blood pressure during second trimester, returns to normal by term. During periods of stress, the mother will maintain vital signs at the expense of the fetus. The mother can maintain stable vital signs and adequate perfusion with a 30 to 35% (1500 ml) gradual blood loss and a 10 and 20% acute blood loss | Fetus may be in distress even when the mother is not. Hypovolemia decreases uterine blood flow. The uterus is normally a nonvital organ, prone to orthostatic changes. Sustained hypertension during pregnancy is never normal but is associated with toxemia |
| Increased venous pressure in lower extremities secondary to pressure on inferior vena cava by the uterus | Increased bleeding in leg injuries |
| Increased pelvic vascularity | Increased risk of maternal hemorrhage, hematoma formation, and formation of deep vein thrombi |
| Increased uterine size leads to shift in left electrical axis of the heart by 15° | T-wave flattening or inversion in leads III, and Q waves in lead AVF not indicative of ischemia |
| *Hematological* | |
| Physiological hypervolemia of approximately 50% by 34 weeks gestation. | Improves maternal tolerance to hemorrhage |
| Physiological anemia of pregnancy is a result of expansion of plasma, up to 45% by term, rather than red cell volume in which there is only slight increase | Confuses interpretation of lab studies, particularly those evaluating blood volume. Decreases colloid oncotic pressure |
| Physiological leukocytosis of pregnancy | Confuses picture of infection |
| Physiological increase in fibrinogen and Factors VII, VIII, and IX, and increase in plasminogen activator | Potential maternal benefit if hemorrhage occurs, but increased risk of thromboembolic disease associated with pelvic or extremity fracture or immobilization |
| Uterine and placental injury can result in hematoma and amniotic fluid embolism. The placenta contains large amounts of thromboplastin, and the uterus is a major source of plasminogen activator | May produce consumptive coagulopathy |

**Table 36.1.** Physiological changes in pregnancy[a] (continued)

| Changes | Implication |
|---|---|
| *Hematological (continued)* | |
| Increased sedimentation rate due to increased fibrinogen | Can confuse diagnosis of true infectious process |
| *Respiratory* | |
| Decreased functional residual capacity by 20% at term | Decreased oxygen reserve, predisposes to hypoxia |
| Increased respiratory rate (by 15%) plus increased tidal volume (by 40%) results in an increased minute ventilation by 50%, "hyperventilation of pregnancy" | Consider when interpreting diagnostic and lab studies. Chronic compensated respiratory alkalosis and decreased buffering ability. Altered response to inhalation anesthetics, more rapid induction, and decreased tolerance |
| Increased oxygen consumption, but measured $PaO_2$ not affected unless patient is supine, then it is decreased | Hypoxemia leads to decreased uterine blood flow |
| Engorgement of upper airways | Increased risk for nosebleeds and obstruction |
| *Gastrointestinal* | |
| Distension of abdominal wall by enlarging uterus results in decreased guarding and rebound tenderness | Diagnosis of abdominal injuries and intraperitoneal bleeding more difficult |
| Relative physiological ileus and decreased emptying of stomach and bowel | May mimic silent abdomen. Increased risk of aspiration. Decreased tolerance of enteral feedings |
| Lateral and upward displacement of small bowel by enlarging uterus | Varies anatomical location, which alters pattern of injury. Enlarged uterus makes palpation of viscera or masses more difficult but also may shield them from injury |
| The spleen is displaced downward from its natural position behind the ribs, and it is more engorged | More prone to rupture and hemorrhage |
| *Genitourinary* | |
| Bladder is usually full because of decreased capacity from enlarging uterus; is elevated out of the pelvis, becoming an "abdominal" organ | More prone to rupture or injury |
| Relative hydroureter and hydronephrosis | Not to be confused with urinary obstruction. More prone to urinary tract infection |
| Relative bladder atony leads to incomplete bladder emptying | More prone to urinary tract infections |
| Bladder more hyperemic, as is the uterus | Increased blood loss if injured |
| Increased glomerular filtration rate | Decreased creatinine and BUN results |
| *Musculoskeletal* | |
| Laxity of pelvic ligaments; wide gait and decreased balance | More prone to falls |
| Vessels of retroperitoneum dilated | Increased retroperitoneal hemorrhage if injured |

[a]*Sources:*

Smith LG. The pregnant trauma patient. In: Cardona VD, Hurn PD, Bastnagel-Mason PJ, et al, eds. Trauma nursing: from resuscitation through rehabilitation. Philadelphia: WB Saunders, 1988:643–663.

Haycock C. Emergency care of the pregnant traumatized patient. Emerg Med Clin North Am 1984;4:843–851.

Crosby W. Traumatic injuries during pregnancy. Obstet Gynecol 1983;4:902–912.

Patterson R. Trauma in pregnancy. Clin Obset Gynecol 1984;1:32–38.

Crosby W. Trauma in the pregnant patient. Community Med 1986;4:251–258.

Stuart G, Harding P, Davies E. Blunt abdominal trauma in pregnancy. J Canad Med Assoc 1980;8:901–905.

Straffor P. Protection of the pregnant woman in the emergency department. J Emerg Nurs 1981;7:97–102.

**Table 36.2.** Laboratory values in pregnancy[a]

| Test | Normal Value | Value during Pregnancy |
|---|---|---|
| *Hematology* | | |
| White blood count | 4500–10,000/mm$^3$ | 18,000–25,000/mm$^3$ by third trimester, no change in differential |
| Hemoglobin | 12–14 gm/dl | Decreased due to hemodilution |
| Sedimentation rate | 0–20 mm/hr | 30–90 mm/hr |
| *Coagulation* | | |
| Fibrinogen | 250–400 mg/dl | >400–600 mg/dl |
| Platelet count | 150,000–300,000/mm$^3$ | Same or slightly decreased |
| Factors VII, VIII, and IX | | Increased |
| *Chemistry* | | |
| Sodium | 135–145 mEq/liter | Slight dilutional hyponatremia |
| Potassium | 3.5–5.0 mEq/liter | Within normal limits |
| Chloride | 100–105 mEq/liter | Within normal limits |
| Blood urea nitrogen | 10–20 mg/dl | 4–10 mg/dl |
| Albumin | 3.5–5.0 gm/dl | 2.0–4.5 gm/dl |
| Lipids | 450–900 mg/dl | >900 mg/dl |
| Total cholesterol | 110–200 mg/dl | 220–250 mg/dl |
| *Urine* | | |
| Specific gravity | 1.010–1.030 | Below normal |
| Glucose | Negative | Occasionally spills |
| Creatinine clearance | 3.5–5.0 ml/minute | 2.0–3.5 ml/minute |
| *Arterial Blood Gases* | | |
| pH | 7.35–7.45 | 7.40–7.48 |
| PaCO$_2$ | 35–45 mm HG | 25–30 mm Hg |
| PaO$_2$ | 95–100 mm Hg | 100–110 mm Hg |
| Bicarbonate | 24–30 mEq/liter | 17–22 mEq/liter |

[a]*Sources:*
Smith LG. The pregnant trauma patient. In Cardona VD, Hurn PD, Bastnagel-Mason PJ, et al, eds. Trauma nursing: from resuscitation through rehabilitation. Philadelphia: WB Saunders, 1988:643–663.
Haycock C. Emergency care of the pregnant traumatized patient. Emerg Med Clin North Am 1984;4:843–851.
Strange J. Shock trauma care plans. Springhouse, PA: Springhouse, 1987:99–106.

redistribution of blood to fetal vital organs and decreased fetal oxygen consumption. The fetus seems to be able to tolerate maternal asphyxia more readily than maternal hypovolemia (4). In the case of maternal hypovolemia, the fetus may be in serious jeopardy, whereas the mother appears to be in no acute distress.

When abdominal trauma is suspected, open peritoneal lavage should be performed as with nonpregnant patients (2, 4, 11, 12). The following values are indicative of a positive minilap necessitating surgical intervention: red blood cells >100,000/mm$^3$; white blood cells >500/mm$^3$; presence of gastrointestinal contents; and elevated amylase supporting presence of small-bowel injury (12).

Pelvic trauma is also a frequent complication of blunt trauma in motor vehicle accidents (13). The dilated vessels of the retroperitoneum are frequently injured, and 10 to 15% of pelvic fractures are complicated by injury to the lower urinary tract. Venous thrombosis associated with pelvic fractures is further exacerbated by the normal hypercoagulation of pregnancy.

**Table 36.3.** Effects of vasopressors in pregnancy[a]

| Vasopressor | Effect on Mean Arterial Pressure | Effect on Uterine Blood Flow |
|---|---|---|
| Dopamine | | |
| ≤5 µg/kg/minute | Increases | Neglible effect |
| >10 µg/kg/minute | Increases | Decreases |
| Ephedrine | Increases | Increases |
| Epinephrine | Increases | Decreases |
| Mephentermine | Increases | Increases |
| Levophed | Increases | Decreases |

[a]*Sources:*
Patterson R. Trauma in pregnancy. Clin Obstet Gynecol 1984;1:32–38.
Barnhart E, et al. Physicians desk reference. 43rd ed. Oradell, NJ: Medical Economics Books, 1989.

## 2. What are the nursing diagnoses of highest priority?

A. Potential for altered tissue perfusion, maternal
B. Potential for altered tissue perfusion, fetal
C. Potential for injury, fetal
D. Potential for injury, maternal
E. Fear, anxiety, and anticipatory grief

### A. Nursing Diagnosis

Potential for altered tissue perfusion related to maternal cardiovascular instability, emboli formation, and abnormal clotting secondary to normal physiological changes of pregnancy

### Goal of Care

Maternal vital signs will remain within normal limits, and patient will experience no abnormal clotting phenomenon.

### Nursing Interventions

- Position patient in left lateral decubitus position as much as possible.
- Follow vital signs, hematocrit, and hemoglobin closely.
- Follow maternal coagulation profile.
- Observe for signs and symptoms of microemboli formation: Check calf tenderness every shift; observe for signs and symptoms of pulmonary embolus, such as blood in sputum, sudden onset of respiratory distress, tachycardia, anxiety, and cyanosis.
- Maintain thromboembolic stockings and pneumatic compression devices as ordered.

### Rationale

Positioning the patient in left lateral decubitus position decreases inferior vena caval pressure by the enlarging uterus, which can decrease venous return and lead to profound hypotension. If the patient cannot be placed on her left side, her left hip should be elevated with a pillow and the uterus manually displaced to the left. If injuries do not preclude its use, a low-airloss bed may enable prolonged positioning on the left, decreasing the risk of skin breakdown. The patient should still be turned to the right side every 2 to 3 hours for 30 to 60 minutes, minimizing the supine position as much as possible.

If anticoagulant therapy is necessary, heparin intravenously is the drug of choice, as it does not cross the placental barrier (14). Abdominal subcutaneous injections of heparin may not be feasible because of a taut abdominal wall from an enlarged uterus (14).

## B. Nursing Diagnosis

Potential for altered tissue perfusion of fetus related to alterations in maternal oxygenation or perfusion

### Goals of Care

- FHTs will remain within normal limits, 130 to 150.
- Maternal $PaO_2$ will remain $\geq 80$.

### Nursing Interventions

- Monitor FHTs with maternal vital signs.
- Monitor fundal heights every shift.
- Monitor fetal activity every 4 hours.

### Rationale

Assessment of fetal well-being can be achieved by monitoring FHTs. During periods of maternal or fetal instability, more frequent determinations of FHTs are warranted, and continuous fetal monitoring is advisable. Changes in FHTs will often be the first indicator of a decrease in maternal blood volume (4).

Fundal height is a determinant of fetal growth; however, a sonogram is a more accurate predictor of fetal development and may be periodically used, particularly with prolonged maternal hospitalization (Fig. 36.1).

## C. Nursing Diagnosis

Potential for injury of fetus related to maternal exposure to x-ray procedures and/or drugs

### Goal of Care

Fetus will be protected from unnecessary exposure to x-rays and toxic drugs.

### Nursing Interventions

- Only necessary x-rays should be taken after initial evaluation.
- Shield the mother's abdomen when all but abdominal films are taken and when x-rays are taken in adjacent nonshielded rooms.
- Inform all nursing and x-ray staff that there is a pregnant patient in the unit so that she is protected from procedures.
- Check all maternal drugs ordered for their use during pregnancy.
- Monitor maternal drug levels routinely and keep at lowest therapeutic level possible.

### Rationale

If maternal condition is stable, routine daily chest x-rays may be re-evaluatd and other means of assessing respiratory status emphasized. The nurse must be cognizant of the effects of drugs on fetal development and status. Few drugs have been established as safe for use during pregnancy; some have known deleterious effects to the fetus (Table 31.4). Drugs with a high molecular weight, such as heparin, do not cross the placental barrier. A general rule for antibiotic use during pregnancy is that penicillins, cephalosporins, and aminoglycosides are generally safe, whereas sulfonamides, chloramphenicol, and tetracycline should be avoided (Tables 36.4 and 36.5) (15–17 [pp. 77–101]).

The teratogenic effect, or the potential to produce anomalies, of any agent is dependent on:

- *The agent itself.* Some cause abnormal development in all cases, others less consistently, some not at all.

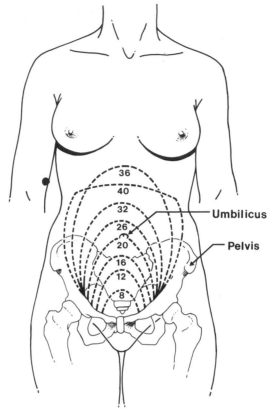

**Figure 36.1.** Uterine size and location showing gestational age. (From Cardona VD, Hurn PD, Bast-nagel-Mason PJ, Scanlon-Schilpp Am, Veise-Berry SW, eds. Trauma nursing: from resuscitation through rehabilitation. Philadelphia: WB Saunders, 1988.)

- *Pharmacogenetics of mother and fetus.* Not all embryos will be affected. This is influenced by rate of absorption, maternal metabolism, placental transfer, and fetal metabolism.
- *Exposure during particular time in gestation.* The time during embryogenesis when cells of a given organ system divide most rapidly is the period of greatest teratogenic susceptibility. Once developed, an organ system is relatively resistant to teratogenic effects. Usually by 14 weeks gestation, organ systems have been formed.
- *Dose.* Low doses may have no effect, intermediate doses may cause a specific malformation pattern, and high doses may lead to death of embryo (17 [pp. 77–101]).

Because drugs have the most deleterious effects early in pregnancy, all women of childbearing age who have sustained trauma should be considered pregnant until pregnancy is ruled out (1). The patient herself may not be aware that she is pregnant or may not be able to communicate this information at the time of initial assessment.

**Table 36.4.** Effects of drugs on fetus and neonate[a]

*Documented Relative Safety in Pregnancy[b]*

| | |
|---|---|
| Aldactone | Lasix |
| Aldomet | PAS |
| Apresoline | Penicillins |
| Benedictin | Phenobarbital |
| Caffeine | Procholorperazine |
| Cephalosporins | Reserpine |
| Dextromorphan | Rifampin |
| Digoxin | Steroids |
| Ethambutol | Theophyllin |
| Erythromycin | Thyroid hormone |
| Flagyl | Tobramycin |
| Heparin | Tricyclic antidepressants |
| Isoniazid | |

*Suspected Teratogenic Effects*

| | |
|---|---|
| Amphetamines | LSD |
| Bactrim | Phenothiazides |
| Haldol | Propanalol |
| Insulin | Pyrimethamine |
| Lithium | |

*Known Teratogenic Effects*

| | |
|---|---|
| Antineoplastic agents | Narcotic addiction |
| Diethystilbestrol | Smoking |
| Dilantin | Streptomycin |
| ETOH | Tetracycline |
| Environmental toxins | Thiourea agents |
| Biphenyls, magnesium naphthalene (moth balls) | Valium |
| Kanamycin | Vitamins A and D in excess |
| Lead | Warfarin |
| Associated with low birth weight | |

*Documented Neonatal Hazardous Effects*

| | |
|---|---|
| Compazine | Steroids |
| Chlorampohenicol | Sulfonamides |
| Magnesium sulfate | Thiazides |
| Oxytocin | Warfarin |
| Propanalol | |

[a]*Sources:* Adapted from
Barnhart E, et al. Physicians desk reference. 43rd ed. Oradell, NJ: Medical Economics Books, 1989.
Wise R. Antibiotics. Br Med J 1987;294:42–46.
Ellis J, Beckmann C. A clinical manual of obstetrics. Norwalk, CT: Appleton-Century-Crofts, 1983:77–101.
Kremkau F. Biological effects and possible hazards. Clin Obstet Gynecol 1983:395–405.
[b]Avoid use 48 to 72 hours prior to delivery if possible; may have deleterious effect on neonate.

## D. Nursing Diagnosis

Potential for injury to mother related to complications of pregnancy such as toxemia, abruptio placenta, premature rupture of membranes, and premature labor.

## Goal of Care

Mother will be monitored closely for possible complications of pregnancy.

## Nursing Interventions

- Observe for signs of toxemia of pregnancy: hypertension; nondependent edema of face and upper extremities; proteinuria (check urine every shift); cerebral or

**Table 36.5.** Common infectious conditions in pregnancy and recommended treatment[a]

| Condition | First Choice | Second Choice |
|---|---|---|
| Bacteruria or cystitis | Broad-spectrum penicillin, ampicillin, or cephalin P.O. | Nitrofurantoin |
| Acute pyelonephritis | Broad-spectrum drug such as cefuroxine, ampicillin | Gentamicin |
| Pharyngitis | Procaine penicillin I.M. | Erythromycin |
| Aspiration pneumonia | Ampicillin, penicillin | Erythromycin |
| Endocarditis prophylaxis | Amoxacillin P.O. | Erythromycin |
| Endocarditis treatment | Gentamicin, penicillin | Vancomycin |
| Chlamydia | Erythromycin | |
| Abdominal operation prophylaxis | Cefazolin | Gentamicin |
| Tuberculosis | Rifampin, isoniazid, ethambutal | Gentamicin |
| Undiagnosed sepsis[b] | Gentamicin, penicillin, possibility Flagyl | Broad-spectrum cephalosporin— Cefuroxime or Ceftazidime |

[a]*Sources:*
Physicians desk reference. 43rd ed. Oradell, NJ: Medical Economics Books, 1989.
Wise R. Antibiotics. Br Med J 1987;294:42–46.
Ellis J, Beckmann C. A clinical manual of obstetrics. Norwalk, CT: Appleton-Century-Crofts, 1983.
[b]Treat before causative organism is identified.

visual disturbances, such as headache, decreased level of consciousness, blurred vision, scotoma, and seizures (late).

- Observe for signs of placental abruption: vaginal bleeding, uterine tenderness, rapid increase in fundal height, fetal distress, uterine rigidity, maternal shock, constant low back pain, generalized abdominal tenderness, consumptive coagulopathy (late hallmark).
- Observe for sign of premature rupture of membranes or premature labor: rhythmic uterine contractions, sudden gush of vaginal fluid with a pH between 7 and 7.5, positive fern test of vaginal fluid, slight vaginal bleeding (show), increased agitation in unconscious patient.

### Rationale

Preeclampsia occurs almost exclusively in primigravida patients, particularly those younger than 20 or older than 35. It is occasionally seen in multiparous patients with underlying renal and/or vascular disorders. Diagnosis is based on a classic triad of symptoms: hypertension, proteinuria, and edema after the 20th week of gestation. Eclampsia is characterized by grand mal seizures, one third of which occur antepartum, one third during labor and delivery, and the other third up to 18 hours postpartum.

Abruptio placenta normally occurs in 1 to 2% of all pregnancies, with a previous history of abruption in 10% of cases. There is, however, an increased risk associated with blunt abdominal trauma. It is the most common cause of fetal death following motor vehicle accidents (20). In 20% of abruptios, vaginal bleeding is not present (17). A placental separation of ≥50% greatly endangers fetal viability and greatly increases the risk of consumptive coagulopathy in the mother (17, 20 [pp. 575–589]). Treatment is emergency C-section.

Premature rupture of membranes (PROM) is a common obstetric complication occurring in 3 to 14% of pregnancies, but incidence also increases when associated with maternal injury (19 [pp. 557–567]). The goal of treatment is to prevent neonatal and maternal infection while maximizing fetal survival. Minimum viable gestational age in high-risk neonatal centers today is 26 to 28 weeks. Before 36 weeks gestation, labor usually begins within 24 hours of PROM in 35 to 50% of patients (17 [pp. 557–567]). The latent period between PROM and delivery can be prolonged; the decision to do so is based on fetal gestational age and maternal risk. The greatest hazard to the fetus before 33 weeks gestation is prematurity; after 33 weeks, the risk of infection is more significant (18).

The fern test for determining the presence of amniotic fluid is performed by allowing suspect vaginal fluid to dry on a slide and examining the fluid under a microscope. Crystallization in a fern-like pattern is a positive test, due to the high NaCl and protein concentrations found in amniotic fluid (17).

An obstetrical consultation is advised for the treatment of the above complications of pregnancy, as this content is beyond the scope of this text.

### E. Nursing Diagnosis

Fear, anxiety, and anticipatory grief of family and patient related to potential or actual loss of fetus secondary to fetal trauma, hypoxia, or maternal complications

### Goal of Care

Patient and family will display effective coping.

### Nursing Interventions

- Allow family to express feelings.
- Allow family members and patient to listen to FHTs and feel fetal movements.
- If live baby is born prematurely, have the nurse caring for the baby visit and give update, take pictures of the infant, contact the LaLeche League if mother planned to breastfeed.
- If baby is stillborn, offer family and patient the opportunity to view and hold the infant if desired; provide information about local support groups.

### Rationale

Remember that the family is concerned for two individuals. If the pregnancy was unplanned or even unwanted, feelings of guilt or grief may be heightened.

The LaLeche League is a support group in most areas that can assist mothers with problems related to breastfeeding. Milk flow in a nonnursing mother can be maintained by use of a breast pump every 2 to 4 hours. Breast engorgement postdelivery is a source of patient discomfort and a potential source of infection. Ice packs can be helpful, as well as frequent manual expressions of milk.

In conclusion, women today are enjoying more active lifestyles, participating in work and recreational activities frequently up until the time of delivery. Such increased mobility, however, increases the risk of injury. Early in pregnancy, when the mother is more prone to fainting and fatigue, she is more at risk from falls. Minor blunt trauma involving the pregnant abdomen frequently occurs as a result of falls, but is rarely associated with serious morbidity for mother or fetus. As pregnancy progresses, the wide gait, relaxed pelvic ligaments, and diminished balance due to the gravid uterus further increase the risk of falls (1, 9, 13, 15).

No one knows the exact incidence of trauma in pregnancy. Various reports show a rate of 0.4 to 6% of deliveries sustained a trauma during pregnancy requiring hospitalization (11, 17). Auto collisions, gunshot wounds, stab wounds, and physical assault accounted for nearly all of these. Maternal trauma is the leading cause of nonobstetric maternal death (3, 14). Head injury is the leading causative factor in these cases; however, intra-abdominal injury is nearly as frequent (3). Maternal

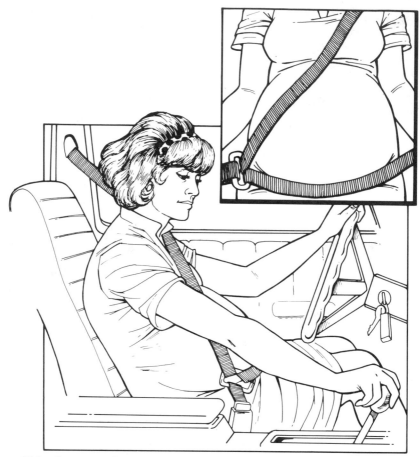

**Figure 36.2.** Proper use of a seat belt during pregnancy. (From Cardona VD, Hurn PD, Bastnagel-Mason PJ, Scanlon-Schipp AM, Veise-Berry SW, eds. Trauma nursing: from resuscitation through rehabilitation. Philadelphia: WB Saunders, 1988.)

death is the leading cause of fetal death, followed by abruptio placenta. Direct injury to the fetus as a result of blunt trauma is uncommon because of the shock-absorbing effects of amniotic fluid. A wide variety of fetal injuries have been reported, however: Intracranial injuries predominate, followed by fetal extremity fractures (7). There have been reported cases of maintaining a maternal vegetative state for up to 14 weeks and successfully delivering a normal, healthy baby at 34 weeks gestation (19). These cases may present some ethical concerns to some practitioners.

The increased size of the gravid uterus predisposes this organ to a higher injury rate. Immediately on impact, intrauterine pressure may increase to values 10 times those found in labor. This probably accounts for uterine rupture, the treatment for which is hysterectomy. This can have serious implications for the patient who wishes to have more children. Such is also the case for the patient who required C-section delivery because of maternal injury or complications.

As is the case for most vehicular trauma, the use of safety restraints greatly reduces the severity of injury in most circumstances. They must, however, be worn properly (Fig. 36.2). The use of a lap belt without a shoulder belt is inadequate protection (1, 20–22).

## ASSOCIATED NURSING DIAGNOSES

A. Ineffective airway clearance
B. Alteration in comfort
C. Impaired physical mobility
D. Alteration in nutrition
E. Altered patterns of urinary elimination
F. Altered bowel elimination

### REFERENCES

1. Smith LG. The pregnant trauma patient. In Cardona VD, Hurn PD, Bastnagel-Mason PJ, et al, eds. Trauma nursing: from resuscitation through rehabilitation. Philadelphia: WB Saunders, 1988:643–663.
2. Haycock C. Emergency care of the pregnant traumatized patient. Emerg Med Clin North Am 1984;4:843–851.
3. Baker D. Trauma in the pregnant patient. Surg Clin North Am 1982;2:275–289.
4. Crosby W. Traumatic injuries during pregnancy. Obstet Gynecol 1983;4:902–912.
5. Newkirk E, Fry M. Trauma during pregnancy: nursing assessment in the emergency department. Focus Crit Care 1985;6:30–39.
6. Bremer C, Cassata L. Trauma in pregnancy. Nurs Clin North Am 1986;4:705–716.
7. Foster C. The pregnant trauma patient. Nursing 84 1984;11:58–63.
8. Patterson R. Trauma in pregnancy. Clin Obstet Gynecol 1984;1:32–38.
9. Physicians desk reference. 43rd ed. Oradell, NJ: Medical Economics Books, 1989.
10. Crosby W. Trauma in the pregnant patient. Community Med 1986;4:251–258.
11. Stuart G, Harding P, Davies E. Blunt abdominal trauma in pregnancy. J Canad Med Assoc 1980;8:901–905.
12. Dunham CM, Cowley RA. Shock trauma/critical care handbook. Rockville, MD: Aspen, 1986:299–312.
13. Lavin J Jr, Polsky S. Abdominal trauma during pregnancy. Clin Perinatol 1983;10:423–438.
14. Wagner M, et al. Drugs. Nursing 82 books. Springhouse, PA: Springhouse, 1982:15.
15. Wise R. Antibiotics. Br Med J 1987;294:42–46.
16. Eisenberg M, Furukawa C, Ray C. Manual of antimicrobial therapy and infectious diseases. Philadelphia: WB Saunders, 1980:239.
17. Ellis J, Beckmann C. A clinical manual of obstetrics. Norwalk, CT: Appleton-Century-Crofts, 1983.
18. Kremkau F. Biological effects and possible hazards. Clin Obstet Gynecol 1983:395–405.
19. Hill L, Parker P, O'Neill B. Case report: Management of maternal vegetative state during pregnancy. Mayo Clin Proc 1985;60:469–472.
20. Strange J. Shock trauma car plans. Springhouse, PA: Springhouse, 1987:99–106.
21. Attico N, Smith R III, Fitzpatrick M, Keneally M. Automobile safety restraints for pregnant women and children. J Reprod Med 1986;3:187–192.
22. Fakhoury G, Gibson J. Seat belt hazards in pregnancy. Br J Obstet Gynaecol 1986;4:395–396.
23. Golan A, Sandback O, Teare A. Trauma in late pregnancy: A report of 15 cases. South African J Med 1980;5:161–165.

# CHAPTER 37

## The Trauma Patient with Acquired Immunodeficiency Syndrome

Nancy J. Hoyt, MA, CIC
Christy L. Crowther, RN, MS, ANP-C, CCRN

## Clinical Presentation

A 31-year-old man was admitted to the hospital following a motor vehicle accident. On admission, he was combative, spontaneously opening his eyes, and moving all extremities. He had bruising over the frontal area of his head and several lacerations on his chin and face, including a 2-cm laceration over the bridge of his nose. He also had a 5-cm open fracture of his right mandible and a 6-cm intra-oral laceration.

Admission vital signs were blood pressure 100/70; pulse 98; respirations 24; and temperature 37°C (98.6°F). Facial x-rays demonstrated multiple facial fractures; a computerized tomography (CT) scan of his head showed a fracture of the anterior and posterior walls of the frontal sinus and left frontal lobe contusions. The rest of his physical examination was benign. Past medical history was significant for a seizure disorder, which he had had since childhood.

He was taken to the operating room, where a tracheostomy was performed, an intracranial pressure (ICP) bolt was placed, and his facial fractures were repaired with intramandibular fixation (IMF) and arch bars.

During his first 7 days of hospitalization, his behavior was noted to be severely agitated. He had several episodes of fever ranging from 39° to 40°C. Multiple fever workups were done, which included chest x-ray, blood, urine, and sputum cultures, and complete blood counts with differential. No clear source for the fevers could be identified; therefore, they were attributed to his closed head injury and inflammatory processes related to his underlying injuries.

His neurological status gradually improved. On the eighth day of admission, he was noted to have significant facial swelling and some erythema over the right side of his face. The following week he developed elevated liver function enzymes associated with complaints of right upper quadrant and epigastric pain; however, no etiology was found. During the third week, it was noted that his intra-oral laceration was not healing. Near the beginning of the fourth week, his mandibular implanted hardware was found to be exposed, and he returned to surgery for cleaning of his oral cavity and adjustment of his IMF.

He was discharged from the hospital to a rehabilitation facility after 34 days; he returned 4 days later for surgery to repair his nonhealing mandibular fracture, an orocutaneous fistula, and an infected right lower canine tooth. At that time, he revealed that he had tested positive for human immunodeficiency virus (HIV) antibody 6 months prior to his accident. Two months after discharge, he returned to the hospital, was admitted for sudden onset of swelling and tenderness over his right zygoma, and was taken to surgery where he underwent removal of infected facial hardware.

### 1. What is the pathophysiological basis for this patient's problem?

Acquired immunodeficiency syndrome (AIDS) is the most severe manifestation resulting from infection with a retrovirus known as human immunodeficiency virus (HIV). Retroviruses are those viruses that, during the first stage of replication, transcribe the genetic

**Table 37.1.** Progression sequence in HIV infection manifestation

1. Infection with the human immunodeficiency virus (HIV)
2. HIV-antibody response: Period from the time of infection to the production of detectable antibodies, usually within 3 months of infection, with range from 6 weeks to 6 months.
3. Induction phase: Period from the time of HIV antibody positivity to the presentation of clinical signs and symptoms of disease, ranging from 6 weeks to 7 years.
4. Acquired immunodeficiency syndrome (AIDS)
5. Death

information from ribonucleic acid (RNA) to deoxyribonucleic acid (DNA). This transcription is a reversed process of replication, which normally proceeds from DNA to RNA, and it is facilitated by the enzyme reverse transcriptase (1, 2).

Attachment of the HIV to the host cell requires the presence of a surface receptor. In humans, a protein surface marker, the CD4 antigen complex, found on helper T-lymphocytes and other cells, is thought to be such a receptor (3, 4). After attachment, the virus enters, or infects, the host cell by a mechanism that is not completely understood (4) and begins replication mediated by the reverse transcriptase. Once a cell becomes infected, it can fuse with healthy cells bearing the CD4 antigen complex and bind to them. The result is a cluster of nonfunctional joined cells known as synctia; the nonfunctional syncytium then eventually dies (3). As helper T-4 lymphocytes die, there is a resultant decline in the host's immune response, which allows opportunistic and other pathogens to invade the host.

The spectrum of HIV infection ranges from asymptomatic HIV antibody seropositivity to the final stages of immunodeficiency known as AIDS. The progression sequence is shown in Table 37.1.

At this time it is not known if all persons who are HIV antibody positive will eventually develop AIDS or what the eventual upper limit of the induction phase will be. It is also important not to confuse the amount of time required to mount an antibody response with the amount of time to induce disease.

T-lymphocytes play an important role in cellular immunity, which is a key immune response for combating viral, fungal, parasitic, mycrobacterial, and bacterial diseases. Other white blood cells affected by the virus include monocytes and macrophages. Various cells in the skin, brain, liver, spleen, and mucous membranes are also affected. Therefore, a person with HIV infection is susceptible to infectious diseases (5) as well as a number of different kinds of cancer, such as Kaposi's sarcoma and lymphoma, and a decline of central nervous system (CNS) cells, manifesting as AIDS dementia and a variety of CNS dysfunctional disorders (6). These disorders are the clinical manifestations of AIDS, and all will ultimately progress to death.

Although there is much yet to be learned about HIV infection and AIDS, there have been no new modes of transmission discovered since the advent of the AIDS epidemic in 1979. The modes of transmission are delineated in Table 37.2.

When one examines the demographic data of persons with HIV infection, some characteristics common to trauma patients can be seen (7). Namely, more than 90% of all AIDS cases occur in people between the ages of 20 and 49 years. More than 93% of these cases are male, with about 15% of these being intravenous (IV) drug abusers (8). Similarly, trauma is the leading killer of Americans under the age of 38; most victims are male, and drug and alcohol abusers seem to have higher trauma rates. Of these patients, those sustaining gunshot wounds resulting from situations related to IV drug abuse or drug dealing occur more frequently within large metropolitan areas and surrounding communities than in rural settings. Similarly, studies describing the seroprev-

**Table 37.2.** Modes of HIV transmission

1. *Injection with human immunodeficiency virus (HIV) contaminated blood.* These mechanisms include sharing of needles and syringes during the injection of illicit drugs; injury from a sharp object contaminated with HIV-infected blood, primarily occurring in the prehospital and inhospital phases of patient care; tranfusion with HIV-contaminated blood and blood products (unlikely or rare since May 1985).
2. *Unprotected sexual intercourse with infected partner.* The primary mode is through anal sex performed by homosexual or bisexual men, or heterosexual partners; vaginal intercourse between women and men infected from high-risk behaviors, such as intravenous drug abuse or unprotected sex. Risks of infection are enhanced if underlying sexually transmitted diseases are present.
3. *Mother to child.* Transmission is thought to occur via three mechanisms: vertical transplacental spread from HIV-infected mother to fetus; traumatic birth from HIV-infected mother; or in some rare cases, infants suckling breast milk from HIV-infected mother or drinking infected mother's milk.
4. *Contact of blood on abnormal skin or mucous membrane.* This mode was suspected as being a means of infection of a health care worker who was not complying with appropriate infection control guidelines.

alency rates of HIV antibody positivity among trauma patients reflect the demographic patterns of HIV infection within the community (9–12). For example, the emergency department of a large metropolitan inner-city hospital reported a seropositivity rate of 18% of IV drug abusers treated in the emergency room at 10.6% of patients admitted for penetrating trauma (11). On the other hand, a hospital approximately 2 miles away, whose trauma population is mostly referred from outside of the same city limits, reported a seropositivity rate of 1.7% of admissions (12).

Little has been written about HIV or AIDS in the trauma patient. A primary reason for this paucity of documentation is that the major reason the patient is admitted to the hospital is to treat conditions unrelated to HIV infection, and most patients admitted with this infection are in the asymptomatic, carrier phase of the illness. The clinical presentation of HIV infection can be masked by the underlying effects of trauma; that is, both trauma and HIV infection can make the patient more susceptible to infection and cause CNS dysfunction.

Identification of HIV-infected patients admitted for trauma may be difficult. Routine screening of admissions has little, if any, value (13). Detection of carriers cannot be guaranteed by either the enzyme-linked immunosorbent assay (ELISA) or the Western blot electrophoresis. Both have intrinsic flaws, and both detect only the antibodies to HIV and not the virus itself (14, 15). The ELISA is a highly sensitive test for antibody response; however, it is not specific. Reactivity with similar antigens can give positive results. Western blot electrophoresis is a highly specific test for HIV antibody proteins, which are identified on the basis of molecular weight. Adequate concentrations of antibody proteins must be present before the results are considered positive. Therefore, the most widely accepted criteria for HIV antibody positivity require that both tests be performed and both be positive (or reactive) (6).

Because these are antibody tests, newly infected individuals may test negative because their bodies have not had adequate time to mount an antibody response. These individuals may have viral particles in their blood that can infect a health care worker who sustains a percutaneous or mucocutaneous exposure to the blood. Another factor that may influence HIV antibody results is the massive fluid replacement often necessary for the resuscitation and stabilization of trauma patients. In this situation, the fluid replacement can dilute any antibodies that may be present and result in a falsely negative HIV antibody test (16). Therefore, the single most important measure that can be taken to prevent the occupational acquisition of HIV infection is to observe universal precautions and consider all blood and body fluids as infectious (13, 17). In addition, because HIV antibody tests performed on a patient's blood may not determine whether a health care worker sustaining a misadventure has been exposed, the most prudent postexposure treatment is to document the event and test the health care provider's blood at the time of exposure and 6 weeks, 3 months, and 6 months postevent (13).

It is important to note that informed consent is mandatory for HIV antibody testing in many states. This requirement exists because HIV antibody-positive persons have been severely discriminated against as a result of public awareness of their infection. Informed consent is particularly important for trauma patients, since the reason for their admission is not HIV infection. For this reason, substitute consent of unconscious or cognitively impaired patients may not be legal unless formal legal guardianship is established (18).

## 2. What are the nursing diagnoses of highest priority?

A. Potential for infection: opportunistic and nosocomial
B. Potential for infection: HIV transmission to others

## 3. What are the goals of nursing care?

### A. Nursing Diagnosis

Potential for opportunistic and nosocomial infection related to dysfunction of the body's immune system

### Goal of Care

Decrease risk of opportunistic and nosocomial infection.

### Nursing Interventions

- Use aseptic techniques for invasive procedures such as dressing changes and for handwashing.
- Observe patient for signs and symptoms of infection:
  - changes in temperature, white blood cells, mental status
  - complaints of fever, chills, sweating, nausea, or malaise
  - nonhealing or delayed healing of wounds
  - increase or change in wound drainage
  - localized pain, redness, heat, or tendency to fluctuation

### Rationale

Trauma patients are at increased risk for developing infections because of the nature of the underlying injuries; the multiple necessity for invasive procedures and mechanical support devices; the loss of the anatomical host defenses; the microorganisms of the body's resident flora and those of the hospital environment; the use of antibiotics; the clinical scenarios of resuscitation; and the amount of attention paid to infection control guidelines (19). Of those trauma patients who survive their initial injury, infection is second only to severe head injury as the leading cause of death (20, 21). The individual with a pre-existing immunodeficiency is particularly at risk for developing nosocomial infections. Initial signs of infection may be subtle; therefore, changes in wound appearance or laboratory values may provide the first clue of a beginning infection.

### B. Nursing Diagnosis

Potential for infection: HIV transmission to others

## Goal of Care

Prevent transmission of HIV infection to others.

## Nursing Interventions

- Use universal precautions for contact with blood or bloody body fluids:
  - gloves
  - eyewear, gowns, and masks if splashing might occur
  - remove as soon as procedure is complete
- Observe aseptic handwashing technique
  - before and after patient care
  - after removal of gloves
- Dispose of sharps properly
  - do not recap needles
  - use puncture-resistant containers
- Counsel patient regarding modes of transmission in community setting.

## Rationale

Preventive strategies to reduce the transmission of HIV infection must be directed against the occupational acquisition of disease and against the spread of the disease in the community. As the HIV epidemic emerged, nurses and many health care providers became increasingly more concerned over their possible occupational acquisition of HIV infection. Despite the extremely low probability that this could occur (22), both the Centers for Disease Control (CDC) (13, 23) and the Occupational Safety and Health Administration (OSHA) (24, 25) recommended and mandated the use of universal precautions in health care settings.

Clients who have been infected with HIV can infect others if they participate in activities demonstrated to cause infection, such as unprotected sexual intercourse or the sharing of syringes for the injection of illicit drugs. Education and counseling have been among the best methods to thwart the spread of HIV infection in the community. Nurses should support and facilitate such education and counseling.

## REFERENCES

1. Baltimore D. DNA polymerase in Rous sarcoma virus. Nature 1970;226:1211–1231.
2. Mitsuta H, Broder S. Strategies for antiviral therapy in AIDS. Nature 1987;325:773–778.
3. Levy JA. The human immunodeficiency virus and its pathogenesis. Infect Dis Clin North Am 1988;2:289.
4. Weber JN, Weiss RA. HIV infection: the cellular picture. Sci Am 1988;259:101–109.
5. Redfield RR, Burke DS. HIV infection: the clinical picture. Sci Am 1988;259:90–98.
6. Centers for Disease Control. Revision of the CDC case surveillance definition for acquired immunodeficiency syndrome. Morbid Mortal Weekly Rep 1987;36(1S):3S–13S.
7. Meythaler JM, Cross LL. Traumatic spinal cord injury complicated by AIDS related complex. Arch Phys Med Rehabil 1988;69:219.
8. Ward JW, Hardy AM, Drotman DP. AIDS in the United States. In: Worman GP, ed. AIDS and other manifestations of HIV infection. Park Ridge, NJ: Park Ridge, 1987:18–35.
9. Aprahamian C, Olson D, Gottschall JL, et al. Potential risks of human immunodeficiency virus in critically injured patients. J Trauma 188(28):1081.
10. Kelen GD, Fritz S, Quiqish B, et al. Unrecognized human immunodeficiency virus infection in emergency department patients. N Engl J Med 1988;318:16445–16450.
11. Baker JL, Kelen GD, Sivertson KT, et al. Unsuspected immunodeficiency virus in critically ill emergency patients. JAMA 1987;257:2609–2611.
12. Soderstrom CA, Furth PA, Glasser D, et al. HIV infection rates in a center treating predominantly rural blunt trauma victims. (In press)
13. Centers for Disease Control. Recommendations for prevention of HIV transmission in health care settings. Morbid Mortal Weekly Rep 1987;36(2S):1s–18S.
14. Weiss SH, Goedret JJ, Sarngadharan MG, et al. Screening test for HTLV-III (AIDS agent) antibodies: specificity, sensitivity, and applications. JAMA 1985;253:221–225.
15. Council on Scientific Affairs Report. Status reports on the acquired immune deficiency syn-

drome: human T-cell lymphotrophic virus type III testing. JAMA 1985;254:1342–1345.

16. Lane TW, Ivey FD, Falk PS, et al. False negative human immunodeficiency virus (HIV): testing an organ donor [abstract]. Am J Infect Control 1987;15:87.

17. Hoyt NJ. Infection control and emergency medical services: facts and myths. Maryland Med J 1988;37:551–557.

18. 73 Opinions of the Attorney General at 34 (1988) [Opinion No. 88-046 (October 17, 1988)] Maryland.

19. Hoyt NJ. Infection and infection control. In: Cardona VD, Hurn PD, Bastnagel-Mason PJ, et al. Trauma nursing: from resuscitation through rehabilitation. Philadelphia: WB Saunders 1988:224–262.

20. Caplan ES, Hoyt NJ. Infection surveillance and control in the severely traumatized patient. Am J Med 1981;70:638–640.

21. Trunkey DD. Infectious complications following trauma. In: Root RK, Trunkey DD, Sande MA, eds. New surgical and medical approaches in infectious diseases. New York: Churchill Livingstone, 1987:175–187.

22. Vlahov D, Polk FB. Transmission of human immunodeficiency virus within the health care setting. Occupational Medicine: State of the Art Reviews 1987;2:429–450.

23. Centers for Disease Control. Update: Universal precautions for prevention of transmission of human immunodeficiency virus, hepatitis B, and other bloodborne pathogens in health-care settings. Morbid Mortal Weekly Rep 1988;37:377–387.

24. Federal Register. Joint Advisory Notice: Department of Labor/Department of Health and Human Services. HBV/HIV 1987;52(210):4181–4223.

25. Federal Register. Occupational exposure to hepatitis B virus and human immunodeficiency virus (proposed rules). 1987;52(228):45438–45441.

# CHAPTER 38

# Suicide Attempt

Barbara Panariello, RN, BSN

## Clinical Presentation

Mr. W., a 22-year-old man, was admitted to the hospital following a race-car accident in which he was the driver. Friends at the scene reported that he was driving recklessly and had not performed the required safety check of the car prior to the race. On arrival at the emergency department he was awake, with no history of loss of consciousness at the scene; however, he was agitated, combative, and yelling, "Let me die!" Although uncooperative, he was moving all extremities and following commands appropriately. He complained only of a severe headache. A large amount of serosanguinous drainage was oozing from a pressure dressing on his head, and further examination revealed a large, deep, frontal scalp laceration. His blood pressure (BP) was 186/104, pulse was 120, and respiratory rate was 30/minute, rapid and regular. Neurological exam was normal.

The frontal laceration was cleansed and sutured after the area was anesthetized with lidocaine. A tetanus shot was given after the patient reported he had never received one. A computerized tomography (CT) scan of the head was negative for skull fracture and hematoma. The patient was medicated with an intramuscular injection of Thorazine 50 mg after ascertaining a history of no drug allergies. He became calm and subdued within 30 minutes. He was admitted to the intensive care unit (ICU) for neurological and psychological observation. His vital signs were BP 130/70, pulse 104, respiratory rate 20 breaths/minute. There was an intravenous catheter in his left forearm with fluids infusing at 100 cc/hr. Suicide precautions were instituted. The siderails on his bed were padded, and the bed was moved to the center of the ICU in front of the nurses' station for closer observation. The room window was locked; needles and other sharp objects were removed from the bedside supply stand; and restraints were placed at the bedside. Liquids stocked in his cubicle, including alcohol, povidone-iodine, hydrogen peroxide, and benzoin, were removed. The staff was notified of the potential for suicide, and a psychiatry consult was ordered.

The following day the patient was interviewed by the psychiatric nurse who found him sullen, lethargic, and withdrawn. After some time he confided that on the day before his accident, his wife, from whom he had been separated for a year, announced she wanted a divorce. They had been married for 4 years, and, although they were having problems, he stated he couldn't live without her. His wife was interviewed later that day and told the psychiatric nurse that in the past, Mr. W. had been diagnosed as "depressed" and had been noncompliant with psychotherapy and medications. Elavil, a tricyclic antidepressant, had been prescribed, but he had never had the prescription filled. She said Mr. W. was a very pessimistic, jealous, and angry man. He had been physically and verbally abusive toward her, and when she suggested they see a marriage counselor, he refused. She said he coped with problems by becoming depressed and apathetic. He also drank heavily. His father had committed suicide when Mr. W. was 13 years old.

## 1. What is the pathophysiological basis for this patient's problems?

This patient is depressed, as evidenced by his past history and his suspicious accident. Depression is an altered mood state consisting of despair, gloom, foreboding, and emptiness (1). This morbid sadness or melancholy may be a transient stage of grief, a symptom of a psychoneurotic or psychotic disorder, or there may be no apparent cause. All deeply depressed people are potentially suicidal (2). The suicidal impulse appears to arise in many cases from a combination of hate, anger, guilt, and intolerable frustration. It is an effort to communicate the need for attention and help (3), as well as a release from unbearable pain. Depressed persons sometimes feel there is no alternative except to take their life. Suicide often appears to be an act in which individuals express toward themselves the anger they feel toward others or the world in general. They punish themselves for their own shortcomings. A variety of perceived or actual events may precipitate depression, including a recent loss of close or important persons through death or divorce. The loss of a job, financial problems, or alterations in health may lead to a diminished self-image and depression. A family history of depression and/or suicide attempts is also a risk factor (4).

Psychological symptoms of depression include feelings of melancholy, apathy, irritability, anxiety, helplessness, and hopelessness. Isolation from family and friends, obsessive thoughts, and contemplating suicide or death are also signs. A poor memory, inability to concentrate, and delusions or hallucinations may also occur. Physical symptoms may take the form of a change in sleep patterns, anorexia, decreased libido, and/or constipation. Observable manifestations of depression may include a sad or anxious expression, lethargy, a slowed response, and psychomotor agitation such as foot tapping, pacing, and nail biting (5).

Suicide attempts may be overt or covert. Overt attempts include self-inflicted gunshot wounds, stabbing, cutting or mutilation of self, drug overdose, hanging, or carbon monoxide poisoning. Covert attempts may be single car accidents, "accidental" falls from high places, burns, "accidental" gunshot wounds, and drownings (6). It is very important for the caregivers to obtain a thorough psychosocial assessment of the patient and to be suspicious of questionable accidents, as depression or suicidal thoughts cannot be treated until they are recognized.

The majority of suicidal persons do not want to die, they merely want to be relieved of psychological pain (4). Their suicidal thoughts are ambivalent, and their death wish is usually temporary (7). Most people are suicidal for only a limited time. Eight out of 10 persons who commit suicide have given definite warnings of their intent (5). There is a high incidence of repeated attempts in those who are initially unsuccessful (5). People with chronic illnesses are more likely to commit suicide than those with terminal illnesses (5). Incidence is highest in adolescents aged 15 to 24 and individuals over age 50. Men have a higher incidence of suicide than women (5); however, women in their twenties and thirties make the most nonlethal attempts (8).

## 2. What are the nursing diagnoses of highest priority?

A. Potential for further self-harm
B. Potential for high anxiety
C. Alterations in family coping

## 3. What are the goals of nursing care?

### A. Nursing Diagnosis

Potential for further self-harm related to maladaptive coping skills secondary to suicide attempt or suspected suicide attempt

### Goal of Care

Prevent self-destructive behavior.

### Nursing Interventions

- Implement suicide precautions as needed and according to institutional policy.
- Document suicidal or depressive behaviors.
- Inform staff of need for maintaining suicide precautions.
- Inform patient of staff's concern over possible self-destructive behavior and of precautions to be instituted to prevent such behavior.
- Initiate psychiatric consult in collaboration with physician.
- Provide continual observation with suicidal patient.
- Remove potentially harmful objects from patient's immediate environment (e.g., razors, needles, belts, gauze, antiseptic solutions, plastic bags).
- Observe patient closely when taking oral medications.
- Inform patient's family of suicide precautions so hazardous objects are not inadvertently provided to the patient.
- Administer tranquilizers or sedatives as needed and document patient's response to them.
- Use restraints judiciously, according to hospital policy.

### Rationale

Suicide is the ultimate self-destructive act. It is a destructive, aggressive act turned inward. Self-destructive behaviors may be manifestations of inner conflict, self-hatred, and anger. These extreme behaviors are seen in people who are unable to identify and communicate their needs and feeling. They are unable to cope effectively with loss, depression, illness, disappointment, rejection, and stress (4). These maladaptive coping skills usually develop in childhood and without intervention form future abnormal patterns of coping.

To prevent further self-harm, observe these patients closely for previously identified verbal and nonverbal signs of depression and/or suicide intent. Report any identified signs to other members of the health care team. Implement suicide precautions and administer medications as needed. Suicides have been prevented when the staff responds appropriately (9).

### B. Nursing Diagnosis

Potential for high anxiety related to depression, helplessness, and hopelessness secondary to suicide attempt

### Goal of Care

Assess patient for self-destructive thoughts, feelings, and behaviors.

### Nursing Interventions

Psychological Interventions:
- Listen actively to the patient.
- Encourage ventilation of needs, thoughts, and feelings.
- Question patient directly when appropriate.

Nursing Approach with a Suicidal Patient:
- Be calm.
- Convey empathy by gentle touch, frequent eye contact, and supportive responses.
- Demonstrate an accepting, nonjudgmental attitude by spending time with the patient, listening, validating feelings.
- List issues patient is dealing with in care plan.
- Ask the patient what the nursing staff could do to reduce distress.

## Rationale

The suicidal patient may have difficulty communicating suicidal thoughts, and it is important for the nurse to develop a trusting, therapeutic relationship by being open and honest. Use of touch, if it relaxes and supports, can communicate caring and concern (9). "Normalizing," or giving permission to a patient for a wide range of feelings to be normal or expected, makes it easier for patients to expose their uncomfortable feelings (1). Normalizing communicates to the patient that the nurse expects various positive and negative feelings (10). These patients may elicit fear and anxiety in the caregiver (4). To be effective, one must recognize anxiety in one's own self and develop control over one's own responses by not becoming anxious reciprocally. If suicide conflicts with a nurse's religious or philosophical beliefs, value judgments must be avoided. Developing a personal awareness will curtail this. The nurse should convey the attitude that a constructive solution can be found.

## Goal of Care

Help patient identify anxiety.

## Nursing Interventions

Identify patient's anxiety:
- Provide feedback in behaviors that indicate anxiety, such as foot tapping.
- When appropriate, help patient identify anxiety by asking questions such as, "Are you uncomfortable right now?"
- Help patient clarify and understand the nature of his problem.

## Goal of Care

Help patient reduce anxiety.

## Nursing Interventions

- Explain procedures and hospitalization.
- Keep pad and pencil at bedside.
- Provide for means of getting nurse's attention.
- Mutually develop a daily schedule of activities.
- Offer support including use of nonverbal behavior such as quiet presence and touch.
- Employ comfort measures such as warm baths and rest periods.
- When appropriate, engage in recreational and diversional activities to decrease anxiety.
- Allow patient to work at own level and pace in solving problems.
- Provide consistency in information given to patient by all caregivers.

Nursing Approach with highly anxious patient:
- Use short, simple sentences.
- Speak in a calm, firm voice.
- Avoid requests requiring decision making.
- Refrain from asking for cause of behavior.
- Recognize and intervene early to prevent increase of anxiety to severe levels.
- Encourage ventilation of feelings, considering readiness of patient (don't probe if patient is experiencing severe or extreme anxiety).

## Goal of Care

Teach patient about anxiety.

## Nursing Interventions

- Instruct in self-observational skills.
- Teach problem-solving skills.
- Teach validation and assertiveness skills.
- Assist with progressive relaxation techniques.

## Rationale

Anxiety is a feeling of uneasiness, apprehension, or dread (11). Anxiety may be rational, and almost everyone experiences some anxiety during changes in one's life. Irrational or unrealistic anxiety, to a certain degree, is also common for many people. However, when anxiety is severe, or when it interferes with life, intervention is required.

The patient must be educated about anxiety; some anxiety is a part of living, and enduring mild anxiety can enhance learning and growth. Teach the patient to observe what is happening in a given situation, to describe the situation, and to analyze his or her expectations concerning how this differs from the actual situation. Guide the patient in developing alternatives to solving problems or changing expectations. This educational process is long term, and the nurse can lay the groundwork for it.

## C. Nursing Diagnosis

Alteration in family coping

## Goals of Care

- Support the family.
- Increase family awareness.

## Nursing Interventions

- Interview family and/or significant other.
- Explain suicide precautions.
- Refer to social services as needed.
- Teach family about anxiety, depression, and self-destruction.
- Instruct them about patient's emotional needs.
- Explain need for hospitalization and/or medications.

## Rationale

It is important to include the family in the care plan because they are important to the patient, they are his primary support, and they will be with him after discharge.

Ongoing assessment and evaluation of the patient's emotional state is very important. The patient's interactions with others, his behavior, physical appearance, emotional state, and thought content must be documented and communicated to others caring for the patient to ensure high-quality care. Two criteria useful in evaluating patient progress include increasing the patient's ability to communicate problems, thoughts, and feelings, and increasing the patient's willingness to listen to healthy alternatives (4).

# ASSOCIATED NURSING DIAGNOSES

A. Alterations in comfort
B. Impaired adjustment
C. Impairment of skin integrity
D. Potential for infection
E. Sleep pattern disturbances

## REFERENCES

1. Saunders JM, Valente SM. The withdrawn response. In Riegel B, Ehrenreich D, eds. Psychological aspects of critical care nursing. Rockville, MD: Aspen, 1989:92–108.
2. McAlpine DE. Suicide: recognition and management. Mayo Clin Proc 1987;62:778–781.
3. Schmidt T. Psychiatric evaluation of self-poisonings. In: Beyer MJ, Rumack BH, eds. Poisonings and overdose. (Topics in Emergency Medicine). Rockville, MD: Aspen, 1989;1(3):121–127.
4. Seremet S. Needs of the attempted suicide patient in the ICU. CCQ 1984;6:40–46.
5. Hyman S. Manual of psychiatric emergencies. Boston: Little, Brown, 1984.
6. McMahon B. Self-inflicted wounds. Philadelphia: Bailliere Tindall, 1986:222–224.
7. Hendin H. Suicide in America. New York: WW Norton, 1982:264.
8. Bhagat M, Shellital R. Attempted suicide: nursing mirror. 1978;146(6):26–27.
9. Kleck HG. ICU Syndrome: onset, manifestations, treatment, stressors and prevention. CCQ 1984;6:21.
10. King AC, Morrell EM. Helping the hospitalized depressed client. In: Backer BA, et al, eds. Psychiatric mental health nursing. 2nd ed. Monterey, CA: Wadsworth, 1984:107–120.
11. Webster's new collegiate dictionary. Springfield, MA: G & C Merriam Company, 1983.

# CHAPTER 39

# A Patient with a "Do Not Resuscitate" Order

Barbara J. Daly, RN, MSN, CCRN, FAAN

## Clinical Presentation

Mr. C., a 68-year-old retired machinist, was replacing some loose shingles on the roof of his house when he lost his balance and fell two stories to the ground. His fall was heard by his wife, who immediately called the local emergency squad. The paramedics took Mr. C. to the local community hospital. On arrival at the emergency department he was unconscious but breathing, with a blood pressure of 146/62 and a pulse of 94. X-rays revealed a fractured right clavicle, fractured right hip, open femur fracture, and skull fracture. When his respirations slowed and his blood pressure began to fall, he was intubated and started on a dopamine drip. His fractures were stabilized with splints, and he was then air transported to the nearest medical center.

A computerized tomography (CT) scan and an arteriogram were performed at the medical center, revealing a tear in the middle meningeal artery. Mr. C. was immediately taken to the operating room. A craniotomy was performed and an epidural hematoma evacuated; his hip and femur fractures were also pinned.

Mr. C. was admitted to the intensive care unit (ICU) approximately 12 hours after the injury occurred. He remained on the ventilator for the next 5 days, with acceptable blood gases on an $FiO_2$ of 0.50 and an assist/control rate of 16/minute. He did not regain consciousness, although brain-stem reflexes, including a gag reflex and corneal reflex, remained present. He had been started on broad-spectrum antibiotics in surgery because of his open fractures, but he remained febrile throughout this period, spiking fevers as high as 40.2°C (104.4°F) at times.

Mr. C.'s family remained at the hospital almost continuously. His wife and two daughters stayed in the ICU waiting room overnight for the first 48 hours, but were persuaded by the nursing staff to go home on the third night to get some rest. His wife, daughters, and sons-in-law visited each evening.

On Thursday evening, a conference was held with the family to explain the results of a repeat CT scan and discuss further treatment options. On hearing that there was significant tissue damage to the left cerebral hemisphere and that recovery of speech and reasoning ability was unlikely, Mrs. C. began to shake her head and say quietly, "He'd hate this; he would just hate this." Mr. C.'s daughter asked if there were any chance that her father could regain "normal function." The physician explained that it was almost certainly impossible that Mr. C. would ever improve to the point of being able to be independent in daily living, but that it was possible that he might gain some improvement in level of consciousness.

On Friday, the day after the conference, Mrs. C. and her daughters told Mr. C.'s nurse they wanted to talk with the physician. They stated that they had discussed the situation the previous night after the meeting and all agreed that Mr. C. would not want to live this way. They wanted the "machines" removed and wanted to let him "die in peace." They were in favor of a "Do not resuscitate" (DNR) order.

## 1. What are the pathophysiological basis and the theoretical framework for this patient/family situation?

This patient sustained a severe neurological injury. Epidural hematomas, such as those he suffered, are associated with the highest mortality rate of all complications of head injury. Displacement of brain tissue occurs as the collection of blood beneath the skull expands, causing further damage to brain tissue not injured in the initial fall (1, 2). Lack of improvement by the fifth or sixth postoperative day when some of the cerebral edema should have resolved, and the continued evidence of sepsis, are poor prognostic signs.

Decisions to limit or withdraw treatment have become the subject of a great deal of attention in the nursing, medical, legal, and philosophical literature over the past 10 to 20 years. As technology generates increasing ability to maintain and, in some cases, restore biological survival, caregivers are increasingly confronted with situations in which patients, families and health care professionals must consider quality-of-life issues.

There are numerous values and principles involved in situations such as Mr. C.'s, in which life can be maintained, but at a level or quality so different from the individual's previous state that questions regarding the benefit or desirability of maintaining life are inevitable. Although the values and beliefs of all individuals involved in the situation must be considered, the most important consideration is the choice or wish of the patient. The principle underlying the imperative to act according to patient wishes is that of autonomy.

Autonomy is accepted in our culture as the right of individuals to self-determination, to make choices regarding their own life, and to be free from restraint or interference in those choices. It is limited only by the requirement of competence and the prohibition from infringing on the rights of others. This principle has been repeatedly recognized by the courts, which have upheld the right of patients both to refuse treatment and to decide on the cessation of treatment (3–5).

In cases in which the patient cannot express an opinion, there are several ways in which decisions can be made consistent with the commitment to foster patient autonomy. The most desirable of these is the use of advance directives. Advance directives are any form of communication from the patient in which specifications regarding decisions are made in advance of the time when they are needed (6). A Living Will is an example of a written advance directive, but unrecorded conversations with family members or physicians are also forms of advance directives. In the absence of such explicit expressions from the patient, health care providers most often rely on substituted judgment, such as occurred in Mr. C.'s situation. Substituted judgment refers to the use of the judgment of someone close to the patient, usually a family member, of what the patient would have wanted were he or she able to make a decision. It depends on the knowledge and judgment of the significant other regarding the patient's values and life choices.

Conflicts between family members and health care providers, or among health care providers, regarding decisions to limit or withdraw treatment can be related to a variety of nonethical factors, such as disagreements regarding prognosis or communication problems. Moral dilemmas may occur when health care providers perceive conflicting obligations, such as the obligation to follow patient wishes (withdraw treatment) and the dictates of the principle of beneficence (7). The principle of beneficence is one of the most fundamental to health care providers. It is the duty to do good and prevent or minimize harm, and is often interpreted as the obligation to promote life and prohibit any act that could lead to death.

Resolution of the potential moral dilemmas involved in the decision to withhold or withdraw life-supporting treatment is a complex issue, beyond the scope of this case study. In general, recognition of both the moral appropriateness and the legal appropriateness of treatment limitation hinges on two principles. First, is the primacy of autonomy, which is grounded in the nature of humans as rational beings. Willingness to withdraw or limit treatment requires the recognition that there is neither a moral obligation nor a legal obligation to provide treatment in which the burdens outweigh the benefits, as judged by the patient.

There have been attempts in the past to consider such distinctions as ordinary treatments versus extraordinary treatments and active euthanasia versus passive euthanasia, to provide guidance concerning acceptable options in cases such as Mr. C.'s. However, such distinctions have proved to be artificial. There are few interventions in today's health care world that can truly be said to be "ordinary" in terms of natural ways of functioning. The only meaningful interpretation of "extraordinary" is the consideration of whether *the patient* would judge the treatment to be excessive in regard to its burdens and benefits.

Similarly, attempts to justify the withholding or omission of treatment as "passive euthanasia," as compared to the withdrawal of treatment as "active euthanasia," have rested on confusion regarding the requirements of moral behavior. A single act, such as the decision not to begin a patient on mechanical ventilation, or the decision to discontinue the ventilator after it has been started, cannot be judged in terms of the extent to which it requires overt action. Rather, the morally significant considerations relate to the context of the decision, the justification for the action, and the extent to which the action is in accord with moral principles (4).

These considerations emphasize the importance of the process used in reaching treatment limitation decisions. Even in situations such as Mr. C.'s, in which the family members reached a consensus and initiated the consideration of withdrawing treatment, it is essential to manage all aspects of the process carefully. All individuals involved in the patient's care must have the opportunity to have input into the decision to limit treatment measures. The goal of the treatment plan must be communicated to and understood by all. Because of the many treatment options in today's critical care units, all life-supporting treatments should be considered and decisions regarding them clearly documented (8). For example, if the treatment goal is to continue to provide comfort measures while death is allowed to come as quickly and peacefully as possible, then it would be consistent to have orders to withhold the use of vasopressors, antiarrhythmics, antibiotics, and parenteral nutrition, as well as to not resuscitate. If, however, the goal is to continue to provide aggressive support until an event that is viewed as irreversible (i.e., a cardiopulmonary arrest) occurs, then it would be appropriate to use a DNR order without limiting the use of any other treatment modalities.

If there is disagreement among caregivers regarding the justification or morality of the decision, outside resources should be used. Both the Ethics Committee of the American Nurses' Association and the American Medical Association have written guidelines that can be helpful to practitioners in dealing with these issues (9, 10). Many hospitals have ethics committees that serve an advisory function for caregivers struggling to make treatment decisions. As a last resort, if individual nurses or physicians are not able to support the decision reached because of their own moral code, arrangements must be made that will permit them to withdraw from that patient's care without fear of reprisal.

## 2. What are the nursing diagnoses of highest priority?

A. Alteration in family process
B. Grieving

## 3. What are the goals of nursing care?

### A. Nursing Diagnosis

Potential for alteration in family process, related to the crisis of the patient's illness and the decision to limit treatment

### Goal of Care

Assist the family to cope with the crisis effectively and return to precrisis level of function.

### Nursing Interventions

- Assess the usual coping patterns.
- Foster use of previously existing strengths.
- Use planned, consistent communication techniques.
- Acknowledge feelings.
- Provide active, anticipatory guidance.

### Rationale

The life-threatening illness of a family member will create a potential crisis in any family. The need to make a decision regarding life-support therapy is an additional intense stressor that will threaten the usual coping abilities of even the strongest family. *Crisis* may be defined as a sudden situation in which the individual's usual ability to manage through problem solving is threatened, and feelings of helplessness, anxiety, and defeat predominate (11). The nurse's goal in working with a family that is normally able to function in a productive fashion is to support their usual methods and provide the additional assistance needed to help them cope in this vulnerable period.

The crisis for the family begins with the initial injury and is usually evident on their arrival to the ICU. The abrupt onset of illness or injury inhibits the ability of the family to make any kind of psychological preparation, and the nurse's initial focus is on guidance, explanation, and direction until the family can regain some equilibrium (12). The usual nursing actions of accompanying the family to the bedside and providing explanations of equipment, updating them on patient status, and answering questions are all especially important in the first 24 to 48 hours.

To foster the use of previously existing strengths, the nurse makes observations regarding the family's interactional style and use of resources. Recognition of their overwhelming emotions is helpful and can lend some structure to the situation. It may be appropriate to be fairly direct in asking about other supports the family has found useful in the past and to arrange these, such as involving the family priest or minister; letting the family remain together as a group in visiting; arranging for the wife to have time alone with her husband; or arranging for the family to use the conference room for quiet discussions.

For the family to use any problem-solving methods, they must have adequate information. Because both their cognitive resources and their emotional resources are already under stress, the communication must be structured and consistent. Individuals with little prior experience in a threatening situation or those with limited intellectual resources are the most likely to misinterpret reality (13). The high degree of anxiety typically present for everyone is crisis situations limits the ability to see alternatives and make decisions (14), and the family needs to have a limited number of caregivers who can provide clear, consistent information. Designation of a primary nurse or primary team is most helpful in addressing this need.

In addition to acknowledging feelings, providing information, and guiding the family in using previously established resources, the nurse can provide anticipatory guidance at the time of decision making. Most families have not had the experience of a loved one dying in an intensive care unit, and rarely have they been in the situation of requesting withdrawal of treatment. They need explicit discussion of the probable course of events, and the nurse can be most helpful in clarifying the options and questions to be asked. For example, most lay persons, unfamiliar with critical illness, do not have the knowledge to recognize the many alternatives, such as establishing a DNR decision; choosing to limit or withhold additional treatments, such as further antibiotics or dialysis; or actually withdrawing treatment, which may include the withdrawal of IV fluids and nutritional support. Whichever decision the family reaches, the nurse can provide anticipatory guidance by telling them what to expect realistically. It is not uncommon for families who have made the decision to remove mechanical ventilation to assume that the patient will die peacefully and quickly, only to have the patient continue to breathe. This leaves the family unprepared to confront the need for another decision regarding further treatment withdrawal several days later.

## B. Nursing Diagnosis

Anticipatory grieving: A state in which the individual or family responds to the realization of a future loss

## Goal of Care

To assist the family in their grief work.

## Nursing Interventions

- Acknowledge feelings.
- Assist in dealing with and resolving ambivalence.
- Identify/provide supportive resources.

## Rationale

The interventions indicated for this diagnosis are similar to those the nurse used with the previous diagnosis of potential alteration in family process. Mr. C.'s sudden injury and hospitalization initiated a crisis situation; recognition of his irreversible condition and the decision to limit treatment (i.e., not to resuscitate) will initiate a process of grieving in anticipation of his death. The intervention of acknowledging the common emotions of shock, anger, and sadness assists all family members in proceeding through the stages of grief, as well as supporting previous coping mechanisms.

Anticipatory grief, the first stage of the bereavement process, serves as a kind of preparation or rehearsal for the actual event of the death (15). This kind of grieving can occur in any situation in which it is perceived that a loss will occur sometime in the future. The conclusiveness of a DNR order often initiates this process as family members and health care providers alike acknowledge that resuscitative efforts are contraindicated, either because these aggressive treatment efforts would be futile or because the patient or family believes they would cause an unreasonable burden and suffering to the patient.

The period of time between the writing of a DNR order and the actual death of a patient provides family members with the opportunity to work through their feelings and reach a degree of acceptance of what has happened. However, it also prolongs the time during which destructive emotions and behaviors can occur as family members become exhausted and coping abilities are overwhelmed. In prolonged terminal illnesses, family members may reach the point where they wish for the death to happen as an end to the suffering of both the patient and themselves

(16). Especially problematic in DNR situations is the ambivalence, which is usually a part of anticipatory grieving.

Ambivalence normally results from the attempts of the individual to deny the reality of what is happening and to accept the inevitable. As the person moves toward acceptance, she may begin to question her motives, her willingness to "give up" rather than maintain hope. She may become angry with caregivers who cannot provide a cure (17). It is essential that the nurse recognize this ambivalence, allow family members to express their anger, and provide consistent reassurance, as family members begin to question whether or not they made the right decision. Reinforcement that they are acting in the patient's best interests must be repeatedly provided. Although we accept the family's decision-making authority, it is helpful to discuss treatment decisions as *shared* decisions, to share the burden of the decision-making responsibility with the family, and to lessen their fear that they have made the wrong decision.

Family members may also be ambivalent about making preparations for the patient's death and need reassurance from the nurse that this is appropriate. The nurse can do this by helping the family think about the usual roles played by the patient and the implications of his or her absence. It may be appropriate to offer referrals to financial or insurance counselors. This kind of help has been found to be espeically important to younger patient/family units who are less likely to have had experience with the death of a family member and in which the patient may be the sole wage earner (18).

In some circumstances it may be appropriate for the nurse to refer the family to a psychiatric social worker or to family services, if available. This may be especially useful if the nurse assesses that he/she has been unable to establish rapport for whatever reason, or if it would be beneficial to have follow-up services available for the family.

## ASSOCIATED NURSING DIAGNOSES

A. Impaired adjustment
B. Anxiety
C. Fear
D. Hopelessness
E. Powerlessness

### REFERENCES

1. Karb V. Care of the patient with neurological problems. In: Daly BJ, ed. Intensive care nursing. New York: Medical Examination Publishing, 1985:301–386.
2. Davis JE, Mason CB. Neurologic critical care. New York: Van Nostrand Reinhold, 1979:123–125.
3. Clarke DB. Euthanasia and the law. In: Monagle JF, Thomas MA, eds. Medical ethics. Rockville, MD: Aspen, 1988:217–233.
4. President's Commission for the Study of Ethical Problems in Medicine and Biomedical and Behavioral Research. Deciding to forego life-sustaining treatment. Washington, DC: US Government Printing Office, 1983.
5. Veatch RM. A theory of medical ethics. New York: Basic Books, 1981:190–213.
6. Lo B. The clinical use of advance directives. In: Monagle JF, Thomas MA, eds. Medical ethics. Rockville, MD: Aspen, 1988:209–216.
7. Flynn PAR. Questions of risk, duty, and paternalism: problems in beneficence. In: Fowler MDM, Levine-Ariff J, eds. Ethics at the bedside. Philadelphia: JB Lippincott, 1987:62–78.
8. Youngner SJ. Do-Not-Resuscitate orders: no longer secret but still a problem. Hastings Center Report 1987;17:24–33.
9. American Nurses' Association. Code for nurses with interpretive statements. Kansas City, MO: American Nurses' Association, 1985.
10. American Medical Association. Judicial council opinions and reports. Chicago: American Medical Association, 1977.
11. Williams RA. Crisis intervention. In: Longo DC,

Williams RA. Clinical practice in psychosocial nursing: assessment and intervention. New York: Appleton-Century-Crofts, 1978:191–210.

12. Chavez CW, Faber L. Effect of an education-orientation program on family members who visit their significant other in the intensive care unit. Heart Lung 1987;16:92–99.

13. Clark C. Nursing diagnosis: ineffective coping. Heart Lung 1987;16:670–674.

14. Williams RA. Crisis intervention. In: Longo DC, Williams RA, eds. Clinical practice in psychosocial nursing: assessment and intervention. New York: Appleton-Century-Crofts, 1978:205.

15. Arkin AM. Notes on anticipatory grief. In: Schoenberg B, Carr AC, Kutscher AH, Peretz D, Goldberg IK, eds. Anticipatory grief. New York: Columbia University Press, 1974:10–13.

16. Martocchio BCM. Living while dying. Bowie, MD: Robert J Brady, 1982.

17. Aldrich CK. Some dynamics of anticipatory grief. In: Schoenberg B, Carr AC, Kutscher AH, Peretz D, Goldberg IK, eds. Anticipatory grief. New York: Columbia University Press, 1974:3–9.

18. Burns N, Carney K. The caring aspects of hospice: a study. In: Paradis LF, ed. Hospice handbook. Rockville, MD: Aspen, 1985:249–282.

# CHAPTER 40

## The Pediatric Trauma Patient

### Patricia A. Moloney-Harmon, RN, MS, CCRN

## Clinical Presentation

A 5-year-old girl was admitted to the hospital after being struck by a fast-moving automobile in the parking lot at the apartment complex where she lived. On admission to the emergency department, she had a blood pressure of 70/40, heart rate of 160, no spontaneous respirations, and a Glasgow Coma Scale score of 7. Her right pupil was larger than her left, and she was reacting sluggishly. She was intubated with a 5-mm endotracheal tube and resuscitated with Ringer's lactate. Chest x-ray films were obtained to rule out cervical spine fractures; a computerized tomography (CT) scan revealed diffuse brain swelling associated with a closed head injury. Her other injuries included left pulmonary contusion, fractured left femur, and multiple abrasions.

On admission to the intensive care unit (ICU), she was attached to a volume-cycled ventilator on an intermittent mandatory ventilation (IMV) mode of 15, a positive end-expiratory pressure (PEEP) of 5, and an $FiO_2$ of 0.60. A subarachnoid screw, inserted for intracranial pressure monitoring, revealed an initial pressure of 35 mm Hg. A right radial arterial line was inserted, and the pressure readings were 110/60, with a mean of 80 on insertion. Her other vital signs were a heart rate of 100 and a temperature of 38.0°C (100.4°F). She had an indwelling Foley catheter in her bladder, a single-lumen catheter in her right external jugular vein, and a left-hand peripheral line. She had no spontaneous respirations and responded only to painful stimuli.

She was given a dose of mannitol, and her IMV was increased to 20. Her arterial blood gases showed a $PaO_2$ of 65, so her PEEP was increased to 8 and her $FiO_2$ increased to 0.70. Her intracranial pressure (ICP) decreased to 18 mm Hg, where it remained for 30 minutes before increasing acutely to 32 mm Hg. She was hyperventilated manually and given another dose of mannitol, which decreased her ICP to 22 mm Hg. A pentobarbital drip was started to induce a barbiturate coma. Her medication orders also included furosemide (Lasix), lidocaine before suctioning, epinephrine and dobutamine drips, pancuronium bromide (Pavulon), and fentanyl.

Her parents are in the waiting room, obviously distraught. Her mother had been shopping and had left her with her father. Her mother is alternating between expressing feelings of guilt about leaving her child and anger at the father for not watching the child more closely.

## 1. What is the pathophysiological basis for this patient's problem?

Pediatric trauma is the leading cause of mortality and morbidity in children between the ages of 1 and 14 years. Multiple organ injuries are common, since the majority of childhood accidents involve blunt trauma (1). A typical pattern of injury for pedestrian trauma is named Waddell's triad, a combination of injuries to the head, thorax, and extremity. This pattern can occur, for example, when a child is struck by a car and sustains injuries to the thorax and femur. The child is thrown by the impact, landing on his or her head, and receives a closed head injury.

Head injury is common in childhood trauma. Authorities report that 75% of all children experiencing multiple trauma suffer head injury, and 80% of all trauma deaths in children are associated with significant head injury (2). Children are at higher risk for brain injury because the head makes up a larger proportion of the body weight. Their brains are less myelinated and more easily injured than adults' brains. The cranial bones are thinner and less developed than the adult cranium, offering less protection to the brain.

Children's responses to brain injury differ from those of adults. Children have a much lower incidence of intracranial mass lesions following head trauma. However, intracranial hypertension is more common in the child. Children suffer from "malignant brain edema," which consists not actually of edema but of significant cerebral hyperemia in the immediate postinjury period (3). Because mass lesions do not occur commonly and because intracranial hypertension and cerebral hyperemia occur frequently, children are more susceptible to secondary brain injury. Secondary brain injury is partially more treatable than primary head injury, so a child's outcome following head injury is significantly better than an adult's (4, 5).

Respiratory failure develops in children after injury from a number of causes, including pulmonary contusion, flail chest, rib fractures, pneumothorax, and cardiac injuries. Blunt thoracic injuries are the result of the rapid deceleration accidents so common with children. The incidence of rib fractures is less because their chests are more compliant; however, a serious thoracic injury can still exist even if no chest wall injury is obvious. Respiratory failure can also result from pulmonary changes in response to the injury—the adult respiratory distress syndrome (ARDS). Hypotension and extensive tissue damage appear to predispose the child to the development of ARDS (6).

## 2. What are the nursing diagnoses of highest priority?

A. Alteration in cerebral tissue perfusion
B. Impaired gas exchange
C. Decreased cardiac output
D. Fear
E. Family coping: potential for growth

## 3. What goals of care and nursing interventions are appropriate for the above diagnoses?

### A. Nursing Diagnosis

Alteration in cerebral tissue perfusion related to head injury and cerebral hyperemia

### Goal of Care

Maintain cerebral perfusion at a level to support cerebral metabolism.

### Nursing Interventions

- Assess airway, breathing, and circulation.
- Assess perfusion.
- Assess level of consciousness, pupil size and responsiveness, reflexes, verbal and motor ability, vital signs.
- Monitor for posttraumatic seizures.
- Maintain cerebral perfusion pressure (CPP) at greater than 50 mm Hg.
- Maintain $PaCO_2$ at 25 to 30 mm Hg.
- Position child with head midline and head of bed elevated to 30 degrees.
- Plan nursing care activities to provide rest periods.
- Limit duration of suctioning to less than 10 seconds.
- Administer appropriate medications and monitor response.

### Rationale

Children with head injury who are inadequately ventilated will experience an increase in their $PaCO_2$, which can lead to intracranial hypertension. Signs of changes

**Table 40.1.** Modified Glasgow Coma Scale for infants

| Activity | Best Response | Score |
| --- | --- | --- |
| Eye opening | Spontaneous | 4 |
| | To speech | 3 |
| | To pain | 2 |
| | None | 1 |
| Verbal | Coos and babbles | 5 |
| | Irritable cries | 4 |
| | Cries to pain | 3 |
| | Moans to pain | 2 |
| | None | 1 |
| Motor | Normal spontaneous movements | 6 |
| | Withdraws to touch | 5 |
| | Withdraws to pain | 4 |
| | Abnormal flexion | 3 |
| | Abnormal extension | 2 |
| | None | 1 |

in perfusion such as cool, mottled extremities; slow capillary refill; cyanotic nailbeds and mucous membranes; and weak peripheral pulses may indicate developing shock in the child and will often be observed before a dropping blood pressure. Head injury rarely causes hypovolemic shock; if shock is present, the child needs to be assessed for other causes of bleeding.

Level of consciousness can be assessed by using the Glasgow Coma Scale (GCS). Table 40.1 presents the modified GCS that takes into account age-appropriate behaviors. Assessing motor and verbal ability is a useful means of evaluating cognitive function. If the child is able to respond, he or she may claim not to remember the accident for fear of being punished. It is important to distinguish between this fear and true posttraumatic amnesia, since the latter may indicate concussion.

In looking at vital signs, respiratory rate and pattern are valuable parameters, since abnormalities may indicate the level of the lesion. Abnormalities may also alter the $PaO_2/PaCO_2$ relationship and alter cerebral blood flow and intracranial pressure. Cushing's phenomenon (consisting of bradycardia, hypertension, and alterations in respirations) is not often seen in young children and should not be relied on to detect early deterioration.

Posttraumatic seizures occur in about 10% of head-injured children. There is a correlation between seizures and severe head injury (GCS scores 3 to 8), diffuse cerebral edema, and acute subdural hematoma (7). If seizures do occur, diazepam (0.1 to 0.3 mg/kg) or phenobarbital (20 to 30 mg/kg) may be given for immediate control. Posttraumatic seizures may occur up to 1 to 2 years after injury.

ICP monitoring is necessary in head-injured children. The subarachnoid screw and ventricular catheter are the most common monitoring tools in children. Methods of treating increased ICP include hyperventilation to keep $PaCO_2$ between 25 and 30 mm Hg, diuretics, fluid restriction, barbiturates, and expert nursing care. An important nursing action is to monitor the $PaCO_2$ before hyperventilating the patient, since $PaCO_2$ values of less than 20 mm Hg can have a negative effect on cerebral blood flow.

Loop diuretics are useful in children, since cerebral hyperemia may be exacerbated by osmotic diuretics such as mannitol. Mannitol is not recommended in the initial management of head-injured children, but it may be used later to reduce brain bulk and ICP. A dose of 0.25 mg/kg is recommended. Loop diuretics, such as furosemide, are administered at dosages of 0.5 to 1.0 mg/kg every 4 to 6 hours. Fluids may be restricted to two-thirds to one-third of the child's normal maintenance, depending on severity of the injury and cardiac output.

The use of barbiturates to control intracranial hypertension in children is controversial. When this therapy is chosen, pentobarbital is most commonly used in children. A loading dose of 2.0 to 5.0 mg/kg is given followed by a continuous infusion of 1.0 to 3.0 mg/kg/hr to maintain a serum level of 20 to 40 μg/ml.

Positioning the child with the head midline and elevated promotes venous drainage from the head. Nursing care activities need to be planned to provide rest periods; various studies have demonstrated that nursing care activities have a cumulative effect on ICP (8, 9). These studies recommend that 5 to 10 minutes be allowed between nursing care activities to provide rest and prevent cumulative effects.

Suctioning causes increased ICP in children (10). Along with limiting duration of this procedure, hyperinflation and/or hyperoxygenation should be performed before suctioning. Drugs such as thiopental or lidocaine may be administered to control ICP during suctioning.

Steroids may be administered, although their use remains controversial for treatment of cerebral edema. If they are used, the recommendation is dexamethasone at 0.25 to 1.0 mg/kg or methylprednisolone at 10 to 15 mg/kg (2).

Children who die as a result of traumatic brain injury do so because of airway compromise, bleeding, and/or irreversible central nervous system injury. Because hypoxia is the final common pathway by which these three cause death, it is important to prevent this from occurring. If the child develops respiratory and/or circulatory failure, resuscitation must begin immediately. Proper equipment sizes and drug dosages are listed in Tables 40.2 and 40.3.

## B. Nursing Diagnosis

Impaired gas exchange related to pulmonary contusion and development of ARDS

### Goal of Care

Maximize gas exchange so that arterial blood gases are within normal limits for child.

### Nursing Interventions

- Monitor for hypoxemia that does not respond to oxygen; respiratory alkalosis; respiratory distress; diffuse, bilateral infiltrates on chest x-ray film; and poor pulmonary compliance.
- Monitor breath sounds, chest wall movement, ventilator settings, arterial blood gases, $O_2$ saturation, and end tidal $CO_2$.
- Monitor vital signs and level of consciousness.
- Administer appropriate medications, such as steroids, antibiotics, and bronchodilators.
- Maintain airway.
- Use two people to suction patient.

### Rationale

The child with a severe pulmonary contusion or ARDS will show the defining characteristics of hypoxemia: unresponsiveness to $O_2$, respiratory alkalosis, dyspnea, tachypnea, and changes in x-ray studies and pulmonary compliance. These children require volume ventilation with high levels of PEEP. The nurse must assess constantly for signs of a tension pneumothorax related to high ventilator pressures. These include diminished breath sounds on the affected side, decreased chest wall

**Table 40.2.**  Appropriate sizes of resuscitation equipment for children[a]

| Age | Weight (kg) | Resus. Mask | Laryngoscope | ET Tube | Suction Catheter (mouth/tube) | Chest Tube | NG/Foley | BP Cuff (cm) | Trach |
|---|---|---|---|---|---|---|---|---|---|
| Newborn | 3–5 | 0–1 | 0 Miller | 3.0 | 10/6 | 10–12F | 8F/5F | 5 | 00 |
| 6 mo | 7 | 1 | 1 Miller | 3.5 | 10/6 | 10–12F | 8F/5F | 5 | 1 |
| 1 yr | 10 | 1–2 | 1 Miller | 3.5 | 10/8 | 16–20F | 8F/8F | 5 | 1 |
| 18 mo | 12 | 2 | 1 Miller | 4.0 | 10/8 | 16–20F | 8F/8F | 5 | 1–2 |
| 3 yr | 15 | 3 | 2 Miller | 4.5 | 14/10 | 16–20F | 10F/10F | 7 | 2–3 |
| 5 yr | 20 | 3 | 2 Miller | 5.0 | 14/10 | 20–28F | 10F/10F | 7 | 3 |
| 6 yr | 20 | 3 | 2 Miller | 5.5 | 14/10 | 20–28F | 10F/10F | 7 | 3 |
| 8 yr | 25 | 3 | 2 Miller | 6.0 | 16/10 | 20–28F | 10F/10F | 9.5 | 4 |
| 10 yr | 30 | 3 | 2 Miller | 6.0 | 16/10 | 28–32F | 12F/12F | 9.5 | 4 |
| 12 yr | 40 | 4 | 2 Miller / 2 Mac | 6.5 | 16/14 | 28–32F | 12F/12F | 9.5 | 5 |
| 14 yr | 50 | 4–5 | 3 Miller / 3 Mac | 7.0 | 16/14 | 32–42F | 14F/12F | Adult | 6 |

[a]*Source:* Reprinted with permission from Widner-Kolberg MR. Maryland Institute for Emergency Medical Services Systems, 1989.

**Table 40.3.** Emergency medications for cardiac arrest in children

| | |
|---|---|
| Epinephrine (1:10,000) | 0.01 mg/kg |
| Atropine | 0.02 mg/kg (minimum, 0.1 mg) |
| Sodium bicarbonate | 1 mEq/kg |
| Calcium chloride | 20 mg/kg |
| Lidocaine | 1 mg/kg |
| Glucose | 2–4 ml/kg $D_{25}W$ |
| Isoproterenol | 0.05–1.0 µg/kg/minute |
| Dopamine | 1–20 µg/kg/minute |

movement, increasing ventilator pressures, worsening blood gases, and decreased $O_2$ saturation. Bradycardia and hypotension indicate worsening respiratory distress in the child; these are very late signs. Level of consciousness changes occur with increasing $PaCO_2$ or decreasing $PaO_2$. Medications such as steroids, antibiotics, and bronchodilators may be used to produce therapeutic effects at lower doses. The child's airway must be maintained for optimal $O_2$ delivery. A child who is receiving such large ventilator pressures is extremely sensitive to sudden decreases in that pressure, particularly when being disconnected from the ventilator for suctioning. Two people should suction to provide the fastest transition from the ventilator to the bag and to avoid hemodynamic instability.

## C. Nursing Diagnosis
Decreased cardiac output related to barbiturate coma and high ventilator pressures

### Goal of Care
Maintain adequate cardiac output to promote perfusion of all tissues.

### Nursing Interventions
- Monitor pulse, blood pressure, systemic perfusion, and core temperature.
- Monitor invasive hemodynamic parameters such as central venous pressure, pulmonary arterial pressure, pulmonary capillary wedge pressures, cardiac output, and cardiac index.
- Monitor systemic perfusion, arterial blood gases, complete blood count, electrolytes, and weight.
- Administer fluids as appropriate.
- Administer medications such as vasopressors and/or vasodilators, noting the child's response.

### Rationale
There are many causes of decreased cardiac output in children, including hypovolemic shock, barbiturate therapy, late sepsis, electrolyte disturbances, and high ventilator pressures. The pediatric trauma victim may experience any or all of these. Observation of vital signs and invasive hemodynamic parameters helps in evaluating the child's degree of decreased cardiac output and helps guide and evaluate therapy. Core temperature is often a more accurate indicator of developing shock, since the child's skin temperature is easily influenced by the environment. Systemic perfusion changes are also reliable indicators of decreased cardiac output and may be seen before overt changes in vital signs. Laboratory values will help determine the presence of metabolic acidosis, electrolyte disturbances, or bleeding.

As mentioned earlier, fluid therapy is critical, since children become hypovolemic more quickly than adults because of their higher metabolic rate and larger body surface area. Maintenance of the child's circulating volume is necessary to maximize cardiac output. The child may also need drugs to improve cardiac contractility, increase heart rate, and reduce afterload.

## D. Nursing Diagnosis

Patient fear related to alien environment, procedures, pain, and separation from family

### Goal of Care

Reduce fear.

### Nursing Interventions

- Provide age-appropriate explanations for all procedures.
- Be honest while providing reassurance.
- Provide the child with toys or other objects of comfort from home.
- Allow the child to play as appropriate.
- Allow the parents to spend as much time as possible with the child.
- Touch the child, conveying a sense of warmth and caring.
- Respect the child's modesty and autonomy.
- Do not allow the child to witness treatment given to another critically ill child or adult.

### Rationale

The intensive care unit is a stressful place for children. They are exposed to foreign sights, sounds, and people and often feel they are being punished. Separation from parents, loss of self-control, and painful and/or invasive procedures induce most of the stress children experience during hospitalization (11). The child's ability to cope is affected mostly by the developmental level. Appropriate nursing interventions are also based on the child's developmental level (12). A summary of essential developmental issues in treating critically injured children is presented in Table 40.4.

The child described at the beginning of this article is at the preschool level. Preschoolers often have well-developed physical and verbal abilities that make them seem more mature than they actually are. They are egocentric and use much magical thinking and fantasy in viewing their world. They have a great need to feel in control (11). Nursing interventions should be based on these aspects of preschoolers. A predominant fear among preschoolers is being alone; having parents or significant others with the child as much as possible is therefore extremely important.

## E. Nursing Diagnosis

Alterations in family process related to the unplanned admission of the child to the critical care unit

### Goal of Care

Promote positive coping within the family system.

### Nursing Interventions

- Be honest and accurate in giving information about the child.
- Allow the parents to be with the child as much as possible.
- Help parents interpret information given to them by the physician.
- Assist parents in finding places to sleep, bathe, and eat.
- Encourage the parents to touch and talk to their child. Also encourage them to participate in their child's care.
- Listen to the parents when they provide information or express concerns about their child.

**Table 40.4.** Developmental approach to pediatric trauma patients

| Age (yr) | Important Developmental Issues | Fears | Useful Techniques |
|---|---|---|---|
| Infancy: 0–1 | Minimal language<br>Feel an extension of parents<br>Sensitive to physical environment | Stranger anxiety | Keep parents in sight<br>Avoid hunger<br>Use warm hands<br>Keep room warm |
| Toddler: 1–3 | Receptive language more advanced than expressive<br>See themselves as individuals<br>Assertive will | Brief separation<br>Pain | Maintain verbal communication<br>Examine in parent's lap<br>Allow some choices when possible |
| Preschool: 3–5 | Excellent expressive skills for thoughts and feelings<br>Rich fantasy life<br>Magical thinking<br>Strong concept of self | Long separation<br>Pain<br>Disfigurement | Allow expression<br>Encourage fantasy and play<br>Encourage participation in care |
| School age: 5–10 | Fully developed language<br>Understanding of body structure and function<br>Able to reason and compromise<br>Experience with self-control<br>Incomplete understanding of death | Disfigurement<br>Loss of function<br>Death | Explain procedures<br>Explain pathophysiology and treatment<br>Project positive outcome<br>Stress child's ability to master situation<br>Respect physical modesty |
| Adolescence: 10–19 | Self-determination<br>Decision making<br>Peer group important<br>Realistic view of death | Loss of autonomy<br>Loss of peer acceptance<br>Death | Allow choices and control<br>Stress acceptance by peers<br>Respect autonomy |

• Allow the parents to express feelings of guilt and anger, but help them to direct those feelings of guilt and anger into positive channels. Do not feed into them or tell them not to feel that way.

• Assure the parents that they are essential in meeting the needs of their child.

## Rationale

Unexpected admission of a child to an intensive care unit is an extremely stressful experience for parents. Suddenly, their healthy child is critically ill, and his or her appearance and behavior have changed radically. Parental stressors following a child's unplanned admission to a pediatric intensive care unit include the environment, procedures, communication with staff, staff behavior, the child's appearance, and changes in the parental role (13). Parental needs include the need to be with their child, information, facilities for sleeping and eating near the unit, participation in their child's care, and assurance that their child is receiving the best posisble care (14). Caring for the family of a critically injured child is an integral part of the child's care plan.

## ASSOCIATED NURSING DIAGNOSES

A. Potential for infection
B. Potential for fluid volume deficit
C. Impaired physical mobility
D. Alteration in nutrition: less than body requirements
E. Alteration in comfort: pain
F. Sleep pattern disturbance
G. Altered growth and development

## REFERENCES

1. King DR. Trauma in infancy and childhood: Initial evaluation and mangement. Pediatr Clin North Am 1985;32:1299–1310.
2. Davis RJ, Dean JM, Goldberg AL, Carson BS, Rosenbaum AE, Rogers MC. Head and spinal cord injury. In: Rogers MC, ed. Textbook of pediatric intensive care. Baltimore: Williams & Wilkins, 1987:649–699.
3. Bruce DA, Alavi A, Bilaniuk L, Dolinskas C, Obrist W, Uzzell B. Diffuse cerebral swelling following head injuries in children: the syndrome of ''malignant brain edema.'' J Neurosurg 1981;54:170–178.
4. Pfenninger J, Kaiser G, Lutschg J, Sutter M. Treatment and outcome of the severely head injured child. Intensive Care Med 1981;9:13–16.
5. Alberico AM, Ward JD, Choi SC, Marmarou A, Young H. Outcome after severe head injury: relationship to mass lesions, diffuse injury and ICP course in pediatric and adult patients. J Neurosurg 1987;67:648–656.
6. Yaster M, Haller JA. Multiple trauma. In: Rogers MC, ed. Textbook of pediatric intensive care. Baltimore: Williams & Wilkins, 1987:1266–1322.
7. Hahn YS, Fuchs S, Flannery AM, Barthel M, McLone DG. Factors influencing posttraumatic seizures in children. Neurosurgery 1988;22:864–867.
8. Bruya M. Planned periods of rest in the intensive care unit: nursing care activities and intracranial pressure. J Neurosurg Nurs 1981;13:184–194.
9. Snyder M. Relation of nursing activities to increases in intracranial pressure. J Adv Nurs 1983;8:273–279.
10. Fisher DM, Frewen T, Swedlow DB. Increase in intracranial pressure during suctioning: stimulation vs. rise in $PaCO_2$. Anesthesiology 1982;57:416–417.
11. Smith JB. Nursing process in pediatric critical care. In: Smith JB, ed. Pediatric critical care. New York: John Wiley & Sons, 1983:1–20.
12. Widner-Kolberg MR, Moloney-Harmon PA. Pediatric trauma. In: Cardona VD, Hurn PD, Bastnagel-Mason PJ, et al, eds. Trauma nursing: from resuscitation through rehabilitation. Philadelphia: WB Saunders, 1988:664–691.
13. Eberly TW, Miles MS, Carter MC. Parental stress after the unexpected admission of a child to the intensive care unit. CCQ 1985;8:57–65.
14. Philichi LM. Supporting the parents when the child requires intensive care. Focus Crit Care 1988;15:34–38.

# CHAPTER 41

## Nutritional Needs of the Trauma Patient

Alyce F. Newton, RD, MS

## Clinical Presentation

A 46-year-old Asian man fell asleep while driving his car and drove into the rear end of a tractor-trailer. Assessment of injuries occurred following helicopter transport to the emergency department. A mild closed head injury, bilateral rib fractures with flail chest, bilateral hemopneumothoraces, and pulmonary contusions were detected. Early adult respiratory distress syndrome (ARDS) and a distal radius fracture were also diagnosed. An exploratory laparotomy revealed a liver laceration and contusions of the gallbladder, duodenum, and pancreas. The patient underwent a cholecystectomy and entered the intensive care unit (ICU) intubated and mechanically ventilated.

Worsening ARDS required pharmacological paralysis with metubine and intravenous (IV) morphine for 2 weeks, resulting in an ileus. Total parenteral nutrition (TPN) was started on day 3 and was continued for 41 days. Enteral tube feedings were started on day 35, 6 days after discontinuation of IV morphine. An oral diet began on the 47th day. Complications during the hospital course included a gram-negative pneumonia, treated with vancomycin and amikacin, and hyperglycemia, treated with an insulin drip. The patient was discharged to home after a hospital stay of 60 days.

### 1. What are the nutritional implications of this patient's injury?

Following trauma, hypermetabolism and accelerated protein breakdown with nitrogen loss occur (1). Abdominal trauma, intestinal ileus, or narcotics administration often prevent early enteral feedings. TPN solutions must contain adequate protein and calories to promote wound healing, meet metabolic needs, and support the immune system to fight infection.

### 2. How would a nutritional assessment be performed on this patient on admission to the ICU?

A. Nutritional assessment begins with anthropometric measurements. Anthropometric measurements are measurements of the human body, including height, weight, limb size, and skinfold measurements to determine fat and muscle stores. This patient's height and weight, reported by the patient's family, were 5'3'' (160 cm) and 145 lb (66 kg). Because of problems with edema, skinfold measurements are frequently inaccurate following multiple trauma.

Harris and Benedict developed the Harris-Benedict equation (HBE) in 1919 from oxygen consumption measurements of healthy men and women (2). The equation provides an approximate basal metabolic rate based on sex, age, height, and weight.

HBE/males: $66.47 + (13.75 \times$ wt in kg$) + (5.0 \times$ ht in cm$) - (6.76 \times$ years)
HBE/females: $655.10 + (9.56 \times$ wt in kg$) + (1.85 \times$ ht in cm$) - (4.68 \times$ years)
Case patient: $66.47 + (13.75 \times 66) + (5.0 \times 160) - (6.76 \times 46) = 1463$ calories/day

The HBE does not reflect the increased caloric needs following multiple trauma. In

**Table 41.1.**  Selected metabolic laboratory values

| Test | Day | | | | | |
| --- | --- | --- | --- | --- | --- | --- |
|  | 1 | 6 | 20 | 32 | 40 | 60 |
| Albumin | 2.5 | 2.4 | 2.8 | 3.2 | 3.3 | 3.6 |
| Glucose | 205 | 202 | 103 | 124 | 135 | 96 |
| Prealbumin |  | 5 |  | 11 |  |  |
| Transferrin |  | 82 |  | 135 |  |  |
| Nitrogen (urine) |  | 21 |  | 20 |  |  |
| Nitrogen balance |  | 1.1 |  | 2.1 |  |  |

1979, Long et al. reported that in multiply-injured trauma patients energy expenditure increased from 25% to 132% over the calculated HBE (3). The injury and activity factors derived from the study by Long et al. are frequently used to adjust the calculated HBE to cover increased needs following trauma. Indirect calorimetry (IC) is the measurement of a patient's oxygen consumption ($VO_2$) and carbon dioxide production ($VCO_2$). Oxygen consumption reflects the degree of caloric expenditure and increases following injury. Recent studies in IC reveal a lower caloric need than reported by Long et al. following multiple trauma. In one study, trauma patients measured a 15 to 16% increase over calculated HBE (4). Studies of multiple trauma patients often suggest a minimum of 20% and a maximum of 30% additional calories over HBE (5).

*Calculated Energy Needs*
HBE $\times$ 1.25 = estimated calorie needs/day
1463 $\times$ 1.25 = 1829 calories needed/day (case patient)

B.  Protein needs following multiple trauma can be as high as 2 to 3 gm/kg/day (6).

*Calculated Protein Needs*
66 kg $\times$ 2.5 gm/kg = 165 gm protein needed/day (case patient)

## 3. Which laboratory tests are used in the nutritional assessment of the trauma patient?

A.  Albumin
B.  Prealbumin
C.  Transferrin
D.  Nitrogen balance

### A. Albumin

Albumin is a serum protein produced by the liver, with a half-life of 20 to 21 days. Serum albumin maintains plasma oncotic pressure and functions as a carrier protein for enzymes, drugs, hormones, and trace elements. It is a good index of severe malnutrition, but because of its long half-life and sensitivity to fluid shifts, it does not accurately reflect early protein deficiency. Significant losses into the interstitial fluid associated with altered capillary permeability occur following trauma (7, 8). Sepsis and trauma alter distribution of albumin between the intravascular space and extravascular albumin pool. Infusion of blood products may increase albumin levels. Normal albumin levels are 3.5 to 5.0 gm/100 ml. Mild depletion levels are 2.8 to 3.5 gm/100 ml. Moderate depletion levels are 2.1 to 2.7 gm/100 ml. Severe depletion levels are less than 2.1 gm/100 ml (9). Table 41.1 displays albumin levels collected for the case patient.

## B. Prealbumin

Prealbumin is a serum protein also produced by the liver, with a half-life of 2 days. Prealbumin transports thyroxine and is a carrier protein for retinol-binding protein. Thyroxine-binding levels decrease rapidly following trauma or acute infections. Normal levels are 15.7 to 29.6 mg/ml. Mild depletion levels are 10 to 15 mg/ml; moderate depletion levels are 5 to 10 mg/ml; and severe depletion levels are less than 5 mg/ml. Prealbumin levels, depressed by sudden demands for protein synthesis, may not reflect nutritional repletion efforts (9, 10). Table 41.1 contains prealbumin values of the case patient.

## C. Transferrin

Transferrin is a serum protein produced by the liver with a half-life of 8 to 10 days. Transferrin is a carrier protein for iron in plasma. Serum transferrin levels decrease during severe malnutrition, infection, or stress. Because of its long half-life, transferrin is inappropriate for detection of early protein deficiency. Normal levels are 250 to 300 mg/100 ml. Mild depletion levels are 150 to 200 mg/100 ml; moderate depletion levels are 100 to 150 mg/100 ml; severe depletion levels are less than 100 mg/100 ml. Transferrin values increase during iron deficiency (9, 10). Table 41.1 shows the tranferrin levels of the case patient.

## D. Nitrogen Balance

Nitrogen balance measures the net changes in the body's total protein mass. Urine collected for 24 hours is analyzed for urine urea nitrogen (UUN). During the same period, the nitrogen consumed is recorded. The UUN is adjusted to cover non-urea nitrogen present in urine, sweat, and stool. In trauma patients, 25% of the UUN measured is added back to the UUN to account for non-urea nitrogen (11). Refer to Table 41.1 for nitrogen balance data.

Example: UUN = 30 gm: UUN × .25 = 7.5 gm + 30 + 7.5 = 37.5 gm or 38 gm nitrogen lost. Protein intake is 150 gm or 24 gm of nitrogen (6.25 gm protein in 1 gm nitrogen). Nitrogen consumed minus adjusted nitrogen excreted equals the nitrogen balance. This number is either positive, negative, or zero, indicating nitrogen equilibrium; 24 − 38 = negative 14 gm of nitrogen lost per day or 88 gm of protein lost per day. Eighteen additional grams of nitrogen would produce a positive nitrogen balance ( + 4). A total of 42 gm of nitrogen or 263 gm of protein are required daily.

# 4. What is the nursing diagnosis related to nutrition?

A. Alteration is nutrition: less than body requirements

# 5. What is the goal of nursing care?

## A. Nursing Diagnosis

Alteration in nutrition; less than body requirements related to trauma and infection

## Goal of Care

Meet nutritional needs as assessed.

## Nursing Interventions

- Provide nutritional support with:
  - Parenteral nutrition
  - Enteral nutrition
  - Oral nutrition
- Monitor for complications

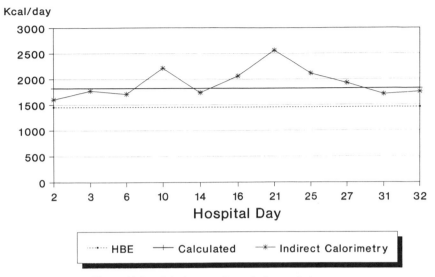

Figure 41.1.  Caloric expenditure: Indirect calorimetry.

## Rationale

**Parenteral Support**: During parenteral support the patient received from 1774 to 2224 calories/day, depending on the calories measured by IC (Fig. 41.1).

The average caloric expenditure measured was 1922 kcal per day. When the patient was no longer mechanically ventilated, a higher calorie level provided energy for the increased work of breathing and ambulation (Fig. 41.2).

During parenteral support, the patient received from 120 to 168 gm of protein per day (19.2 to 26.9 gm of nitrogen). During the period of sepsis/gram-negative

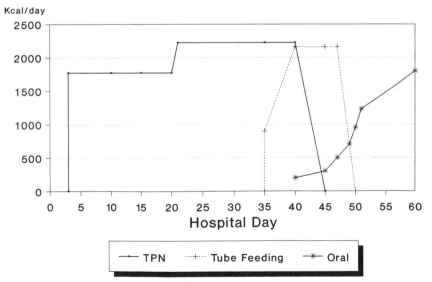

Figure 41.2.  Calories provided during hospitalization.

Grams/day

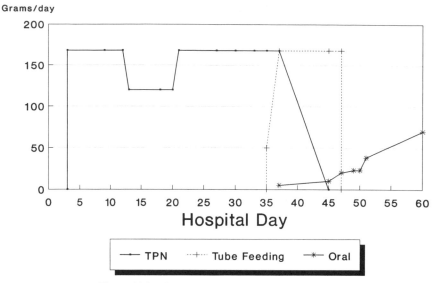

**Figure 41.3.** Protein provided during hospitalization.

pneumonia/ARDS, the patient received a modified TPN solution containing 45% branched chain amino acids (BCAA) (Fig. 41.3) The BCAA leucine, isoleucine, and valine are the preferred amino acids for oxidation by the muscle following trauma (11). Measurements of serum levels of BCAA in septic/trauma patients are often low, indicting preferential oxidation. Decreased nitrogen excretion during the administration of BCAA may occur during sepsis and trauma (12).

There may be mechanical, metabolic, and/or infectious complications of TPN (13). *Mechanical complications* related to the subclavian catheter may include pneumothorax, hemothorax, and hemomediastinum. Injuries may occur to the subclavian artery, brachial plexus, and thoracic duct. Air embolism, catheter embolization, cardiac arrhythmias, subclavian vein thrombosis, and improper catheter-tip placement can also occur. *Metabolic complications* include hyperglycemia, hypopglycemia, carbon dioxide retention, azotemia, hypophosphatemia, hypertriglyceridemia, and electrolyte disorders. Close monitoring of laboratory data and the appropriate TPN solution will prevent many of the metabolic complications. *Infectious complications* are avoided by aseptic catheter placement and proper catheter and IV tubing maintenance.

**Enteral Support**: Tube feedings are provided to patients with intestinal peristalsis, decreased gastric drainage, mechanical ventilation, and inability to eat.

The case patient started tube feedings on day 35. Half-strength Traumacal (Bristol Myers) at 50 cc/hr was advanced to three-fourths strength at 80 cc/hr with 5 scoops of ProMod (Ross Laboratories) protein powder added per liter of tube feeding. This mixture provided 2160 kcal and 168 gm of protein over 24 hours (Figs. 41.2, 41.3). The patient tolerated the feeding well without elevated gastric residuals or diarrhea until day 47; the patient began to eat following a successful swallowing evaluation on that date.

Tube feedings may incur mechanical, metabolic, and infectious complications (14). *Aspiration pneumonia* is a serious complication caused by regurgitation of gastric contents. To decrease the risk of aspiration, the head of the bed is elevated, gastric residuals are checked every few hours, and feedings are held if the residuals exceed twice the flow rate. An intestinal feeding may eliminate this problem.

*Diarrhea* is a common malady and can be associated with administration of various antibiotics, such as nafcillin, clindamycin, and ampicillin. Several medications, such as magnesium-containing antacids, histamine $H_2$ receptor antagonists, theophylline, digoxin, potassium chloride, guanethidine, methyldopa, propanol, and quinidine can cause diarrhea. Diarrhea may be caused by a rapid feeding rate or bacterial contamination of the feeding. Product formulation such as a hypertonic feeding and hypoalbuminemia associated with malnutrition have been reported to cause diarrhea.

*Nausea and vomiting* may occur in patients with gastric retention of formula. Occasionally the smell of the formula may distress the patient and cause nausea. A dilute, low-fat feeding can decrease the gastric retention. Feeding concentration is increased as toleration is demonstrated. Medication may contribute to the problem of nausea and vomiting.

*Dehydration/fluid overload* are often caused by inadequate or excessive free water. In addition to monitoring the intake and output of a patient, the nurse can check the serum electrolytes and the skin and mucous membranes to ensure that adequate free water is provided. A rule of thumb is that one ml of free water is provided for each kcal provided. To achieve this goal, the tube feeding is diluted and administered at a higher rate. If preferred, water boluses can be administered every 4 to 6 hours or as necessary.

*Electrolyte imbalances* and *hyperglycemia* can occur in patients with inadequate monitoring of laboratory data. The formula concentration, sodium, phosphate, magnesium and carbohydrate content can be adjusted to correct imbalances.

*Mechanical complications* may include a clogged feeding tube. The tube can be flushed every few hours with 15 to 20 ml of water or the water boluses. Viokase pancreatic enzyme has been used successfully to clear obstructed feeding tubes (15). Other serious complications include pulmonary placement of the feeding tube, nasopharyngeal erosions, and a knotted feeding tube in the stomach. Placement of a feeding gastrostomy is the preferred method of long-term feeding and can eliminate many complications.

*Pharmacological complications* include the inhibition of phenytoin absorption by continuous nasogastric tube feeding, which should be held for one hour before and after the drug is administered. Serum concentrations should be monitored to ensure that adequate doses are given (16).

**Oral Support**: Once a patient consumes an oral diet, the nurse can evaluate the patient's acceptance of the diet and actual intake. The case patient had calorie count recorded by nurses for 3 days. From days 49 to 51, 23 to 58 gm of protein and 705 to 1230 calories were consumed (Fig. 41.2, Fig. 41.3).

Complications associated with an oral diet include inadequate intake of calories and protein. The case patient's oral intake was less than desired when tube feedings were discontinued. Additional complications related to oral support include dysphagia and aspiration, as evaluated by a speech-language pathologist. Soft foods and thick liquids are easier to control than thin liquids. The case patient drank high-calorie, high-protein supplements and ate Oriental food brought from home before discharge.

## REFERENCES

1. Cerra FB. Hypermetabolism, organ failure and metabolic support. Surgery 1987;101:1–14.
2. Harris JA, Benedict FG. A Biometric study of basal metabolism in man. Carnegie Institute of Washington, 1919; Publication No. 279.
3. Long CL, Schaffel N, Geiger JW, Schiller WR, Blakemore WS. Metabolic response to injury and illness: estimation of energy and protein needs from indirect calorimetry and nitrogen balance. JPEN 1979;3(6):452–456.
4. Stanek GS. Predicting energy expenditure in critically ill trauma patients [Abstract]. JPEN 1986;10(suppl 1):4s.
5. Weissman C, Kemper M, Askanazi J, Hyman A, Kinney JM. Resting metabolic rate of the critically ill patient: measured versus predicted. Anesthesiology 1986;64(6):673–679.
6. Cerra FB, Blackburn G, Hirsch J, et al. The effect of stress level, amino acid formula and nitrogen dose on nitrogen retention in traumatic and septic stress. Ann Surg 1987;205:282–287.
7. Starker PM, Gump FE, Askanazi J, et al. Serum albumin levels indicators of nutritional support. Surgery 1982;91(2):194–199.
8. Fleck A, Colley CA, Myers M. Liver export proteins and trauma. Br Med Bull 1985;41(33):265–273.
9. Grant J. Current techniques of nutritional assessment. Surg Clin North Am 1981;61(3):4367–463.
10. Tuten MB, Wogt S, Dasse F, Leider Z. Utilization of prealbumin as a nutritional parameter. JPEN 1985;9(6):709–710.
11. Konstantinides FN, Konstantinides NN, Cerra FB. Can urinary urea nitrogen be substituted for total urinary nitrogen when calculating nitrogen balance in clinical nutrition? JPEN 1988; 12(1):185.
12. Cerra FB, Upson D, Angelico R, et al. Branched chains support postoperative protein synthesis. Surgery 1982;92(2):192–198.
13. Chiarla C, Siegel J, Kidd S, et al. Inhibition of posttraumatic septic proteolysis and ureagenesis and stimulation of hepatic acute-phase protein production by branched-chain amino acid TPN. Trauma 1988;28(8):1145–1172.
14. Ang SD, Daly JM. Potential complications and monitoring of patients receiving total parenteral nutrition. In: Rombeau J, Caldwell M, eds. Parenteral nutrition. Philadelphia: WB Saunders, 1986:331–343.
15. Marcuard SP, Stegall KL, Trogdon S. Clearing obstructed feeding tubes. JPEN 1989;13(1):81–83.
16. Saklad JJ, Graves RH, Sharp WP. Interaction of oral phenytoin with enteral feedings. JPEN 1986;10(3):322–323.

# APPENDIX

# Nursing Diagnostic Categories

The North American Nursing Diagnoses Association (NANDA) has developed a nursing diagnostic classification framework using nine human response patterns for grouping nursing diagnoses. The following list represents the 1988 NANDA-approved nursing diagnostic categories for clinical use and testing.

## Pattern 1: Exchanging

Altered nutrition: more than body requirements
Altered nutrition: less than body requirements
Altered nutrition: potential for more than body requirements
Potential for infection
Potential altered body temperature
Hypothermia
Hyperthermia
Ineffective thermoregulation
Dysreflexia
Constipation
   Perceived constipation
   Colonic constipation
Diarrhea
Bowel incontinence
Altered urinary elimination
   Stress incontinence
   Reflex incontinence
   Urge incontinence
   Functional incontinence
   Total incontinence
Urinary retention
Altered tissue perfusion (specify type) (renal, cerebral, cardiopulmonary, gastrointestinal, peripheral)
   Fluid volume excess
   Fluid volume deficit
      Potential fluid volume deficit
Decreased cardiac output
Impaired gas exchange
Ineffective airway clearance
Ineffective breathing pattern
Potential for injury
Potential for suffocation
Potential for poisoning
Potential for trauma
Potential for aspiration
Potential for disuse syndrome

Impaired tissue integrity
  Altered oral mucous membrane
  Impaired skin integrity
    Potential impaired skin integrity

## Pattern 2: Communicating

Impaired verbal communication

## Pattern 3: Relating

Impaired social interaction
Social isolation
Altered role performance
  Altered parenting
  Potential altered parenting
  Sexual dysfunction
Altered family processes
  Parental role conflict
Altered sexuality patterns

## Pattern 4: Valuing

Spiritual distress (distress of the human spirit)

## Pattern 5: Choosing

Ineffective individual coping
  Impaired adjustment
  Defenseive coping
  Ineffective denial
Ineffective family coping: disabling
Ineffective family coping: compromised
Family coping: potential for growth
Noncompliance (specify)
Decisional conflict (specify)
Health-seeking behaviors (specify)

## Pattern 6: Moving

Impaired physical mobility
Activity intolerance
  Fatigue
Potential activity intolerance
Sleep pattern disturbance
Diversional activity deficit
Impaired home maintenance management
Altered health maintenance
Feeding/self-care deficit
Impaired swallowing
Ineffective breastfeeding
Bathing/hygiene self-care deficit
Dressing/grooming self-care deficit
Toileting self-care deficit
Altered growth and development

## Pattern 7: Perceiving

Body image disturbance
Self-esteem disturbance
   Chronic low self-esteem
   Situational low self-esteem
Personal identity disturbance
Sensory/perceptual alterations (specify) (visual, auditory, kinesthetic, gustatory, tactile, olfactory)
   Unilateral neglect
Hopelessness
Powerlessness

## Pattern 8: Knowing

Knowledge deficit (specify)
Altered thought processes

## Pattern 9: Feeling

Pain
   Chronic pain
Dysfunctional grieving
Anticipatory grieving
Potential for violence: Self-directed or directed at others
Posttrauma response
   Rape-trauma syndrome
      Rape-trauma syndrome: compound reaction
      Rape-trauma syndrome: silent reaction
Anxiety
Fear

# INDEX

Page numbers in *italics* denote figures; those followed by "t" denote tables